Y0-BYA-208

Health Policy

THE LEGISLATIVE AGENDA

**Timely Reports to Keep
Journalists, Scholars and the Public
Abreast of Developing Issues, Events and Trends**

**CONGRESSIONAL QUARTERLY
1414 22ND STREET, N.W., WASHINGTON, D.C. 20037**

Congressional Quarterly Inc.

Congressional Quarterly Inc., an editorial research service and publishing company, serves clients in the fields of news, education, business and government. It combines specific coverage of Congress, government and politics by Congressional Quarterly with the more general subject range of an affiliated service, Editorial Research Reports.

Congressional Quarterly was founded in 1945 by Henrietta and Nelson Poynter. Its basic periodical publication was and still is the CQ *Weekly Report,* mailed to clients every Saturday. A cumulative index is published quarterly.

The CQ *Almanac,* a compendium of legislation for one session of Congress, is published every spring. *Congress and the Nation* is published every four years as a record of government for one presidential term.

Congressional Quarterly also publishes paperback books on public affairs. These include the twice-yearly *Guide to Current American Government* and such recent titles as *Inside Congress, Second Edition; The Washington Lobby, Third Edition;* and *Congressional Ethics, Third Edition.*

CQ Direct Research is a consulting service which performs contract research and maintains a reference library and query desk for the convenience of clients.

Editorial Research Reports covers subjects beyond the specialized scope of Congressional Quarterly. It publishes reference material on foreign affairs, business, education, cultural affairs, national security, science and other topics of news interest. Service to clients includes a 6,000-word report four times a month bound and indexed semiannually. Editorial Research Reports publishes paperback books in its fields of coverage. Founded in 1923, the service merged with Congressional Quarterly in 1956.

Editor: Margaret C. Thompson.

Major Contributor: Elizabeth Wehr. **Contributors:** Elizabeth Bowman, Harrison Donnelly, Edna Frazier-Cromwell, Martha V. Gottron, Diane C. Hill, Marc Leepson, Suzanne de Lesseps, Peg O'Hara, Brigette Rouson, Winifred Scheffler, Laura B. Weiss.

Editorial Assistant: Carolyn Goldinger.

Index: Claire L. Tury.

Art Director: Richard A. Pottern. **Staff Artist:** Robert O. Redding.

Production Manager: I. D. Fuller. **Assistant Production Manager:** Maceo Mayo.

Book Department Editor: Patricia Ann O'Connor.

Cover Design: Richard Pottern
Cover Photo: Stephen McCarroll, Uniphoto

Library of Congress Cataloging in Publication Data

Congressional Quarterly, inc.
 Health policy.

 Bibliography: p.
 Includes index.
 1. Medical policy — United States.
2. Medical laws and legislation — United States. I. Title.
[DNLM: 1. Health policy — United States — Legislation.
2. Health services — United States — Legislation.
3. Health planning — United States — Legislation. WA33 AA1 C7h]
RA395.A3C696   1980   362.1'0973   80-18847
ISBN 0-87187-199-8

Table of Contents

Editor's Note

Faced with spiraling costs in health services, one of the nation's major industries, citizens and their elected representatives have become increasingly concerned with developing measures and methods to control or reduce inflation in health care. *Health Policy: The Legislative Agenda* provides an overview of health programs and policies being considered by Congress and the executive branch.

This book describes key legislative proposals to enact a national health policy; to control hospital costs; and to provide for the distribution of health services where they are most needed.

Other issues discussed include the following:

● Should there be more competition in the health care industry?

● Should financially troubled hospitals receive more federal assistance?

● Should Congress play a greater role in determining the amount and length of funding for health research programs?

● Should an individual's medical records be protected from scrutiny by others?

● Should victims of environmental health hazards be permitted to seek legal redress?

Chapters on existing or proposed major federal health programs include background on the Medicare/Medicaid programs; the development of prepaid group health plans (health maintenance organizations); the controversy surrounding mental health programs and community mental health centers; proposed changes in child and maternal health and nutrition programs; the continuation of the popular emergency medical services program; revisions in veterans' health programs; and the establishment and performance of state health planning agencies.

Also covered are proposed or existing measures to prevent illnesses and promote good health — disease prevention and workplace safety programs; proposed changes in drug laws and food labeling; and revisions in food laws.

The appendix provides a chronology of major legislation in health care during the period 1973-79. A bibliography and index are also included.

Introduction

One astounding figure tells the story: America's expenditures for health care rose 350 percent between 1965 and 1978.

Moreover, there is no end in sight to the skyrocketing increases. Government figures indicate outlays will rise from the $192 billion level of 1968 to more than $400 billion by the mid-1980s and over $700 billion by the end of the century. *(Box, p. 2)*

Can the nation afford it? That is a key — perhaps *the* key — question of the continuing national debate over America's health care system.

At the center of this debate are such issues as:

● How much health care is "enough?"

● How much are people willing and able to pay for health care?

● Does the system mitigate against cost controls when most people have insurance to cover their medical bills?

● Is it possible to make the existing chaotic system of health care delivery and payment more efficient?

There are a number of reasons for the rapid and continuing rise in health care costs, reasons that are either built into the system or are simply unavoidable. One basic factor has been population growth. Another has been changes in the types of medical goods and services offered and the way they are used. Since enactment of the federal programs of Medicare for the aged and Medicaid for the poor in 1965, health care has been made available to more and more Americans. New programs, new technology, advances in medical research all have expanded the scope of available health care.

Inflation has been a major factor responsible for rising health care bills. Between 1972 and 1978, the medical care share of the consumer price index (CPI) rose 20 percent faster than the CPI for all categories other than health care. Although health care prices are relatively high compared to other services, the need for them is frequently not related to the prices charged. To put it another way, the supply and demand, price competition basic to many other industries, is often absent in the health care field.

Another reason for the nation's escalating health care costs is the growing size and age of the elderly population, which has contributed to rising expenditures in all areas of health care. The elderly spend more time in hospitals, visit doctors more often, purchase more drugs and need more nursing home services than do the rest of the population.

But underlying these inescapable explanations for soaring health care costs is a fundamental problem — the non-competitive nature of the health care industry.

Although the patient chooses his doctor, it is the doctor who largely determines the treatment he needs. The physician is the central decision-maker for more than 70 percent of health care services. Added to this is the fact that 90 percent of hospital bills are paid by private insurance companies or the government, rather than by the patient immediately and out of his own pocket. Payment usually is made on the basis of costs incurred, or fee-for-service, an expensive and, in the opinion of many observers, a generally inefficient way to function. Furthermore, insurance often will cover only inpatient (hospitalization) care for treatment that could be performed equally satisfactorily on a less costly, outpatient (ambulatory) basis.

Some of the dilemmas facing the nation's health care industry and the people it serves are ironic. Advances in health research and technology have made it possible to treat illnesses — such as some forms of cancer, including childhood leukemia, and heart disease — that would have been fatal a decade or more ago. Yet, in many instances, this has been accompanied by installation of very expensive equipment such as the computerized axial tomography (CAT) scanner which is able, through use of a computer, to take detailed X-ray pictures of any part of a person's body, and the establishment of intensive cardiac care units in many hospitals. These services may be duplicative and add considerably to the total U.S. health care bill.

The number of physicians also has grown dramatically in the past 20 years, accompanied by increasing doctor specialization. These developments have produced more and better services, but there are drawbacks: a possible "glut" in certain areas and specialties of doctors who, in competing for business, may charge ever-higher prices for services that might not always be needed.

Hospitals, too, have been able to provide increasingly sophisticated and comprehensive care. Yet they have been criticized for sometimes providing unnecessarily costly services and for maintaining excess capacity — a situation resulting from hospital construction programs of the 1940s that created an excess of expensive-to-maintain beds, estimated at at least 100,000 total, with more than 200,000 empty on any given day.

Maldistribution of doctors and hospitals has continued to plague the nation. Rural and inner-city areas have

Health Industry: An American Giant

The health care industry dwarfs most other enterprises in the United States. Moreover, it is getting bigger fast.

It provided more than 7 million jobs at the end of the 1970s and accounted for almost one-tenth of all goods and services produced in the United States.

National health expenditures grew at a compound annual rate of 12.2 percent from 1965 to 1978, compared to 9 percent for the gross national product (GNP), the total of all goods and services produced in the United States. These outlays increased 350 percent during that period — from $43 billion in 1965 to $192 billion in 1978. They were expected to reach $245 billion in 1980, $440 billion in 1985 and $760 billion in 1990, according to the Health Care Financing Administration (HCFA) in the U.S. Department of Health and Human Services. As a part of GNP, health costs rose from 6.2 percent to 9.1 percent between 1965 and 1978. There was little doubt they would rise more, probably by 10.5 percent by 1985 and 11.5 percent by 1990.

Hospital expenditures were the largest segment: $76 billion in 1978, two-fifths of total health care expenditures. The rate of hospital cost growth also has been spectacular: more than 260 percent from 1968 to 1978. That's an average of 14 percent annually. Hospital spending increases were expected to average 13.1 percent from 1978 to 1990 — somewhat lower than in previous years, according to HCFA. Expenditures have been estimated to reach $335 billion by 1990.

The second largest category of health expenditure has been physicians' services. These outlays quadrupled from 1965 to 1978, increasing at an average annual rate of 11.6 percent. In 1965, payments for doctors' services amounted to $8.5 billion, or $43 per person; by 1978, they had jumped to $35.2 billion or $158 for every man, woman and child in America. Expenditures were projected to grow to $45 billion in 1980, $78 billion in 1985 and $129 billion in 1990.

The third major cause of rising health costs has been nursing home care, where the average annual increase was 16.9 percent between 1970 and 1978, reaching $15.8 billion in the latter year. Expenditures for nursing home care were expected to more than double between 1978 and 1985 and to reach $76 million by 1990.

Spending by government programs accounted for 41 percent of health care outlays in 1978 — $78 billion, or $350 per person. Private spending for health care by patients themselves and private insurance companies was growing at a faster rate than public spending and reached $513 per capita in 1978.

---

significantly fewer health care services than metropolitan and particularly suburban areas.

Also underserved are the elderly and the poor. Federal programs of Medicare for the aged and Medicaid for the poor, passed in 1965, have considerably improved health care for these groups. Nevertheless, Medicare payments, though rising in absolute dollar amounts, have paid less and less of an elderly person's health care bill. At the same time, premiums charged the elderly have almost tripled since the program began. In addition, a large segment of the nation's poor has been excluded from Medicaid coverage because of variations in benefits and eligibility requirements set by the states.

Although there has been some progress in the areas of early detection of childhood disease, immunization, maternity care, infant mortality and child nutrition, these efforts have been faulted for being inadequate. Critics say there has been insufficient attention paid to preventive measures and follow-up treatment. Moreover, the nature and funding of these programs has been controversial.

Teen age pregnancies have persisted at an alarming rate, as have abuses of drugs and alcohol, despite local, state and federal information, counseling and rehabilitation programs. And, although there has been a substantial decline in the number of mental hospital patients — in part as a result of the establishment of community mental health centers and other programs — it is generally agreed that the "stigma" of mental illness remains an obstacle to identifying those in need of help and assimilating them into their communities once they have received or are undergoing treatment.

During the 1960s and 1970s, there evolved a greater awareness of possible environmental hazards to health: air and water pollution; dumping of toxic wastes; and hazardous chemicals and unsafe conditions in the workplace. Although legislation has been enacted to try to control these dangers, they have proved to be stubborn and difficult in some cases to identify.

Moreover, technological break-throughs — new chemicals, new food additives, new drugs — have raised new questions about what is "safe" and "unsafe" and have produced divided opinions about how to monitor these new products.

Along with the growing awareness of the environmental causes of health problems and the increasing burden of paying for illness has been closer focus on preventive health. Physical fitness regimens, anti-smoking campaigns, nutritional education programs, the "health food" boom, information programs to alert citizens to the existence and treatment of high blood pressure have become popular and highly visible. Yet many Americans continue to smoke, drink alcohol, lead sedentary lives and consume too many carbohydrates and too much fat in their diets.

Nature of the Problem

These are only some of the difficulties confronting the health care system in the United States — a system that is extremely complex and fragmented. It is composed of 126 medical schools, more than 6,000 community hospitals in addition to veterans hospitals and state long-term care institutions (such as mental health hospitals); nursing homes; doctors in private practice and doctors in group practices (such as health maintenance organizations); nurses; physician assistants and support staff (including health care administrators); independent laboratories and other suppliers of health care goods and services.

It includes government-sponsored or administered programs such as Medicare and Medicaid; local health sys-

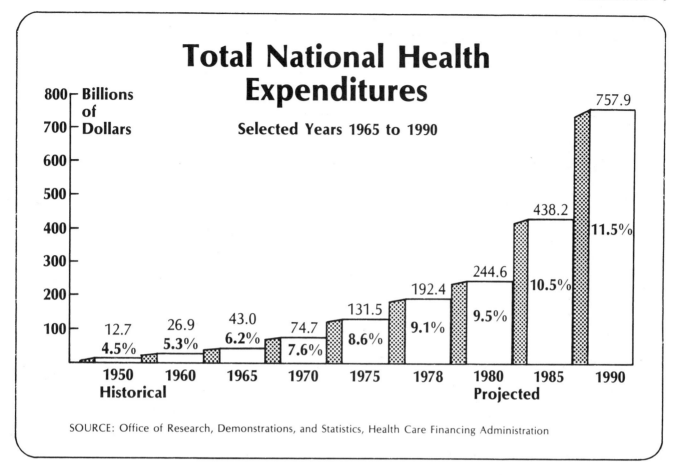

Total National Health Expenditures

Selected Years 1965 to 1990

800 ┌ **Billions**
700 ├ **of**
600 ┤ **Dollars**
500 ┤
400 ┤
300 ┤
200 ┤
100 ┤

12.7 **4.5%** — 1950
26.9 **5.3%** — 1960
43.0 **6.2%** — 1965
74.7 **7.6%** — 1970
131.5 **8.6%** — 1975
192.4 **9.1%** — 1978
244.6 **9.5%** — 1980
438.2 **10.5%** — 1985
757.9 **11.5%** — 1990

Historical   **Projected**

SOURCE: Office of Research, Demonstrations, and Statistics, Health Care Financing Administration

tems agencies (designed to monitor distribution and growth of health services in a region); regional emergency health services programs (which fund ambulances and emergency helicopter services, among other things); professional standards review organizations (established by Congress, these physician groups are intended to function as an oversight body over their colleagues); and a National Health Service Corps (sponsored by the federal government, the program requires students who have received federal aid to serve in physician-short areas for a specified length of time).

Layered onto this are a number of other programs — providing services to Indians and migrant workers, lunches and other meals to children and aid to alcoholics, drug abusers and the mentally ill. The system embraces a massive federal and non-federal health research sector that includes the National Institutes of Health (NIH), the largest research organization of its kind in the world; the pharmaceutical industry that dispensed 1.5 billion prescriptions in 1979; and the federal and private health insurance industry, which paid for $167.9 billion of personal health expenditures in 1978.

Financing Health Care

It is this last feature of the health care system that has been of central concern to many providers, recipients, observers and experts. To them, the prevalence of so-called "third party" financing of health care — whether it be by the federal government through Medicare and Medicaid, or by private insurance companies (including the 87 million member Blue Cross/Blue Shield program) — has been largely responsible for the lack of controls on health care costs. A number of reasons have been cited as explanations for the flaws in this kind of health financing scheme.

First, and most important to some (including the insurance industry itself) is that the traditional method of health care payment in this country has been payment "after the fact." That is, a patient who visits a doctor receives a bill for services rendered rather than having knowledge beforehand of what his procedures will cost. Or, if he does know in advance what the bill will amount to, he will, in all likelihood, agree that the cost is the prevailing one and think no more about it. The doctor then bills the patient's insurance company (90 percent of Americans have one or more health insurance policies) for the fee for his service. Because the insurance company pays "after the fact" for the services, there is less incentive for either the patient or his doctor to economize. The patient, after all, has already paid his insurance premium; the cost of the particular service does not hit his pocket in a direct and immediate way. And the provider of services, knowing that his patient will be sufficiently reimbursed, may have less incentive to charge him a smaller fee.

The same is true for hospitals and their patients. Private insurance companies and the federal government pay hospitals for costs incurred — again, "after the fact," or after they have been provided. Added to the problem — and the dilemma facing the entire health care system — is the fact that many insurance policies will pay only for services rendered by a patient's hospitalization. As a result, doctors often send patients to hospitals for pro-

Health Coalition Lobbying

Every year some 60 health groups, representing victims of specific diseases, the practitioners who treat them, the schools that train the practitioners, and the professional support services, converge on Washington for a sort of shadow budget process of their own.

Members of the 10-year-old Coalition for Health Funding estimate how much federal money they will need in the following year — for treatment facilities, for research in "their" disease at the National Institutes of Health (NIH), and for support services. Coalition board members weigh these "requests" and draft a budget. Groups that think they have been shortchanged can appeal board decisions. Finally, a hefty, 100-page "alternative budget" is submitted to the Appropriations committees of Congress. It requests more money than the president does, details accomplishments of modern medicine, prints names and telephone numbers of group officials interested in each federal program, and carries such politically apt observations as, "The financial burden of cancer approximates $30 billion annually in the United States."

The group ignores authorizing committees, focusing instead on the appropriations process and, increasingly, on the Budget committees.

The coalition does not deal with Medicare or Medicaid — only the discretionary programs. The lobbying of member groups has been an important ingredient in the success of NIH in evading massive budget cuts in the past.

But in 1980 the coalition was unhappy. The discretionary programs were big losers in the revised Carter budget submitted in March. Grants to states for alcohol and drug abuse programs took sizable cuts. A $9 million "adolescent health" program — to prevent teenage pregnancies or ensure adequate prenatal care for young mothers — disappeared entirely. So did major chunks of money for preventive health initiatives such as anti-smoking campaigns and grants to states. Community health centers and the National Health Service Corps both came out with no-growth funding — sharply down from increases in the January budget, when administration officials stressed the need for new medical services in doctor-short areas. NIH programs also took some losses, although the final cut was only about one-third of the original, rumored $300 million.

"The membership's up in arms," said coalition president Jay Cutler, of the American Psychiatric Association, "but nobody's got a real answer."

"Members [of Congress] are going to be hearing from the nurses, the doctors, the patients, the families of patients, everybody," he said, adding that he had urged all these groups to talk about national priorities — not just their particular disease.

But the classic "disease-of-the-month" approach, enlisting individual members of Congress on behalf of specific causes, still had its uses. "You get members behind doors. One insists on money for disease X, another for disease Y, another for disease Z," said Cutler. Sooner or later, he hoped, these members would have to compromise and provide some money for all.

cedures that could be performed in their own offices or in an outpatient setting in order to spare their clients the out-of-pocket cost that might be incurred otherwise.

A closely related factor in the dilemma of health care financing has been the simple fact that more and more Americans have been able to obtain more extensive health care coverage — primarily under the federal programs — and that more and more of them have been demanding, and have received, the high quality expensive treatment that technological and medical advances are now able to offer. For example, an article in the Jan. 10, 1979, *Washington Post* documented the experience of one District of Columbia resident whose 20-day stay at Georgetown University Hospital cost $26,000. Involved in the effort to repair the patient's failing heart were more than 200 persons, ranging from orderlies to the surgeon; use of expensive machines (including a $179,135 Philips Cardio-Diagnost machine to take image-intensified X-rays, and a $72,709 Menner-Greatbatch Physical Sentinel to monitor the patient's heartbeat); major heart surgery and other special and intensive care (including a stay in a $400,000 Coronary Unit and in Surgical Intensive Care, another $400,000 unit). The patient's insurance company paid all but $1,681 of his bills. "This is the kind of comprehensive insurance coverage called a blessing by patients who have it, and a 'disincentive' to economy by those who think Americans should have to pay a larger share of their medical bills in cold cash to avoid saddling the country with so large a tab," wrote reporters Victor Cohn and Peter Milius.

The Health Care Financing Administration cited another factor that has contributed to the growth in insurance coverage and the corresponding rise in health care costs — the provision of tax subsidies for health insurance, namely "the exclusion from taxable income of employer contributions to employee health insurance plans and the deductibility of health insurance premiums ... [which] provide an incentive to purchase more insurance than would otherwise be the case. The additional insurance then encourages further use of medical care."

Paradoxically, however, the prevalence of third-party health care payments has masked another failing of the financing system. In fiscal year 1978, about 26 million people, or 12 percent of the population, had no medical insurance coverage whatsoever through either private or federal programs. Moreover, numerous others who were eligible for federal Medicare and Medicaid payments or who did possess private insurance policies had inadequate, but sometimes overlapping, coverage, lacking provision for major medical expenses and long-term and pharmaceutical coverage (the latter two were particularly important for the elderly). It could be concluded that the existing system has provided too much — and too little — for those it was intended to serve.

An HCFA study of projected future trends in the health care industry (published in the Winter 1980 HCFA *Review*) concluded:

"There seem to be few incentives or constraints to retard the growth of health expenditures under current institutional arrangements. As health costs increase, so does the risk of financial burden to consumers with inadequate health insurance coverage. As this risk increases, the demand for public programs and private health insurance also rises.... As the coinsurance rate (proportion paid out-of-pocket by consumers) declines with the additional insurance, both consumers and providers increasingly tend to treat health care services as a free good at the time of purchase. The ensuing increased demand for medical care interacts with our fee-for-service and cost-based reimbursement systems to further increase costs. . . ."

Other Reasons for High Costs

Although the system of financing health care has often been castigated as the primary reason for the escalating costs of keeping Americans healthy, there are numerous other causes for the system's deficiencies. Most of them, however, are closely linked with the health care financing situation, interacting in both a cause and effect relationship. Among them are:

Manpower Problems. Heeding warnings of a doctor shortage, the United States, starting in the 1960s and spurred by congressional legislation, began turning out M.D.s in record numbers. Meanwhile, the costs of a medical education zoomed; and, as a consequence, so did private and federal scholarships in an effort to prevent the profession from becoming a "rich man's turf." Somewhat paradoxically, however — and defying the law of supply and demand — as the number of doctors swelled, so too did their average salaries. Would-be doctors increasingly entered lucrative specialty fields and chose to practice in areas — usually metropolitan centers — where they could be close to the latest information and technology via consultation with colleagues and proximity to up-to-date medical and research facilities. Another reason for the metropolitan preference of many doctors was that they could command prices for the same service that were higher than they could obtain elsewhere. Remote rural and inner-city locations were, understandably, less attractive to many. So, too, was the practice of primary care (general medicine, pediatrics and obstetrics/gynecology). While the federal government and states were providing Medicare and, particularly, Medicaid payments to persons in need of medical help, those persons frequently could not take advantage of that assistance since they lived in medically underserved areas, and travel to the nearest center often proved too costly — or sometimes nearly impossible.

Hospital Costs. Hospital costs, too, rose in a vicious circle. As with doctors, overall inflation in equipment and labor, as well as for construction costs, added to the soaring prices of hospital stays. Government encouragement to build new and expanded hospitals from the 1940s through the early 1970s — as mentioned above — led to what many observers have described as a maldistribution or at least underutilization of hospital services. But another factor contributing to the hospital cost surge was the fact that it is usually the doctor who determines whether hospitalization is necessary (sometimes on the basis of the kind of insurance his patient carries; that is, whether the insurance will pay only if the service is performed in the hospital, which is frequently the case).

And the hospital to which the doctor sends his patient may be the one that provides the most up-to-date and expensive equipment — CAT scanners, special coronary units and so forth. To attract doctors and patients to utilize their facilities, hospitals may try to obtain more such equipment, which may be duplicated by other hospitals in the area, with the result that those services may not be utilized sufficiently or efficiently. This, of course, adds to the overall cost of hospital care. While the inventory of expensive equipment increases, countless hospital beds in the United States are unfilled on

---

From HEW to HHS

President Carter's first HEW secretary, Joseph A. Califano Jr., wasted little time in pushing forward internal changes at HEW in an attempt to get a handle on one of the government's largest bureaucracies, a task that had stymied many before him.

In both the policies and procedures of his department Califano made a number of changes. In March 1977, he announced a restructuring of the bureaucracy that he said was expected to save $2 billion a year in the long run. He consolidated administration of the Medicare and Medicaid programs in a new Health Care Financing Administration. In July he announced a reorganization of the department's regional offices and in September he pledged an overhaul and review of the department's voluminous regulations — 6,000 pages in 13 volumes. The overhaul was labeled Operation Common Sense.

A much more dramatic upheaval in the department came in 1979. First, Califano was fired by Carter in a July Cabinet shakeup, reportedly because he had made enemies on the White House staff and because his strong advocacy of controversial policies, such as anti-smoking programs, had made him a political liability to the president as the 1980 election approached. He was replaced by Housing and Urban Development Secretary Patricia Roberts Harris.

Then HEW, largest of the executive departments in terms of spending and labeled "unmanageable" by many critics, was ordered to split up. After an 18-month battle, Congress acceded to the wishes of President Carter and the National Education Association and voted to consolidate the education functions of HEW and several other Cabinet departments in a separate Department of Education. Backers of the move said education was overwhelmed by the massive health and welfare programs that dominated the 27-year-old department, and would get more attention with its own secretary in the Cabinet.

HEW officially went out of existence May 4, 1980, and was replaced by two departments: the Department of Health and Human Services (HHS) and the new Department of Education.

---

any given day. To take up the slack, many patients are assigned to acute care (expensive) beds when they could just as feasibly be taken care of in a less expensive long-term care ward.

Malpractice Insurance. For a large number of doctors and hospitals rising expenses have been encountered in the form of costly malpractice insurance as the number of malpractice suits has risen. Doctors' fees have been increased to account for the added costs of carrying this insurance; moreover, the rising incidence of malpractice claims may have encouraged doctors to practice what has been called "defensive" medicine — that is, prescribing more X-rays, tests and other diagnostic examinations than might be called for. This, in turn, impinges on hospital costs, since the patient is frequently sent to the hospital for these services.

Medicare/Medicaid Problems. Beginning in 1965, the government assumed substantial responsibility for paying the health care bills of the elderly and poor. But federal programs have been plagued by problems similar to those confronting the private health sector — primary among them, rising costs. As with private insurance, Medicare and Medicaid provide payments to providers after costs have been incurred, and this, as noted, means there is less incentive on the part of both provider and patient to keep costs down.

On the other hand, as costs have risen, the share the government will pay for health care under the two programs has fallen relative to the amount the patient must pay out of pocket (a phenomenon known as "Medigap"). And because Medicare reimburses doctors and hospitals on the basis of "reasonable" charges — the prevailing rate in a particular locality — costs and payments for the same service often vary considerably from region to region.

Another problem besetting the two government programs has been fraud and abuse, primarily on the part of providers but also on the part of customers, with the government being billed for services not rendered, for patients not seen or, if they were seen, for highly inflated charges; and patients' giving fraudulent information about their eligibility status.

Proposed Solutions

Many of these and other problems that challenge the nation, its legislators and the health care industry itself are discussed more fully in the following chapters. But, despite the complexities and sometimes apparently unsolvable difficulties facing the rather unique economic sector of health care, many innovative proposals have been offered and are under consideration. Moreover, there have been many suggestions that the existing system may well be able to take care of its own problems, to reshape itself into an equilibrium wherein costs are kept under control without sacrificing the quality of medical care.

Among the proposals under consideration, either in legislative, administrative, or simply "idea" form:

Hospital Cost Control

The Carter administration began in 1977 to press for hospital cost control legislation that would set a mandatory cap on hospital revenues. Although the idea has appeal to many for its potential to cut health care inflation, the fact that hospitals have experienced the same, or greater, increases in expenditures for goods and services — costs over which they have little direct control — as have other sectors in the economy has been a central argument mitigating against enactment of a mandatory cost gap. Congress has been reluctant to legislate such controls, preferring instead that the hospitals themselves monitor their expenditures and profits. A voluntary effort to do so was initiated by the hospitals in 1978. As of 1980, the effort seemed to have had an impact in lowering the rate of hospital cost inflation, but only time would tell whether the program would be successful. Some observers felt that, without the threat of possible mandatory controls, hospitals — like other industries — would become less and less willing to practice the self-disciplinary measures embodied in the effort.

Hospital construction and distribution is another issue that has confronted legislators and those in the health care industry. During the mid- and late-1970s, Congress enacted a number of laws designed to cut down on unnecessary hospital construction and purchase of equipment (requiring, among other things, that local health systems

agencies approve "certificates of need" for costly equipment and give prior approval for additional construction). But these programs were still only fragmentary as of 1980, and they had not yet gone far enough in solving the problems of rural hospital shortages and the plight facing many inner-city community hospitals that cared for the indigent.

Physician Distribution and Fees

The distribution of doctors and regulation of their fees may prove more difficult to control in the long run than regulation of hospital costs — although, as mentioned above, the two are closely dependent upon one another. As hospital costs have risen, doctors' fees have risen as well. Again, this is related to the prevalence of third-party insurance, the fee-for-service system, increasing specialization and the installation of new, expensive equipment.

Despite the incentives to encourage medical school graduates to practice in underserved areas, these regions have continued to experience a doctor shortage. In establishing the Health Service Corps in 1972, Congress sought to correct this maldistribution, but questions have arisen as to how well the corps has performed and whether it has provided sufficient incentive to encourage young practitioners to enter the urban ghettos or the outlying regions of the country.

One encouraging sign is that there appears to be a slight trend toward renewed interest in primary care fields on the part of medical school graduates. And the over-supply of doctors on the East and West coasts also seems to be diminishing.

Encouragement of Prepaid Group Practices

Another trend that some observers view as a promising method of controlling costs has been the growth of prepaid group practices that provide a wide range of services to customers for a set, prepaid fee — an incentive to providers to keep costs down. Congress gave its approval to these plans in 1973 by enacting legislation to assist the formation and operation of prepaid groups, called health maintenance organizations (HMOs), after they had been officially certified by the government. Because it was felt that the initial requirements for HMOs were too stiff, the act was amended in 1976 to allow HMOs greater leeway in their start-up operation.

Although the record of group practices has shown general success in controlling costs, HMOs in 1980 still had only a small share of the health care market, and some health care economists expressed doubts as to whether they would become a dominant force in the industry anytime soon. Meanwhile, however, the administration proposed legislation designed to encourage HMOs to provide services for citizens enrolled in Medicare and took administrative steps to stimulate formation of the prepaid practices in inner-city areas.

'Competition' Theory

The problem of escalating health care costs has given a great deal of prominence to a type of "anti-insurance" theory among some academic economists. In hearings and congressional offices, these economists have been urging — with some success — a "free market" or "competitive" approach to cost control and delivery of health services. Some economists contend that widespread private health insurance and excessive government regulation make the medical marketplace "non-competitive" and unnecessarily expensive. Prepaid group medical practices figured prominently in the theory. The economists felt that the prepaid plans had strong incentives to control costs and practice preventive medicine because they must live within a fixed budget each year.

A second and equally important part of the theory was that the existing tax breaks for private health insurance should be cut back to make consumers, doctors and hospitals more cost-conscious.

National Health Insurance

American presidents since Franklin Roosevelt have decided against pressing for a comprehensive, universal national health program because of its cost and because it involved major changes in the federal government's role in regulating health care. "The last time health insurance was really a presidential issue was in 1964, just before enactment of Medicare/Medicaid," recalled Irving Wolkstein, a Washington, D.C., health consultant.

Since then, the existence of Medicare and Medicaid and the rapid growth of private health insurance have somewhat muted or eliminated major sources of political pressure for national health insurance.

Nonetheless, the persistence of health insurance as a political and legislative issue suggests a chronic American anxiety about doctor and hospital bills. A poll taken for the health insurance industry in 1979 found that 72 percent of Americans thought medical care was too expensive and 53 percent thought that most Americans did not have adequate health insurance. But that same poll found, paradoxically, that a plurality of Americans thought they were personally well insured against illness.

Few political figures or economists in 1980 were discussing a British-style public health plan. Most of them generally limited their proposals to the comparatively modest options that dominated congressional discussions of health insurance in 1979.

President Carter, key congressional Democrats and the House Republican leadership all focused on catastrophic health insurance. Moderates in both parties who favored catastrophic coverage said it would take care of the last remaining constituency for a national health plan — the middle class, which feared massively expensive illness. This type of insurance would pay medical bills after individuals had paid substantial "deductibles" — of as much as from $2,500 to $5,000 a year — out of their own pockets or through supplementary health insurance.

Catastrophic health insurance was the only option under active consideration in Congress in 1980. In 1979, the Senate Finance Committee had tentatively decided to require employers to insure their workers against catastrophic costs of major illnesses. The Republican congressional leadership in February 1980 endorsed catastrophic coverage through employers on a voluntary basis.

Carter, however, said he would not sign any national health plan unless it mandated strict cost control measures, including those for hospital costs. Many agreed that any national health insurance program would have to be accompanied by legislation designed to put the brakes on health care costs.

In sum, it appeared that controlling increases in health care costs had pushed aside what had been the principal issue of health care debate for decades — access to services. Conservatives argued that high costs were a reason not to enact new benefits, while some liberals responded that the only way to put a lid on costs was to organize health care nationally.

Meanwhile, as Daniel Greenberg, publisher of the "Science and Government" report, noted in the Dec. 18, 1979, *Washington Post,* "Any disinterested look produces the same conclusion: we've got too many hospitals, too many medical schools, and we're producing too many doctors, most of whom continue to shun the rural and inner-city areas where they are most needed. But little gets done about it. And despite the mounting costs of medical care — yearly health insurance premiums now average about $1,000 per head — it's not likely that anything will get done until the costs become so unbearable that parts of the system will simply go bankrupt."

But a somewhat brighter outlook was offered by Jordan Braverman in his book, *Crisis in Health Care:*

"Despite the many problems which beset this nation today, the future resolution of these issues can be considered optimistically. Society is aware of the problems, is debating the most feasible solutions for them, and realizes that in health care, whether it be in the medical or environmental sense, what is at issue is the survival of society itself. . . . Thus, looking into the future, it may not be long until this nation will have a rational health insurance program in which all of its population, generally, will be protected against the costs and incidence of ill health. . . . The health care professions will enlist the assistance of paramedical personnel in increasing numbers. These personnel will be authorized to provide simple diagnosis, prescriptions and prevention of disease. . . . Prepaid group practices will continue to grow, being stimulated by public funding and the support of the private health insurance industry, as ways are sought to reduce costs and bring a greater efficiency and coordination into the health care system. . . .

"Alternatives to hospital care, such as home care services, will continue to expand. Emphasis will be on the continuing development of such institutions as extended care facilities and out-patient or ambulatory clinics. . . . Health care, both in concept and practice, is an evolutionary process. But the public conscience that health care is a right and not a privilege has been awakened. An enlarging society demands that this basic right be applied in fact rather than in theory. . . . If the present battle for maintaining this society in as good a state of health as possible is lost . . . then society will have lost the basic element for its future existence, namely a healthful life itself."

Margaret C. Thompson
July 1980

National Health Insurance Proposals Debated

To many Americans, national health insurance is seen as a government program that would pay the bills for operations, checkups, eyeglasses, drugs and just about everything else the doctor ordered.

But that was not exactly what President Carter had in mind. Under the national health plan Carter announced June 12, 1979, the government would not suddenly begin to pay everyone's medical bills. Middle-class Americans would feel the pinch of doctor and hospital bills directly in their own wallets. Except for the poor and disabled, and workers who could win full coverage from employers, Americans would have to pay for part of their insurance premiums and part of their medical expenses. The strategy was popular with economists who said it would discourage overuse of doctors and hospitals and save money.

The other two major proposals that were debated in 1979, the health plans sponsored by Sens. Edward M. Kennedy, D-Mass., and Russell B. Long, D-La., also adopted this strategy. Kennedy's comprehensive plan would require much less cost-sharing than Carter's, while Long's "catastrophic" insurance proposals would require more out-of-pocket payments before benefits would begin.

Catastrophic insurance was the core of Carter's "first-phase" national health plan. However, Kennedy and his allies, principally organized labor, opposed catastrophic coverage for fear it would reduce pressure for a more comprehensive national health program. Catastrophic insurance would cover only "catastrophically" high medical bills, those remaining after a family had already paid several thousand dollars out of its own pocket in a year, or after private insurance coverage had been exhausted.

But many in Congress and the administration believed the country could not afford a comprehensive health plan and opted to go for "50 percent of something," rather than hold out for "100 percent of nothing," as Sen. Abraham Ribicoff, D-Conn., a longtime backer of catastrophic insurance, put it.

Senate Finance Committee Chairman Long opened the 1979 action in February, when he announced that he planned to "push and agitate a bit" for catastrophic insurance — "about as much as we can afford to enact in this Congress." He introduced legislation and began hearings and markup in March.

The Finance Committee worked on the legislation off and on throughout the year, and seemed on the verge of reporting it in November. But several committee members and the administration insisted on substantial new health benefits for the poor; Long and some other members objected, and further action was postponed so that committee staff could try to work out an acceptable compromise. No further action had been taken by the committee as of mid-1980.

Kennedy had unveiled his comprehensive national health plan May 14, 1979. He made several concessions to Carter administration positions, and called on the president to join him and the coalition of labor, black, religious, elderly and farm groups that supported comprehensive

national health care, in an effort to guarantee complete health coverage for all Americans.

President Carter announced his plan one month later. It was considerably scaled down from his 1976 campaign commitment to comprehensive national health insurance, but Carter said the United States could only afford a gradually phased in program.

Without naming his opponents, he noted that 30 years of "rigid" pursuit of "the idea of all or nothing at all" had failed to get a comprehensive health plan out of Congress. It was time, he said, to "rise above the differences that have created that stalemate and act now" on his first-phase program.

Carter's plan would increase federal health care spending, in the first year of benefits, by about $18 billion over existing levels, and private (employer) expenses for health care by $6 billion, the administration estimated. Kennedy said his plan would add about $29 billion to the federal budget and $11 billion to expenditures by businesses and workers the first year.

Background

Critics of the existing health care system in the United States have contended that a major restructuring job clearly was in order. Many viewed national health insurance as the best way of controlling costs and guaranteeing everyone the same coverage.

But in discussing the specific design of a national program, supporters of national health insurance have often parted ways.

One divisive issue has been the role of the federal government. Organized labor would like the federal government, instead of private insurance companies, to run the program. Labor groups have been opposed by hospitals, doctors and private health insurers who would like the private insurance industry to run a program of standardized health benefits for all who want to participate.

Proponents of various health insurance proposals also were divided on the most realistic methods of controlling costs. Basically, there were three general methods of financing that, according to research and experience, had the potential for containing health-care inflation. The first would rely on tight public controls and the second on a restructuring of the private medical system to provide doctors, hospitals and other health-care providers with incentives to hold down costs. The second method would mean, for example, encouraging the development of health maintenance organizations (HMOs) and other prepaid delivery systems. "Prospective reimbursement," whereby fees are established before a service is rendered rather than after it has been provided (the so-called "fee-for-service" system), would also be part of this cost-control approach.

The third approach focused on cost-sharing — that is, the amount of a medical bill that the patient was required to pay out of pocket. Supporters of cost-sharing have said that under the existing insurance system of third-party payment, the patient has had little incentive not to overuse health services. They maintained that a national health insurance program should require patients to pay something to avoid overuse and to make them aware of the costs involved. This could be done through "deductibles" or "coinsurance." (A deductible is the amount a patient must pay before insurance begins. Under coinsurance, a patient pays a fixed percentage of the bill.)

Existing Health Care System

"With public spending accounting for some 40 percent of all health expenditures and something like two-thirds of private costs being met through health insurance, the typical consumer seldom comes face to face with his share of the national health bill," Charles C. Edwards, a former commissioner of the U.S. Food and Drug Administration," wrote in the May 17, 1976, *American Medical News,* a publication of the American Medical Association (AMA). "Yet for a family of four that share is approaching $2,500 a year. For most Americans that would be catastrophic if it came in the form of doctor or hospital bills they had to pay out of current income or savings."

Unlike most other goods and services for which the consumer usually pays directly, health care costs are most frequently handled by a "third party." By 1978, according to the Health Care Financing Administration, more than two-thirds of the funds spent for personal health care were supplied by financial agents, principally private health insurance companies or public agencies acting as insurers. Methods of payment varied: the private health insurance company might reimburse the provider in whole or in part for the service cost, or the consumer might be reimbursed for money he had already paid out for insured services. Public agencies might employ the private insurance industry to disburse provider payments on behalf of beneficiaries, or government agencies might provide health care services directly to selected segments of the population.

Third-party involvement has grown substantially. In 1965 only 47 percent of all personal health care funds were handled by third parties, as compared to 67 percent in 1978, according to the Health Care Financing Administration. In 1978 third parties financed $112.6 billion of the total $167.9 billion in personal health expenditures or 67 percent of the total with state, local and federal governments financing $65.0 billion, or 39 percent, of that amount. Health care paid for by private philanthropic organizations and by industry for maintaining in-plant health services accounted for slightly over 1 percent of the total.

In 1978 private insurance companies and the government paid 90 percent of hospital care costs, with government payments increasing from 39 to 54 percent of all hospital care during the period 1965-78, and the share paid by private insurance organizations declining from 42 to 35 percent during the same period.

Although physicians' services have not been reimbursed to as great an extent as hospital care, the overall growth since 1965 has been greater. Government payments rose from 7 to 27 percent of doctors' bills in that period, with all third-party payments for doctors rising from 39 to 66 percent of the total.

The share of personal health care expenses not paid for by third parties ("out-of-pocket" costs) declined from 53 percent in 1965 to 33 percent in 1978 (in 1978, direct payments amounted to $55.3 billion). Although total per capita personal health spending increased fourfold between 1965 and 1978, direct payments per person increased only two and one-half times, from $101 to $248. According to the Health Care Financing Administration, the direct payment increase was only 1.3 percent annually in terms of constant dollars.

In 1978, consumers directly paid only 10 percent of hospital expenses, an average of $34 per person. They paid 34 percent, or an average of $54 each, for doctors' services.

Private Health Insurance

Commercial health insurance owes its beginnings to the development of accident insurance during the mid-19th century, when traveling businessmen began to suffer from frequent railroad and steamboat accidents. Before long, coverage was offered for accidents of all descriptions. Generally, policyholders were reimbursed for pay lost due to disability. Likewise, the early health insurance policies offered protection against the loss of income as a result of a number of diseases, including typhus, scarlet fever, smallpox and diphtheria. At the end of the 19th century a handful of casualty companies began to offer very limited coverage of hospital expenses in conjunction with the income-loss disability policies.

"Modern health insurance was born," according to a 1975 report by the Health Insurance Institute, "in the Great Depression of the 1930s as a means of helping people cope with the costs of health care, and of bringing financial relief to hospitals faced with empty beds and declining revenues." The movement was launched in 1929 when Baylor University Hospital took over a local public school teachers' "sick benefit plan." Using the teachers' experience as a guide to premiums and benefits, and spurred by the hospital's need for a regular source of income, the new plan began to enroll other groups, and the first local Blue Cross was born. Just as the American Hospital Association had encouraged the development of Blue Cross for the payment of hospital fees, Blue Shield programs received a boost in 1938 when the American Medical Association approved the concept of voluntary health insurance — largely to ward off the threat of "socialized medicine." Blue Shield reimbursed surgeons and physicians for specified services either directly or through the patients.

The private health insurance industry continued to grow after World War II, aided in part by a 1948 Supreme Court decision which held that fringe benefits — including health insurance — were a legitimate part of the bargaining process by which labor negotiates its contracts with management. Another stimulus was the sharply escalating cost of health care, which prompted the public to find a way to protect itself against the expense. A third stimulus, according to Jordan Braverman in his book, *Crisis in Health Care* (1978), was the "ability of the private health insurers to introduce new kinds of coverage and broaden existing benefits."

Beginning in the early 1950s, insurance companies began to offer major medical expense coverage, or "catastrophic" coverage. "From its start, major medical has grown rapidly in response to the family's need for protection against swiftly escalating hospital, medical and surgical costs," Braverman wrote.

Braverman also noted that, following World War II, insurance companies increasingly began to offer long-term disability benefits to replace lost income. "Thus, it appears that the health insurance industry has come full circle since its early beginnings when the industry emphasized income replacement rather than health care service benefits in its insurance policies," he wrote.

The private health insurance industry grew rapidly during the 1950s. By 1960, 21 percent of personal health care was covered by private insurance; by 1965 the share had increased to 23 percent. With the passage of Medicare and Medicaid in 1965, the government stepped into the insurance picture, and the growth of the insurance share of the private sector began to slow, stabilizing at about 27 percent by the end of the 1970s.

Hospital care was the first kind of health care service to be extensively covered by private insurance. In 1960, private insurance covered 36 percent of hospital care expenditures; in 1965, it covered 42 percent; by the late 1970s, it averaged around 35 percent. Extensions of coverage beyond surgical procedures led to a higher share of physicians' services being reimbursed by private insurance — 39 percent in 1978 as compared to 29 percent in 1967.

Private insurance coverage has been extremely limited for other health care services, however. Dental care has been the only other service w   ny substantial private insurance coverage — with about 19 percent of dental services being covered in 1978.

Private insurers, which include the Blue Cross and Blue Shield Associations, commercial insurance companies and independent prepaid group and self-insured health plans, paid benefits of $45.4 billion, or 27 percent of personal health care expenditures, in 1978 and collected $53.0 billion in premiums.

A study by Marjorie Smith Carrol and Ross H. Arnett III, in the fall 1979 *Health Care Financing Review* showed that in 1977, 168 million people were covered by private hospital insurance and 164 million carried surgical insurance. About 70 percent of the population had private insurance to help cover costs of out-of-hospital X-ray and laboratory examinations, prescribed drugs and nursing services. However, the authors pointed out, "Coverage and enrollment statistics do not provide a total picture of health insurance protection. Coverage can mean a narrow or a comprehensive range of benefits, a large deductible and co-payment or 100 percent reimbursement by the insurer for health care costs. The range of services and the degree to which benefit payments meet the cost of these services provide a measure of the quality of insurance coverage. For some, the source of payment of insurance premiums is also an indicator of coverage quality."

According to the authors, an estimated 38 million people under age 65 had no private insurance against the costs of hospital-related illnesses. An estimated nine million of the aged had no private hospital insurance; 13 million had no private surgical insurance. However, virtually all persons age 65 and over had coverage for these services under Medicare. For prescription drugs or private duty nursing, more than 19 million (80 percent) of the aged had no insurance protection, either through private insurance or through the Medicare program.

A January 1980 study by Stephen Sudovar and Patrice Hirsch Feinstein of Pracon Inc., under a grant from Roche Laboratories, found that 85 percent of the population in 1977 was covered by private insurance or public medical programs for basic hospital room and board costs, and 89.5 percent for in-hospital laboratory and X-ray fees. But only 29.4 percent had coverage protecting them adequately against catastrophic or major medical expenses. The study also found that nearly two-thirds of the population was covered by maternity care provisions. Only 40 percent was covered for out-of-hospital doctor costs and 44 percent for required skilled and intermediate nursing home care.

Interest in National Insurance Grows

Besides providing impetus for the growth of private health insurance, the 1930s Depression also stimulated interest in a national health insurance program sponsored by the government. This was the threat of "socialized medicine" that was so feared by the American Medical Association. In 1934, President Roosevelt's Committee on Economic Security endorsed the principle of compulsory national health insurance. But a health insurance program was not included in the Social Security Act of 1935 for fear it would endanger passage of the act as a whole. The act did, however, provide for a broad range of social insurance and public assistance programs.

From 1935 on, compulsory health insurance bills were introduced in Congress annually. After Roosevelt's death in 1945, the new president, Harry S Truman, proposed a comprehensive medical insurance plan for all persons, to be financed through an increase in the payroll tax that finances Social Security. The Truman plan and various other proposals were defeated, however, in a lobbying war that pitted labor unions and liberal organizations against the AMA, private health insurers and conservative business groups.

In 1965 Congress amended the Social Security Act to establish the Medicare and Medicaid programs. Medicare provided persons age 65 and older with insurance to cover most medical costs and was financed by the Social Security trust fund to which employers and employees were required to contribute. The Medicaid section provided federal matching grants to states that chose to make medical services available to welfare recipients and the medically indigent. *(See Medicare/Medicaid chapter)*

While willing to expand categorical health programs and to tackle isolated problems in the health care system, Congress sidestepped action on comprehensive national health insurance proposals in the first half of the 1970s.

Both the Nixon and Ford administrations backed health insurance legislation in 1973 and 1974, but deep policy differences over who should run a health insurance program thwarted movement toward a compromise. Organized labor and its allies favored a federally controlled program, while the administration, insurers and medical groups wanted control to remain in private hands.

When the Democrats greatly enlarged their control of the House in the 1974 elections, action on health insurance was widely expected in the 94th Congress. But, reversing his previous position, President Ford vowed in early 1975 to veto new spending legislation such as national health insurance. *(See appendix for further details)*

Other factors weighed against action in 1975. Two House committees claimed jurisdiction over health insurance and could not resolve their dispute. The new congressional budget procedures made legislators more conscious of the potentially enormous cost of a national

Aggregate and Per Capita Amount and Percentage Distribution of National Health Expenditures by Type of Expenditure, Selected Calendar Years, 1965-1990

Type of Expenditure	Historical Years[1]				Projected Years		
	1965	1970	1975	1978	1980	1985	1990
	Aggregate Amounts (in billions)						
Total	$43.0	$74.7	$131.5	$192.4	$244.6	$438.2	$757.9
Health services and supplies	39.5	69.4	123.2	183.0	234.1	422.7	735.5
Personal health care expense	37.3	65.7	116.3	167.9	215.5	389.1	676.3
Hospital care	13.9	27.8	52.1	76.0	97.3	182.8	334.6
Physicians' services	8.5	14.3	24.9	35.3	45.0	78.2	128.8
Dentists' services	2.8	4.8	8.2	13.3	17.9	33.9	59.4
Other professional services	1.0	1.6	2.6	4.3	5.7	10.1	16.7
Drugs and drug sundries	5.8	8.4	11.8	15.1	18.1	27.0	38.9
Eyeglasses and appliances	1.9	2.1	3.0	3.9	4.7	7.1	10.2
Nursing home care	2.1	4.7	9.9	15.8	21.6	42.0	75.6
Other health services	1.3	2.1	3.7	4.3	5.2	8.1	12.2
Expenses for prepayment and administration	1.5	2.3	3.7	10.0	11.6	19.6	33.5
Government public health activities	.8	1.4	3.2	5.1	7.0	14.0	25.6
Research and Medical-facilities construction	3.5	5.3	8.3	9.4	10.5	15.5	22.4
Research	1.5	1.9	3.2	4.9	5.2	8.3	12.3
Construction	2.0	3.4	5.1	5.2	5.3	7.2	10.1
	Per Capita Amounts[2]						
Total	$217.41	$358.63	$604.57	$863.01	$1,078.00	$1,846.00	$3,057.00
Health services and supplies	199.91	333.25	566.61	820.68	1,032.00	1,781.00	2,967.00
Personal health care expense	188.41	315.37	534.82	752.98	950.00	1,639.00	2,728.00
Hospital care	70.46	133.39	239.77	340.93	429.00	770.00	1,350.00
Physicians' services	42.84	68.81	114.66	158.08	198.00	329.00	520.00
Dentists' services	14.20	22.79	37.88	59.64	79.00	143.00	240.00
Other professional services	5.22	7.65	12.04	19.17	25.00	43.00	67.00
Drugs and drug sundries	29.18	40.34	54.32	67.71	80.00	114.00	157.00
Eyeglasses and appliances	9.43	10.08	13.71	17.40	21.00	30.00	41.00
Nursing home care	10.48	22.44	45.46	70.63	95.00	177.00	305.00
Other health services	6.60	9.88	16.97	19.43	23.00	34.00	49.00
Expenses for prepayment and administration	7.33	10.97	17.09	44.94	51.00	83.00	135.00
Government public health activities	4.16	6.91	14.71	22.75	31.00	59.00	103.00
Research and medical-facilities construction	17.51	25.38	37.96	42.33	46.00	65.00	91.00
Research	7.40	8.93	14.65	19.22	23.00	35.00	50.00
Construction	10.11	16.45	23.31	23.11	23.00	30.00	41.00
	Percentage Distribution						
Total	100.0	100.0	100.0	100.0	100.0	100.0	100.0
Health services and supplies	91.9	92.9	93.7	95.1	95.7	96.5	97.0
Personal health care expenses	86.7	87.9	88.5	87.3	88.1	88.8	89.2
Hospital care	32.4	37.2	39.7	39.5	39.8	41.7	44.1
Physicians' services	19.7	19.2	19.0	18.3	18.4	17.8	17.0
Dentists' services	6.5	6.4	6.3	6.9	7.3	7.7	7.8
Other professional services	2.4	2.1	2.0	2.2	2.3	2.3	2.2
Drugs and drug sundries	13.4	11.2	9.0	7.8	7.4	6.2	5.1
Eyeglasses and appliances	4.3	2.8	2.3	2.0	1.9	1.6	1.3
Nursing home care	4.8	6.3	7.5	8.2	8.8	9.6	10.0
Other health services	3.0	2.8	2.8	2.3	2.1	1.8	1.6
Expenses for prepayment and administration	3.4	3.1	2.8	5.2	4.8	4.5	4.4
Government public health activities	1.9	1.9	2.4	2.6	2.9	3.2	3.4
Research and medical-facilities construction	8.1	7.1	6.3	4.9	4.3	3.5	2.9
Research	3.4	2.5	2.4	2.2	2.1	1.9	1.6
Construction	4.7	4.6	3.9	2.7	2.2	1.6	1.3

[1] Expenditures for 1965-1978 are reported in Robert M. Gibson "National Health Expenditures, 1978," *Health Care Financing Review*, Summer 1979, pp. 1-36.

[2] Per capita amounts in projections are rounded to nearest dollar.

Source: Health Care Financing Review, Winter 1980

health program. A series of investigations revealing fraud and abuse in the Medicare and Medicaid programs raised questions about whether the country should move to a national health program before it learned to run existing programs.

During the 1976 presidential campaign, Carter had voiced support of a mandatory program that would provide comprehensive benefits. Carter also said he favored the financing of such a program through payroll taxes and general revenues. However, following his election, Carter postponed announcing the details of his plan.

The proposal that finally emerged in June 1979 was viewed by some as a substantial retreat from his campaign promise for comprehensive, universal health insurance. His aides stressed, however, that even before his election, Carter had said that putting a complete plan in place could take many years.

Although Carter issued a statement of general principles on July 29, 1978, it was not until 1979 that Congress began considering substantive legislative proposals for national health insurance.

1979 Finance Committee Action

The Senate Finance Committee started its markup on national health insurance with three bills before it (S 350, S 351, S 760), but essentially the panel made up its catastrophic health insurance plan as it went along. Staff laid out options, the committee made decisions, and the bill was still to be put in finished form.

S 351, sponsored by full committee Chairman Long and Health Subcommittee Chairman Herman E. Talmadge, D-Ga., authorized employers to provide catastrophic coverage for workers, covering doctor bills over $2,000 and hospital bills after 60 days of hospitalization. Persons not covered by employer plans would be covered by the federal government, through a trust fund supported by a 1 percent payroll tax on employers. Employers could subtract premium costs from their payroll tax bill and get a tax credit. Cost of the bill was estimated at $5 billion to $7 billion a year.

To buy conservative and moderate support, Long eliminated from the bill a plan to federalize the state-federal Medicaid program, in order to ensure uniform national eligibility standards and benefits. That was an element of the catastrophic insurance legislation he had cosponsored with Ribicoff since 1971. But it would double the cost of the bill, according to estimates.

Because Long dropped the provision, Ribicoff refused to cosponsor S 351, and introduced a second bill (S 350) including it. Long joined as a cosponsor on that bill, but indicated he would only push for the narrower plan.

Both bills provided for voluntary federal certification of private health insurance plans that met minimum standards. They contained no cost control mechanisms.

Long introduced S 760 on March 26. Drafted to the specifications of a major insurance company, it made these major changes from earlier bills: eliminated the 1 percent payroll tax; made it mandatory for employers to provide catastrophic insurance; provided tax rebates for half their premium expenses for employers with payrolls under $250,000, public and nonprofit employers, and individuals buying their own coverage; imposed a tax penalty on employers failing to provide catastrophic coverage (150 percent of the premiums they would have paid); and required plans to cover employees' dependents up to age

26 and workers for up to six months after they left a job.

Eliminating the payroll tax was seen as a concession to conservatives and to House Ways and Means Committee Chairman Al Ullman, D-Ore., who reportedly was unsympathetic to any more payroll taxes.

Long suggested two ways to pay the costs of a catastrophic insurance program. One would be from "savings" generated by a bill making changes in Medicare and Medicaid (HR 934). Another would be to earmark some of the "windfall" from the pending oil windfall profits tax for health care. *(HR 934, see Medicare/Medicaid chapter)*

Committee Decisions

The Finance Committee had made most of the critical decisions on its catastrophic health insurance program by the end of 1979. It decided to make it mandatory, not optional, for employers to provide catastrophic insurance for workers. It set the deductible at $3,500, but also provided a lower, income-related deductible for lower-paid workers, a proposal advanced by Ribicoff, Robert Dole, R-Kan., and Daniel Patrick Moynihan, D-N.Y.

These were the general specifications of the plan agreed to by the committee:

Benefits, Coverage. All employers would be required to offer full-time employees health insurance covering the same benefits that had been provided by Medicare: physicians' fees and hospitalization; limited drug, durable medical equipment and mental health benefits; home health visits; and up to 100 days of nursing home care.

Outpatient drugs and extended nursing home care, the two major exclusions of Medicare, would also be excluded from the minimum benefit package. The committee also excluded prenatal, maternity and infant care in the first year of life, with no cost-sharing — a feature the administration especially wanted included.

The plans would pay for specified benefits after an individual or family had spent a substantial amount themselves, either out of pocket or under a supplementary insurance policy, on medical bills.

All full-time employees (those working 25 hours a week or more) would have to join their employers' plans unless they were already covered through a second job or a spouse's or parent's job. No one could be excluded because of pre-existing health conditions. The plans also would have to cover children, students and other dependents of insured individuals; dependent survivors, for at least one year after the insured person's death; a spouse and other dependents, for 30 days after divorce or legal separation from the insured; unemployed former employees, for a certain period after they left a job; and employees of employers who had failed to pay their premiums, for at least 30 days. All these persons with temporary coverage would have the option to convert to individual coverage if they wished.

Self-employed individuals would not be required to buy coverage, but could do so if they wished from an industry "pool." State and local governments also could have their employees covered by the pool.

Cost-Sharing. Individuals or families earning $14,000 a year or more would have to pay up to $3,500 of medical bills annually before insurance coverage began; the deductible would be adjusted periodically for inflation. Workers earning less than $14,000 a year would pay 25 percent of their annual income as a deductible, or $3,500, whichever was less. Insurance carriers would fully pay claims for these persons, periodically billing the federal government for their costs.

Employees could also be required to pay up to one-fourth the cost of their insurance premiums, although employers could pay the full cost or reduce the employees' share if they wished.

Medicare beneficiaries would not have to pay more than $1,000 a year in co-payments and deductibles for hospitalization and doctor bills; above that figure, Medicare would pay all "reasonable" costs or charges for covered services, including, for the first time, drugs to treat life-threatening or chronic illnesses.

Employer Subsidy. Employers could get a tax credit for the cost of providing new, mandated benefits. The credit would be a declining percentage of an employer's new costs for the first few years of the program. Employers could also continue to claim the tax deduction currently allowed for existing health insurance plans. State and local governments choosing to upgrade existing plans to conform with the new catastrophic minimum package could get a rebate from the federal government for their new costs.

"Pool" Coverage. To qualify for the catastrophic program, insurance companies would have to participate in state or regional insurance pools, as would health maintenance organizations and self-insured persons. The pools would sell the basic catastrophic plan to any individual or firm, at no more than 150 percent of the average cost for small employer groups. The pools were intended to be a source of insurance for part-time workers, the self-employed, high-risk individuals and others.

Medigap Certification. The committee agreed to create a voluntary federal certification program for so-called "Medigap" insurance — private plans to supplement Medicare. The committee provided penalties of $25,000 or five years' imprisonment for falsifying information to obtain certification, falsely posing as an agent of the federal government to sell the insurance, knowingly selling duplicative policies, or advertising or selling by mail policies not approved by state insurance commissioners. *(Medigap Legislation, p. 78)*

Labor/Kennedy/Waxman Plan

The comprehensive national health insurance legislation, the Health Care for All Americans Act, was introduced Sept. 6, 1979, by Sen. Kennedy (S 1720, HR 5191). Its chief House sponsor was Henry A. Waxman, D-Calif., chairman of the Interstate and Foreign Commerce Subcommittee on Health. Waxman noted it was the first time a chairman of that subcommittee had sponsored a national health plan.

The bill was based on a plan developed by the labor coalition Committee for National Health Insurance (CNHI) and generally followed broad CNHI "principles" announced in October 1978, on which Kennedy had already held hearings.

However, it was modified somewhat to meet objections to earlier versions. Benefits would be phased in over a period of years (although Kennedy insisted the plan must be enacted at one time). It emphasized cost control, and it put greater reliance on the private sector than Kennedy had in previous years. In fact, Kennedy lost support of an earlier cosponsor, Rep. James C. Corman, D-Calif.,

partly because his new plan would be administered by private insurers rather than by a public agency. (Corman and Ronald V. Dellums, D-Calif., introduced all-public national health insurance bills, HR 21 and HR 2969.)

Under Kennedy's bill, a heavily regulated insurance industry would administer much of the plan. Insurance would be mandatory, with all individuals required to be insured for basic medical services. Employees would have to pay up to 35 percent of the cost of their premiums, but would not have to meet any deductibles or make co-payments.

Assuming enactment in 1980, benefits would be phased in over an unspecified period of time, after a two-year lag to put cost control mechanisms in place. "Not one dime" would be added to the federal budget for benefits until 1983, Kennedy said. In the first year of benefits, he said the plan would add $28.6 billion to the federal budget and $11.4 billion to expenditures by business and workers for the mandatory coverage. Costs would climb above those of existing programs for the first four years, Kennedy said, but then there would be a "crossover." After that point, total U.S. spending for health care would be less each year than if the existing system were to continue, he said.

Kennedy rejected any "piecemeal" approach that would "relieve the political pressure from the constituents and defer the tough, central issues of cost controls and systems reforms for another day." The U.S. health care system was already "strained to the breaking point by runaway costs," he said.

Kennedy acknowledged that selling his plan would be an "uphill battle." Among other problems, two of the four congressional health subcommittee chairmen did not support it. Talmadge was a cosponsor of Long's catastrophic coverage legislation, while Charles B. Rangel, D-N.Y., House Ways and Means Health Subcommittee chairman, had several problems with Kennedy's plan, including its heavy reliance on the private insurance industry, and became a cosponsor of Carter's health plan.

How Kennedy Plan Would Work

● A National Health Board, appointed by the president, would set policy guidelines, oversee implementation and calculate the annual national health budget. State health boards, appointed by governors, would set state budgets, oversee state operations and resolve complaints from consumers and providers.

● Five national consortia would be formed to market qualified health plans: Blue Cross-Blue Shield nonprofit plans; commercial insurance carriers; health maintenance organizations (HMOs); individual practice associations (a type of prepaid group practice); and self-insurance plans. Individual plans would process claims; the consortia would collect premiums and allocate them among member plans, maintain contingency funds, monitor utilization and payment patterns and participate in annual budget negotiations.

● Every individual would be required to have health insurance coverage. Workers and their dependents would be covered by employers' plans; a Federal Hospital Insurance Trust Fund and a Supplementary Medical Insurance Trust Fund would pay for services provided to aged, disabled or other persons not enrolled in any plan.

● Employees would be liable for up to 35 percent of the cost of their health insurance premiums, depending on their wage level. They would not have to meet any deductibles or make any co-payments for covered services. Some employers, principally small employers, could get a tax credit for their premium costs. The income tax deduction for health insurance premiums would be abolished.

● Costs of the plan would be paid by employer and employee premiums, interest on the trust funds, federal appropriations, state contributions and "such other revenues as the National Health Board may specify."

● Benefits would include full coverage inpatient and outpatient hospital care, physician and laboratory services, X-rays, skilled nursing care, immunizations, pre- and postnatal care and well-child examinations up to age 18; limited mental health, nursing home and home health care; and outpatient drugs for treatment of chronic illness for Medicare patients. Exclusions included routine physical examinations, routine dental care, custodial care and cosmetic surgery.

● Federally administered Medicare for the elderly and disabled and state Medicaid programs for services not in the national health plan (such as chronic care) would be retained.

● A $500-million-a-year Health Resources Distribution Fund would fund new medical centers in medically underserved areas, medical education and other health resource programs.

● The annual budget for the national health program would have to be approved by Congress. Spending could increase at the same rate as the gross national product.

● Doctors' fee schedules would be negotiated; hospital budgets would be set in advance each year. Doctors, hospitals and other providers would be "at risk" for any costs beyond those budgeted. Reimbursement for capital expenditures would be allowed only for approved projects. Unusual, risky or costly medical procedures could be eliminated or restricted to specialists by the national board.

Carter Administration Plan

President Carter's national health insurance proposal was introduced Sept. 25, 1979, (HR 5400, S 1812), with Rep. Charles B. Rangel, D-N.Y., and Sen. Abraham Ribicoff, D-Conn., as chief sponsors.

It mandated coverage for everyone for catastrophic health care costs. But except for the poor and disabled, and workers who could win full coverage from employers, Americans would have to pay for part of their insurance premiums and part of their medical expenses. This strategy was popular with economists who thought it would discourage overuse of doctors and hospitals and save money.

Individuals or families would have to pay up to $2,500 a year in medical bills, plus part of the cost of their health insurance. Organized labor and well-paid professionals who had generous "first dollar" and major medical coverage for all or most medical bills would notice little difference in their coverage or out-of-pocket expenses, but there would be a dramatic cut in the tax deductions they could take in figuring their income taxes.

Agricultural and retail trade workers and others in poorly insured occupations would, for the first time, be covered for a package of basic benefits, since their employers would have to buy insurance for them or face tax penalties. But unless they developed enough clout to get employers to provide more than the minimum requirements, these workers would face new expenses as well.

Private insurance companies, meanwhile, would have "a lot of new business," worth about $10 billion a year, according to Benjamin W. Heineman Jr., assistant secretary of the Department of Health, Education and Welfare (HEW, now Health and Human Services).

Employers would have to absorb about $6 billion in new costs, although there would be some help in the form of subsidies for small employers, and a reinsurance fund that companies could use to back up self-insurance schemes. The plan would cost about $18 billion in federal money. The only addition to the plan from versions floated on Capitol Hill earlier in 1979 was a new program for pregnant women and infants, added largely at the insistence of Corman, according to HEW officials and Corman.

Despite administration denials, several congressional aides close to the situation said that pressure from Kennedy had helped resolve an internal administration debate in favor of a more generous health plan pushed by HEW. The losers were said to be the president's chief economic advisers, James T. McIntyre Jr., director of the Office of Management and Budget (OMB), and Charles L. Schultze, chairman of the Council of Economic Advisers, who wanted a very narrow program. However, the fact that Carter's final plan turned out to be much less than an all-out comprehensive program suggested a certain degree of success for the economists.

How Carter Plan Would Work

● The program would have two parts: Full-time employees and their dependents would be covered by employer-provided health insurance meeting federal standards, while a new federal program, HealthCare (combining Medicare and Medicaid), would cover the aged, disabled, public assistance recipients and individuals with incomes below 55 percent of the official poverty level.

● Private insurers would market both employer plans and HealthCare coverage according to federal regulation; the federal government would administer HealthCare. States would continue to administer skilled nursing and other optional services for Medicaid beneficiaries. Insurance carriers could participate in a voluntary reinsurance fund. There would be a HealthCare trust fund and an insurance standards advisory board.

● HealthCare enrollees and privately insured persons who had met their deductible would be covered for hospital care, doctor services, X-rays, lab tests, prenatal care and delivery, child health care including well-child examinations up to age one, family planning services, immunizations; and limited mental health, nursing home and home health care. HealthCare children would get dental, vision and health screening services. Exclusions included routine dental care, eyeglasses, hearing aids and related examinations, elective surgery, cosmetic surgery and custodial care.

● Employers would pay 75 percent of premium costs, workers 25 percent, plus the first $2,500 a year in medical costs. Non-poor elderly and disabled covered by HealthCare would pay up to $1,250 a year for premiums, first-day hospitalization, a percentage of daily nursing home costs, and certain other charges. There would be no cost-sharing for the poor or for prenatal and infant services in either private plans or HealthCare. Employers would pay the same amount for each employee's premium; employees who chose cheaper coverage would get a cash rebate for the amount saved.

• There would be subsidies for some employers, and a new tax credit for individuals. The existing individual income tax deduction for medical costs would continue, but only for costs above 10 percent of income. (Existing law allowed a deduction for expenses above 3 percent of income.)

• Financing of the plan would be from insurance premiums, part of the Social Security tax, state payments (90 percent of total cost) for HealthCare coverage of the poor, and federal general revenues.

• Hospital reimbursement would be limited by the administration's proposed hospital cost control plan. Physician reimbursement for HealthCare patients would be by negotiated schedule; participating doctors could not charge patients more than the allowed fee. There would be no restrictions on physician payments by private plans. There would be an annual national ceiling on total capital investments for expansion of hospital services, under separate legislation.

• The secretary of Health, Education and Welfare (HEW, now Health and Human Services) could override state or local licensing boards to certify non-M.D. practitioners (nurses, physician assistants or others) to practice and be reimbursed for services in outpatient facilities.

Republican Plan

Three Republican senators, Robert Dole, Kan., John C. Danforth, Mo., and Pete V. Domenici, N.M., introduced their own catastrophic bill (S 748) in 1979, with a deductible of $5,000 and 60 days' hospitalization, and improved Medicare benefits.

The four-part plan would require employers to provide catastrophic coverage for workers; add catastrophic coverage to Medicare; require state Medicaid programs to provide catastrophic coverage; and foster creation of a "residual" market catastrophic program for uninsured persons.

The bill would continue federal administration of Medicare and state management of Medicaid. Private companies would market and manage private plans. Carriers would be permitted to establish insurance pools, but they would be required to establish community-rated premiums. The federal government would certify plans in residual programs and would administer premium subsidies for low-income persons and families, determining eligibility and paying insurance carriers.

Medicare would continue to cover the aged and disabled. Employer-based plans would cover full-time employees and dependents, with the following additional requirements: three months' extension of coverage for surviving or divorced spouses or orphaned children of a covered employee; the right of an employee to convert to individual coverage before leaving his job; and three months' extension of group coverage after an employee left a job.

The bill would provide the following benefits. For Medicare enrollees, hospitalization and nursing home care would be provided without co-payment requirements and without time limits on hospital care. For physician and other services, Medicare would pay for all "reasonable" physician charges, drugs as listed on a special formulary and other services for individuals who had paid the deductible.

Benefits under the employer-based catastrophic program would be similar, except that institutional benefits would be covered only after an individual or family unit was hospitalized for 60 days (per year). Physician and other medical services would be provided for individuals who had paid the deductible.

Employer-based plans would be paid for by employers, with employees paying up to 25 percent of premium costs for catastrophic coverage. There would be a federal subsidy for some employers. Individuals and families would pay for catastrophic coverage under the residual program, with subsidies for the low-income population paid by general revenues. Employers would have to offer a program or face civil penalties. Participation would be optional for employees, who also could sue employers for failing to provide mandated coverage.

Private carriers would determine their own reimbursement and quality control policies. Public programs would continue to pay physicians and doctors "reasonable" charges.

Reactions and Outlook

Testimony before the Finance Committee early in 1979 indicated broad political support for insurance against catastrophic medical costs.

One Republican senator, Bob Packwood, Ore., suggested that passage of catastrophic insurance would help stave off demand for a "British-style, or Kennedy-style, national health service."

There was qualified support from much of organized medicine for catastrophic coverage, if government's role were kept to a minimum. Medical and insurance industry spokesmen also expressed support for an all-federal Medicaid program.

Then-HEW Secretary Joseph A. Califano Jr. made clear that the administration would support catastrophic insurance only if it was accompanied by cost control legislation and improved benefits for the poor and elderly.

A spokesman for the American Association of Retired Persons objected that catastrophic legislation would simply heat up health care inflation further if it did not include meaningful cost controls.

The AFL-CIO flatly rejected catastrophic coverage without other improvements, and the National Urban League said such coverage would do nothing to help the estimated 8 million poor people who had neither private nor public health coverage or the one in five Americans who had inadequate coverage.

Kennedy criticized Carter's plan as both unfair and potentially very expensive. Doctors' fees would be controlled in the public plan for the poor and elderly, but not in the private sector, thus perpetuating "separate and unequal" health care systems in America, he charged.

Another major inequity was that the "deductible" of $2,500 would fall most harshly on low-income families, Kennedy said. A family with a $10,000-a-year income would have to spend 25 percent of that on medical bills before benefits began, while a $50,000-a-year family would lose, at most, 5 percent of its income to the deductible.

Kennedy also criticized Carter for failing to set an overall limit on health spending.

Joining Kennedy in rejecting Carter's plan were representatives of blacks, the elderly and organized labor. Douglas A. Fraser, president of the United Auto Workers and chairman of the Committee for National Health Insurance, complained that Carter's plan "turns over huge new sums to health insurance companies and avoids regulating them on the theory that competition alone will make them public-spirited and socially concerned in a way they have not been up until now."

Most members of Congress were noncommittal on the plan. Businesses were not expected to like the extra expense of mandated coverage, although they would be able to write off much of the extra cost as a business expense, as they did with existing plans. The National Association of Manufacturers protested that "mandating insurance coverage will prove costly to employers at a time when inflation is the number one issue in the country.

New HEW Secretary Patricia Roberts Harris attacked Kennedy's plan Nov. 29, 1979, at a joint hearing of the House Ways and Means and Commerce Health subcommittees.

She called it "a potential $200-billion-a-year pork barrel" whose costs could put as many as a million people out of work. She claimed the plan would have a "shock effect" on the nation's economy, raising the Consumer Price Index by one and one-half percentage points, and "would inevitably result in an arbitrary rationing of health care services." Harris claimed Kennedy's plan would cause an 80 percent increase in employer health insurance premium payments.

Although national health insurance remained on the congressional agenda in 1980, prospects for a comprehensive revamping of the system were dim. Reflecting the sentiments of many of his colleagues, Ribicoff said early in the year that the prevailing efforts to cut the federal budget would make it almost impossible to pass a health insurance plan with large immediate costs in the near future.

"Forty years after national health insurance proposals were introduced into Congress during the 1930s, this mechanism has again been chosen as the possible panacea for bridling our nation's health care problems and for bringing them under control in some kind of orderly and organized manner," Braverman had written two years earlier. "It is only a matter of time before such a program is enacted into law. Whether or not it will be the ultimate answer to our nation's [health care] ills, only history will be the ultimate judge. But one point is for certain — there are now many powerful forces in our society who now believe it to be true." ∎

The Long Battle Over Hospital Cost Control

"Inflation is America's most serious domestic problem.... One of the most important components of inflation is the soaring cost of hospital care, which continues to outpace inflation in the rest of the economy. A decade ago, the average cost of a hospital stay was $533. In just the past two years, the average cost of a hospital stay has increased by $317 to $1,634 a stay — an increase of almost 24 percent.

"Hospital cost inflation is uniquely severe. It is also uniquely controllable.... This year, once again, I ask the Congress to join me in grasping that opportunity by enacting a tough program of hospital cost containment."

But, as it had in the past, Congress refused to respond to Carter's March 6, 1979, request for a cost containment bill. The House emphatically rejected the proposal in November 1979, and the administration did not push for a vote in the Senate, reportedly because it did not have the votes to win. The stalemate had not been broken as of mid-1980.

The battle to control hospital costs had begun in April 1977, when Carter sent his initial legislative proposal to Congress. In that year, hospital costs were increasing at an annual rate of 15.6 percent, compared to an overall inflation rate of 6.8 percent. The Senate passed a mandatory cost control measure late in 1978, but the House Commerce Committee gutted the bill and it was never brought to the House floor that year.

Substantively complex, the bill was difficult to sell. The benefits of hospital cost control legislation were relatively remote; moreover, many members of Congress were sympathetic to its target, hospitals. The administration claimed its plan would save more than $50 billion over five years, but since so many Americans were shielded from massive hospital bills by health insurance, the payoff was hard to dramatize.

Health industry warnings that the bill could lead to "rationing" of sophisticated medical techniques and equipment touched one of the most controversial, underlying issues — the question of quality in health care and implications that cost controls meant service cutbacks.

"The American people demand the best," said Rep. Tim Lee Carter, R-Ky., a physician, during 1979 House debate on the legislation. And Rep. Bill Gradison, R-Ohio, warned that if such a program had been in place in past years, "it's doubtful we would now have intensive care units and recovery rooms and cardiac care units."

The bill was also severely hampered simply because it involved regulation at a time when members of Congress were quick to blame inflation and other economic ills on excessive government meddling in the private sector.

These internal problems were compounded by the skilled campaign against the measure by the hospital lobby, the American Medical Association (AMA) and business groups.

Although the insurance industry, organized labor and groups representing the elderly supported the bill, for them it was only one of many pressing legislative priorities — unlike the hospital lobby, which could focus its full attention on the bill. Although labor wanted soaring health costs controlled, it feared that any hospital savings would come disproportionately from workers' salaries.

Reasons for Rising Costs

"Constraining the rise in health care expenditures" had become the "primary objective of public health care policy" and was "essential to the further refinement and improvement of all public health programs," the House Ways and Means Committee said in its Aug. 1, 1979, report on the hospital cost control bill (H Rept 96-404, Part 1). Problems of access and uneven distribution of services could not be dealt with until hospital spending was brought under control, the committee said.

If existing trends continued, the committee said, the nation would be spending $145.8 billion a year on hospital care by fiscal 1984. That would be a 76 percent increase from an estimated fiscal 1979 figure of $83 billion. That, in turn, compared with $13.9 billion worth of hospitalization expenditures for fiscal 1965, the year Medicare and Medicaid — the federal health insurance programs for the elderly and poor — were enacted.

Between 1969 and 1978, hospital expenditures increased more than twice as much as the consumer price index (198 percent as compared to 80 percent), an indication of the inflationary pressure hospital services had created in the health care system.

According to statistics compiled by the Health Care Financing Administration in the Department of Health and Human Services (HHS, formerly the Department of Health, Education and Welfare, HEW), spending for hospital care had increased by an average of 14 percent a year between 1968 and 1978, but was projected to average 13.1 percent for the period 1978 to 1990. Hospital care expenditures were projected to be almost 42 perent of total health expenditures by 1985 and 44 percent by 1990. Expenditures for hospital care were projected to reach $335 billion by 1990. (See chart, p. 20)

By far the largest share of the increase was attributed to inflation, with the remainder due to population growth and to increased "intensity" — greater use and/or changes in the kinds and amounts of services provided.

Between 1970 and 1978, the number of inpatient days increased 8 percent. The number of laboratory tests nearly doubled in six years, growing from 2.2 billion in 1972 to more than 4 billion in 1977. In addition, surgical operations, which generally require more resources than medical stays, grew nearly 19 percent during that period. The number of outpatient visits also increased dramatically between 1972 and 1977 — by 22 percent.

Only in recent years have health experts and federal officials realized that hospital costs were out of control and attempted to deal with them. Some lowering of hospital cost increases was accomplished during President Nixon's economic stabilization program of the early 1970s,

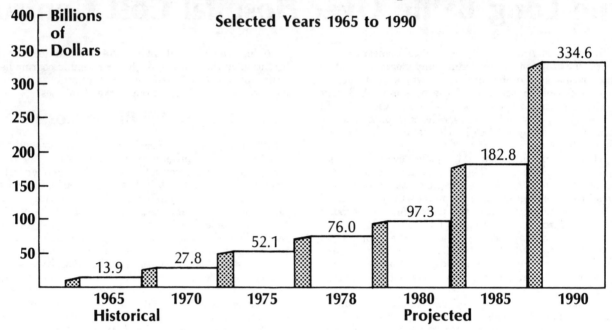

Expenditures for Hospital Care
Selected Years 1965 to 1990

Billions of Dollars

1965 — 13.9
1970 — 27.8
1975 — 52.1
1978 — 76.0
1980 — 97.3
1985 — 182.8
1990 — 334.6

Historical   **Projected**

SOURCE: Office of Research, Demonstrations, and Statistics, Health Care Financing Administration

a program which left bitter memories for many health care providers.

President Ford in 1976 proposed limits on hospital and doctor charges paid out of pocket by elderly Medicare patients as well as reimbursement limits for hospitals and physicians. However, he coupled that proposal with a requirement that the patients pay more of their own bills for short-term care. That provision was uniformly opposed by witnesses, and the whole proposal never got beyond the hearing stage in Congress.

While Congress continued to increase federal spending on health care programs through the years, a growing number of people began to question whether all the spending had made Americans any healthier and whether the country could afford to continue paying the soaring projected costs. Arguments raged as to who was to blame for the rising costs. Bureaucrats blamed doctors, doctors blamed hospitals, and hospitals claimed they were merely providing the "quality care" that Americans demanded.

Hospital Costs

According to administration statistics, the cost of one day's stay in a hospital had risen 1,000 percent between 1950 and 1978. The cost averaged about $175 a day in 1978, compared to about $15 in 1950.

Hospitals noted that the prices they had to pay for the goods and services they bought had been increasing because of inflation — wages paid to employees, food and fuel costs, medical malpractice premiums and equipment costs.

Critics admitted that hospitals had faced rising costs, like the rest of the population, but charged that the

way the system operated had led many hospitals to be inefficient, causing costs to rise unnecessarily.

"Hospitals are unlike any other segment of our economy," noted former HEW Secretary Joseph A. Califano Jr. in 1977. "There is absolutely no competiton among them." Doctors, not the consumers, selected what services were to be given, and in most cases third parties (private insurers or the government) paid whatever bills were submitted, so hospitals had no incentive to control costs. "Hospitals have become over the years, many of them quite obese," said Califano. "They are not trim."

Under the existing "retrospective cost reimbursement" system, hospitals were paid for the bills they submitted to insurance companies or federal or state programs such as Medicare and Medicaid. Thus, there was little incentive on the part of health care providers to resist higher prices and requests for larger quantities of labor or supplies since all bills were reimbursed after the fact.

Excess Capacity. Coupled with this was the problem of excess capacity. In short, there were too many hospital beds in the United States. The administration estimated that of the nation's nearly one million hospital beds, 240,000 were empty at any given time, and 100,000 of them were totally unnecesary.

Part of this problem was due to hospital construction encouraged by federal funding programs such as the Hill-Burton Act of 1946. Hospitals were built with little planning as to whether or not they should be as large as they were, or even whether they were needed at all, critics charged.

Hospitals also had high capital construction costs that must be paid over long periods of time. These costs

Principal Issues in the Hospital Cost Debate

Despite the Carter administration's efforts to tailor its 1979 hospital cost control bill to political realities, the legislation met with sharp criticism from a number of influential congressional Democrats and Republicans. Even administration allies complained that it seemed illogical and unfair for the president to demand standby price controls for the hospital industry while relying on voluntary restraints for the rest of the economy. Among the principal issues were the following:

Health Care: Who Decides? The basic disagreement between the Carter administration and its health industry opponents was over the most emotion-laden question of health policy: how much health care is enough, and who makes that decision?

Michael D. Bromberg of the Federation of American Hospitals (FAH) said that the Department of Health, Education and Welfare (HEW, now the Department of Health and Human Services) was "the last person you want making that decision because they have a conflict of interest — they buy the care."

Hospital officials and the American Medical Association warned that if the federal government interfered with the Voluntary Effort (VE) established by the hospital industry in 1978 to slow spending increases, they would have to arbitrarily cut services, and patients would suffer. "It's rationing, pure and simple," Bromberg warned.

Effectiveness of State Programs. The administration and its supporters insisted that the success of nine existing state hospital rate programs proved that hospitals could cut back spending without short-changing patients. The Maryland state program had shown that "we can contain costs. We can treat people," said Rep. Barbara A. Mikulski, D-Md.

But the experience of the New York state program made Rep. Charles B. Rangel, D-N.Y., wary of the concept. Rangel had seen his Harlem constituents lose needed jobs and access to health care in bankruptcy closings of hospitals in his district. Although he did not directly blame the state program for the closings, he said "the vote was still out" on whether it played an indirect role.

Then-HEW Secretary Joseph A. Califano Jr. said the financial problems of New York City's public hospitals were caused largely by their overload of non-paying patients. The "near poor," who did not qualify for Medicaid, and "undocumented persons" (illegal aliens) who hid their identities to avoid immigration officials, rarely paid hospital bills.

Voluntary Efforts or Mandatory Controls? Bromberg and other hospital industry spokesmen accused the Carter administration of wanting to subvert what Bromberg called "the one shining success" of voluntary industry efforts against inflation. The industry said the VE had more than met its 1978 goal by bringing hospital spending increases down to 12.8 percent nationwide, well under a 13.6 percent target rate.

Only hospital administrators and others familiar with individual and regional needs could make appropriate decisions on where to cut back, the industry contended.

The threat of standby mandatory controls would simply "scare" hospitals into inflationary increases in their charges, Bromberg warned. That was because hospitals would benefit from being locked into relatively high spending levels under mandatory controls. Califano argued that only the threat of mandatory government controls had scared the hospitals into their voluntary cost-cutting efforts, and that without that threat, costs would soar.

A March 13, 1979, Congressional Budget Office (CBO) evaluation of the Voluntary Effort found that it "appeared" to have cut the rate of increase in hospital costs, although data on the program was still so limited that any findings were "quite uncertain." The office also predicted that the VE could not meet its 1979 goal because of rising inflation and because the program was "not powerful enough."

However, data for the first nine months of 1979 appeared to show that the effort had been at least partially successful. During that time, the inflation rate was 11.7 percent after adjustment for rising costs over which hospitals had no control.

In its review of the fiscal 1981 budget, the CBO said the Voluntary Effort might "slacken" if Congress did not enact mandatory controls. "Voluntary approaches depend on institutions and individuals to act in ways contrary to their private interests," said the CBO. "Although this appears to have occurred to some extent, it is not likely to continue indefinitely."

Excessive Regulation? In response to arguments that hospital cost control legislation would lead to additional expensive and time-consuming paperwork, Califano said the program would probably cost about $10 million a year to administer — a good investment to obtain estimated federal savings of as much as $21.8 billion in the period 1980-84 and total savings of $53.4 billion during that same period.

Califano also attacked a study attributing a quarter of New York hospital spending to the cost of complying with federal regulations. In fact, he said, 64 percent of those costs were for record-keeping — charts on patient status and medication, record-keeping requirements of hospital accrediting agencies, medical education programs and the like. Less than one percent of those regulatory costs were caused by federal laws and rules, Califano said.

There were still some unanswered questions about how the program would actually work. Critics argued that hospitals would be "flying blind" because they would not know until after the year's end whether they had come in under their permitted increase. Penalties for noncompliance, denial of Medicaid/Medicare reimbursement and 150 percent excise taxes on both payors and hospitals appeared to some observers to be so harsh that they would never be invoked. And there appeared to be no protection in the bill against what was known as "bundling." Industry spokesmen maintained that hospitals were meeting mandatory state limits with this practice, under which a hospital contracted out services like diagnostic tests so that they were billed separately by the contractor and did not show up as hospital charges.

added on to the other daily costs of a hospital bed, such as labor and food, and had to be paid whether or not a bed was filled. It was estimated that each excess bed cost $10,000 to $20,000 a year to maintain; eliminating 100,000 of them thus would save between $1 billion and $2 billion a year. (It cost about $100,000 to install a single new bed and to provide support equipment; and maintenance of the bed, when occupied, cost $50,000 to $70,000 a year.)

It was not until 1974 that Congress passed legislation (PL 93-641) requiring that hospitals obtain permission, called a certificate of need, from state health agencies before being allowed to build new facilities. However, the program was controversial and was not fully in operation as of mid-1980. (See Health Planning chapter)

Related to the problem of excess capacity were administration estimates that as many as 100,000 of the 700,000 patients in acute-care hospitals could receive adequate, or even better, care at home or in skilled nursing homes at considerable savings to hospitals.

Unnecessarily lengthy hospitalizations, weekend admissions whereby patients often did not receive medical attention until the following Monday, and unnecessary surgery also contributed to escalating hospital costs.

Equipment Costs. Another factor in high-cost hospital care was the tendency of hospitals to buy increasingly expensive and sophisticated equipment. No hospital wanted to have outdated equipment, to be unable to provide "quality" care.

Critics charged that many hospital services might not be needed at all. Because of their desire to attract or keep medical staff members and to enhance the reputation of their institution, hospital administrations bought high-technology equipment and facilities which they did not need or could share with other facilities, it was argued. Examples cited were open heart surgery units and CAT (computerized axial tomography) scanners, which cost as much as $1.2 million to buy and were costly to operate.

Doctors' Fees

Hospital cost increases were not totally responsible for runaway health care costs, however. Physicians' fees accounted for 18 percent of all health care spending in 1978. Expenditures for doctors' services amounted to $8.5 billion, or $43 per person in 1965; in 1978 they had

jumped to $35.3 billion or $158 per person. Physicians' fees were increasing at an average annual rate of more than 12 percent — close to that recorded for hospitals.

Physicians, like hospitals, said they had been beset with rising costs for the goods they had to purchase, the medical malpractice insurance they had to buy, the extra personnel they had to hire to fill out increasing numbers of government regulatory forms.

But physicians were in a unique position of authority in regard to health care in the United States. In most cases, the physician's diagnosis determined the extent to which his or her own services were required, as well as what diagnostic tests and drugs were needed and what hospital to use. "Physicians influence health spending levels to a much greater extent than is indicated by the 18 percent share of spending devoted to their services," noted a 1979 Health Care Financing Administration (HCFA) study. "Physicians are the most important determinant in the process of deciding who will receive hospital care, what care shall be provided, and what the duration of care will be."

A contributing factor to this problem was that many insurance policies only covered medical care performed while the patient was in the hospital. In order to oblige the patient who did not wish to pay for care that could be covered by the insurance company, the physician might admit him to the hospital even if the procedure could be accomplished as an outpatient.

Physicians also were practicing more "defensive" medicine, due to the rapid rise in malpractice claims — ordering more lab tests, X-rays and examinations than might be necessary in order to have protection from liability. Between 1970 and 1978, malpractice insurance averaged a 39 percent annual increase, including a 100 percent rise in 1975 alone.

Other Factors

The public, most of whom were patients at one time or another, also contributed to spiraling hospital care costs. Many persons abdicated much of the consumer savvy they showed in other transactions once they became patients.

Because of their lack of knowledge of relative prices and alternative methods of care, patients tended not to question their physicians' decisions, said Peter H. Schuck of Consumers Union. Since they could not judge what really produced good health, they became preoccupied with the proliferating expensive technology. The result was the belief that " 'first class' care can be delivered only at 'first class' prices," he said.

Health Insurance. Some health experts blamed soaring medical bills on the fact that an increasing number of Americans were covered by health insurance programs in which the majority of the bill was paid not by the patient, but by the third-party intermediary. More than 90 percent of all hospital costs were paid for by someone other than the patients, according to the Health Care Financing Administration.

In addition to private insurance programs, which had been growing rapidly since the 1930s, the federal government stepped into the picture in 1966 with Medicare and Medicaid. These programs expanded the access of large numbers of elderly and low-income Americans to medical care and greatly increased the federal government's share of national health care expenditures. (See Medicare/Medicaid chapter)

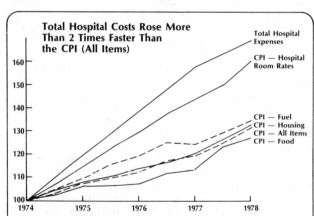

Total Hospital Costs Rose More Than 2 Times Faster Than the CPI (All Items)

Total Hospital Expenses
CPI — Hospital Room Rates
CPI — Fuel
CPI — Housing
CPI — All Items
CPI — Food

1974 1975 1976 1977 1978

To dramatize his argument for hospital cost control, Health, Education and Welfare (HEW) Secretary Joseph A. Califano Jr. presented this chart during congressional hearings. It showed hospital costs increasing far more rapidly than other elements of the Consumer Price Index (CPI) in the 1974-1978 period. Califano said federal hospital spending alone would exceed $60 billion by 1984, nearly double the 1979 level, if Congress didn't pass the legislation.

Economists warned that this increase in third-party coverage, whether through private or government insurance programs, isolated the public from the reality of health care costs. Since the patient did not pay the bill directly, or only a small portion of it, he tended to overuse medical services or did not question services that were ordered for him, it was argued. *(See National Health Insurance chapter)*

Health Habits. Finally the American lifestyle was blamed by some for driving health care costs up. Some health experts warned that until Americans realized that their lack of exercise, their high-fat, high-sugar diet and overuse of cigarettes and alcohol were ruining their health, they would continue to run up doctor and hospital bills for unnecessary physical ailments. *(See Disease Prevention chapter)*

1977 Carter Proposal

President Carter singled out hospital costs as the first target in his drive to put the brakes on skyrocketing health care costs in the United States.

Despite the opposition of much of the hospital industry and a lukewarm reception from Congress, Carter proposed legislation April 25, 1977, to limit hospital cost increases to 9 percent in fiscal 1978, with smaller increases in subsequent years until a different system for paying hospitals could be implemented.

The legislation also would set a $2.5 billion-a-year limit on new hospital building nationwide, to be allocated among the states on the basis of population. Any area with surplus hospital beds — about 80 percent of the nation's hospital service areas — would be prohibited from adding any new ones.

In a message to Congress, Carter called for quick approval of the program so that it could go into effect Oct. 1, the start of the 1978 fiscal year. However, by the end of 1977, only one of the four committees with jurisdiction over the plan had reported the bill — Senate Human Resources.

Meanwhile, then-HEW Secretary Califano said inflation in hospital costs was rising at the rate of $24 million a day, or a million dollars an hour. He did not accuse Congress of deliberate sabotage of the president's program, but he did point out: "Our legislation would take $10 million out of that inflation every day. . . . Not moving the legislation promptly is like throwing money away."

Hospital Cost Controls

As proposed by Carter, controls would be limited to inpatient reimbursement of acute care hospitals only. There would be no cap on outpatient services; the administration said they were less costly and should be encouraged.

HEW said the plan would affect about 6,000 community hospitals. Hospitals for long-term care (mainly mental hospitals) and hospitals operated by health maintenance organizations would be exempt because they were not experiencing high cost increases, HEW said. Hospitals less than two years old and federal hospitals also were not included. Califano said the president would apply the cost controls to Veterans Administration and other federal hospitals by administrative order.

Cap Formula. HEW devised a formula that would permit any hospital included in the plan to increase its revenue from all sources, including private insurance companies, Medicare, Medicaid, and individuals paying their own bills, up to 9 percent during the first year. In subsequent years, the formula would cut back allowable increases.

The formula was based on general price trends in the economy as a whole, plus an additional amount to cover some increase in patient services. The formula would be applied to the dollar total of the hospital's revenue from each payor for 1976, with an adjustment made for 1977, and would be applied on a per-admission basis.

Hospitals with no changes in patient load would have to hold down their charges so that their total annual revenue did not rise more than 9 percent above their base-year earnings. The plan did provide for small changes in patient load, up to a 2 percent increase in patient admissions or a 6 percent decrease.

HEW said that Medicare, Medicaid and Blue Cross already had interim payment schedules in effect that would also be used in the new plan. Should hospital administrators find changes occurring in their patient load during the year, the third-party payors would be readjusting their reimbursements on a per-admission basis to ensure that hospitals stayed within the 9 percent cap.

Penalties. At the end of the year, if total revenue received exceeded the 9 percent limit, hospitals would be required to put the excess amount in escrow and reduce charge increases during the next year by the same amount. Failure to do so would subject the hospital to a tax equal to 150 percent of the violation.

Exceptions. Exceptions to the total revenue limit would be allowed only for hospitals with exceptional changes in patient load or major increases in capacity, types of services or major renovation. Such exceptions would have to be approved by local and state health planning agencies and HEW. The revenue limit could also be adjusted for wage increases to non-supervisory personnel, who Califano said were earning wages about 10 percent below the median wage for other non-agricultural workers.

Hospitals could also be exempted from the program if they were in states that had their own hospital cost containment programs in which 90 percent of the state's hospitals were included, and other criteria were met.

Other Provisions. Other provisions would require hospitals to maintain their share of non-paying charity patients and to make public their current charge schedules and cost-reimbursement reports.

Capital Expenditures

Carter's second major proposal would limit new hospital capital expenditures to $2.5 billion nationally for the first year. The funds would be distributed to states according to population and new projects would have to obtain certificates of need from state planning agencies.

Certificates of need that would result in a net increase in beds would be denied in areas where the number of hospital beds exceeded four per 1,000 persons or where the average hospital occupancy rate was less than 80 percent. HEW said existing bed-shortage areas were mainly in the Southwestern and South Central parts of the nation.

Administration Defense

Carter and Califano defended the plan at a White House briefing April 25 as a necessary and workable program to control spiraling health care costs.

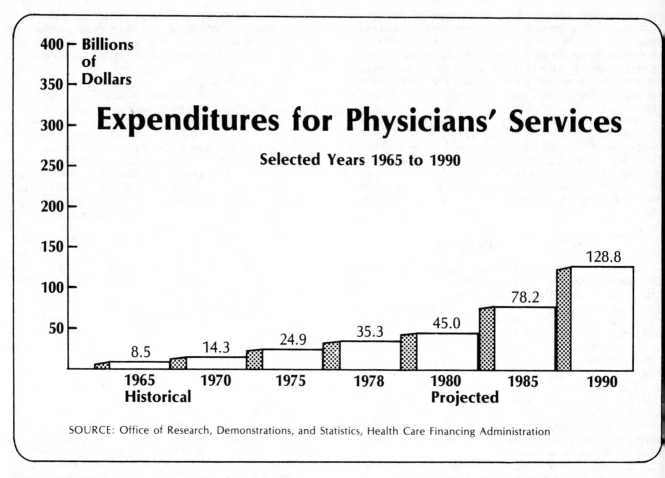

Expenditures for Physicians' Services

Selected Years 1965 to 1990

400 — Billions
of
350 — Dollars

300 —

250 —

200 —

150 —

100 —

50 —

8.5   14.3   24.9   35.3   45.0   78.2   128.8

1965   1970   1975   1978   1980   1985   1990
Historical   **Projected**

SOURCE: Office of Research, Demonstrations, and Statistics, Health Care Financing Administration

They said the program would not result in additional, massive bureaucracy or record-keeping, since HEW could "use essentially the information we are getting on Medicare and Medicaid forms right now."

Califano said the April 25 proposal was "eminently fair" and denied that it was a form of price control.

"We are permitting the hospital administrators to make all the decisions as to what they charge for, what they don't charge for, and how much they charge for it," he said. There would be no item-by-item federal limitation on services, he said.

He added, however, that the program would encourage hospitals to "cut some of the fat" out of their budgets. Califano said hospitals could be more energy-efficient, for example, could share expensive equipment instead of duplicating it, and could cut out excess beds.

"There is no incentive on the hospitals in this country today to operate more efficiently," Califano said. "We hope this legislation will provide that."

Industry Reaction

As expected, the Carter proposal was sharply criticized by members of the health care industry, who generally asserted that the quality of hosptial care would suffer because of the cost cap.

J. Alexander McMahon, president of the American Hospital Association (AHA), said, "The real victims of this bill are the sick and the injured." To McMahon the bill was "wrong in its concept and wrong in its details."

He charged that the revenue-per-admission requirement was "impossible" and would vastly increase the administrative costs of the federal government, private insurance companies and hospitals, contrary to HEW's claim that the plan would need little additional administration.

According to McMahon, hospital accounting practices would make it impossible to find out whether or not a hospital had stayed under the 9 percent ceiling on revenues until the end of the year, when it would be too late. He also opposed the tax penalty imposed "if you guess wrong" in any given year; he said the tax would just make it more expensive to run hospitals.

The director of the Federation of American Hospitals (FAH), Michael D. Bromberg, called the Carter plan "unfair and arbitrary ... nothing more than a camouflaged version of the Nixon Phase IV [economic stabilization] controls."

Bromberg said the FAH, which represented investor-owned rather than community hospitals, supported legislation sponsored by Sen. Herman E. Talmadge, D-Ga., chairman of the Senate Finance Subcommittee on Health. That bill, a revision of legislation introduced in the 94th Congress, would "provide for an incentive payment system offering economic rewards for efficiency," Bromberg said.

The American Medical Association hit strongly at the quality-of-care theme. Its executive vice president, Dr. James Sammons, said April 22, "The medical profession is concerned about the cost of health care, but we cannot be concerned only with the cost in terms of dollars. We must also consider whether the 'lid' or spending means we can buy only second-rate care and whether some care may simply become unavailable for many people."

One of the main arguments against the Carter proposal that was repeated throughout 1977 congressional hearings was that it singled out hospitals to bear the burden of cost control without attempting to control other sectors of the health industry that were contributing to escalating costs.

Bromberg complained that the plan did nothing about patients' lack of concern about the cost of care nor about the lack of competition among hospitals. In addition, said Andrew J. Biemiller of the AFL-CIO, the Carter bill did nothing about the escalating cost of doctors' fees.

Biemiller and others also said the provisions limiting the "dumping" of unprofitable charity patients by private hospitals were too weak. Terrance Pitts of the National Association of Counties said counties would have to pay for much of the care that would result when these charity patients descended on public hospitals run by counties and other local governments.

Biemiller also charged that, although wage increases for non-supervisory employees were not controlled by the plan, the exemption for states that had their own rate control structures could have serious consequences for lower-paid hospital workers in those states. The Carter plan did not require that state rate-setting agencies provide collective bargaining procedures, he said.

Congressional Response, Bills

Although the response from Congress was less antagonistic than from the health care sector, it was also not enthusiastic. Most congressional health care leaders supported the purpose of the legislation — controlling skyrocketing hospital costs — but were cautious about endorsing the specific provisions of the Carter plan.

The bill was introduced in both the House and Senate April 25. The House bill (HR 6575) was introduced by Paul G. Rogers, D-Fla., chairman of the House Interstate and Foreign Commerce Subcommittee on Health and the Environment, and Dan Rostenkowski, D-Ill., chairman of the Ways and Means Subcommittee on Health. The subcommittees shared jurisdiction over the legislation.

The Senate bill (S 1391) was introduced by Edward M. Kennedy, D-Mass., William D. Hathaway, D-Maine, and Wendell R. Anderson, D-Minn. Kennedy's Human Resources Subcommittee on Health and Scientific Research had jurisdiction over parts of the bill. Hathaway was a member of the Senate Finance Committee, whose Subcommittee on Health had jurisdiction over the majority of it.

Most congressional observers agreed that the key person in Congress, whose action, or lack of it, would most directly affect the outcome of Carter's proposal, was Talmadge, who introduced his own bill (S 1470) May 5. *(Details, p. 26)*

While Talmadge claimed his bill was not competitive with the Carter plan, he did make clear that he considered it a "long-term basic structural answer to the problem of rising hospital costs" while the Carter proposal was simply a short-term solution until a permanent program could be implemented.

Talmadge's bill was cosponsored by a high-powered group of Finance Committee members, including the chairman, Russell B. Long, D-La., and the ranking Democrat

and Republican on Talmadge's Health Subcommittee, Abraham Ribicoff, Conn., and Robert Dole, Kan.

Dole spoke in support of the Talmadge bill May 5, calling it "a responsible alternative to the Carter cost containment plan."

Dole said the main problem with the Carter plan was the arbitrary limit it placed on hospital revenue increases without corresponding limits on the goods and services hospitals must purchase. "It is unrealistic and inequitable to expect our health care institutions to bear the entire burden of alleviating the rising health costs problem," he said. The Talmadge bill, on the other hand, would encourage what savings were possible, Dole added, "while maintaining a realistic view of changes which providers are and are not able to make."

While Kennedy introduced the Carter bill in the Senate, he said he had certain reservations about it. For example, he said he thought any cost-control system should have better incentives to encourage greater use of less expensive outpatient facilities, better methods for cutting down on overuse of services and for encouraging physicians to order fewer expensive tests.

On the House side, Rogers said he had many of the same concerns as Kennedy, adding that reimbursement systems should provide hospitals with incentives to be more efficient and to close down facilities that were not needed.

Committee Action

The only committee to act on the proposal was Senate Human Resources which ordered reported a revised version of S 1391 on Aug. 2.

On Sept. 23, HEW issued new national guidelines aimed at holding down the number of hospital beds in the United States. The guidelines, proposed under the authority of the Health Planning Act of 1974 (PL 93-641) and published in the *Federal Register*, set a standard of four general hospital beds for each 1,000 persons and required an average annual hospital occupancy rate of 80 percent, two provisions that were part of the hospital cost control package.

But the guidelines did not sit well with a number of members of Congress who feared that they could lead to closings of rural and small community hospitals. In December, the House unanimously approved a resolution (H Con Res 432) urging that the needs of rural areas be considered in the final version of the guidelines. *(Rural Health story, p. 51; resolution, appendix p. 59-A)*

Compromises in 1978

Attention was refocused on the hospital cost bill early in 1978 by its prominent place in the fiscal 1979 health budget, and by a Feb. 1 announcement by Ways and Means Health Subcommittee Chairman Rostenkowski that he would like to give hospitals a 12-month reprieve to see if they could cut their costs voluntarily.

Throughout the year, however, the legislation was repeatedly pronounced dead. The administration's proposal was gutted by the House Interstate and Foreign Commerce Committee in July and rejected by the Senate Finance Committee in August.

Unexpectedly, the bill was resurrected and passed by the Senate Oct. 12. The Senate-passed bill (HR 5285) was a compromise sponsored by Gaylord Nelson, D-Wis. It would have left cost-cutting to hospitals on a voluntary basis as long as they met certain goals, but mandated strict revenue controls if hospitals failed to reduce the rate at which their spending grew to about 12 percent a year by the end of 1979 and keep it at that level through 1983. It allowed a number of exemptions. The bill also would have converted Medicare and Medicaid to a prospective payment system for hospitals.

Hospitals' 'Voluntary Effort'

On Jan. 30 the industry announced creation of a national steering committee and a network of state "medical and hospital committees." The major goal of the "Voluntary Effort," as the program was called, was to reduce the growth rate of hospital expenditures by 2 percent the first year and by an additional 2 percent the second year. The program's focus on hospital spending differed from the Carter targeting of hospital income. The Voluntary Effort was organized by the American Hospital Association, the Federation of American Hospitals and the American Medical Association. *(See also box, p. 21)*

Besides pruning hospital expenditures, the voluntary program set goals of "no net increases" in hospital beds and "restraint in new hospital capital investment." Implementation was left to the state committees, which were advised to provide technical assistance and use public disclosure and a certification procedure.

It was this program that Rostenkowski proposed to let run for a year. But, he told a Washington meeting of the American Hospital Association Feb. 1, "since nothing stimulates volunteers more quickly than the genuine fear of a draft," he would also push for mandatory "fallback federal controls . . . to assist you" if the voluntary effort failed.

The administration response to Rostenkowski's move was flat rejection. Speaking on behalf of the president, HEW Secretary Califano said Feb. 2 that past performance of the hospitals showed the plan "couldn't work." Although hospitals had promised to hold the line on costs in 1974 when they sought relief from national wage and price controls, "costs have been rolling along" at double the national rate of inflation since then, he said.

The delay proposed by Rostenkowski would "cost the American people $7.5 billion, and the taxpayers almost $3 billion," Califano warned.

Rostenkowski Bill

Concessions to the hospital industry and a lobby fight that pitted the White House against organized labor Feb. 28 dislodged a compromise version of President Carter's plan for controlling hospital costs from the House Ways and Means Subcommittee on Health.

After chewing over the unpopular proposal for nearly a year, the panel voted 7-6 to send to the full committee a substitute bill drafted by Rostenkowski. The outcome was uncertain until the final roll call as unhappy hospital and labor lobbyists sought to tilt the closely divided panel against the compromise.

The committee gave hospitals about a year to trim their spending voluntarily before a mandatory federal limit on revenue increases was imposed. The goal for the voluntary phase was to cut the annual growth rate of hospital spending from the existing 16 percent level to 12 perent within two years, with a constant rate thereafter. The mandatory phase, to be activated if the voluntary program failed, permitted 9 percent growth in the first year, al-

though adjustments could bring that figure to 12 percent. By 1983 the permissible rate of increase under the mandatory program would drop to 10 percent.

While neither the administration nor the hospital industry "warmly embraced" his bill, Rostenkowski said, it might serve as the basis for a compromise. Administration and congressional health sources privately conceded that Rostenkowski's move had bettered the bill's chances politically.

House Commerce Committee Action

The House Commerce Committee finally began marking up the bill in early June, and continued until mid-July, when it voted to scrap the hard-fought, much-amended proposal.

By a 22-21 vote July 18, the panel voted to replace the legislation with a Republican substitute offered by James T. Broyhill, R-N.C. The result of the committee's decision was that the bill (HR 6575) simply endorsed the hospital industry's voluntary efforts to cut back their costs by 2 percent a year. The Broyhill substitute dropped mandatory federal regulations altogether.

Senate Action

A few weeks later, on Aug. 3, the Senate Finance Committee voted 7-11 to reject the administration bill and to approve the more limited version (S 1470) sponsored by Talmadge, that applied only to hospital bills paid by Medicare and Medicaid. The committee added the provisions to a minor, House-passed tariff bill (HR 5285) and reported the measure Aug. 11 (S Rept 95-1111).

Talmadge had begun to move June 20 on his own bill after standing back for more than a year while the other three committees struggled with the administration's hospital cost control proposal.

After the president's plan was shot down in the House Commerce Committee, the administration tried to make Talmadge's bill the vehicle for its hospital cost control effort. President Carter himself reportedly telephoned senators on behalf of the compromise administration amendment, sponsored by Nelson, while heavy lobbying pressure against it was brought to bear by the hospital and medical associations.

The administration and the Kennedy-Nelson forces continued to fight for the compromise after its rejection by the Finance Committee, and it was an amended version of the Nelson amendment that finally passed the Senate Oct. 12, only to die at the end of the session for lack of House action.

Talmadge Bill. The Talmadge bill aimed at replacing the traditional fee-for-service system of paying hospitals with a pre-set, fixed-fee system — but only for bills paid by Medicare and Medicaid.

Talmadge proposed to gradually phase in a "prospective" reimbursement system, with different rates for different types of hospitals. Under the bill, Medicare and Medicaid would reimburse a hospital for routine "bed and board" costs at the average rate for its type, with bonus payments for hospitals with below-average costs. Hospitals whose charges exceeded the average by up to 15 percent would be fully reimbursed, but charges above that level would not be reimbursed.

The administration had two major objections to Talmadge's bill: it was limited to the two federal programs instead of covering all sources of hospital income, and it didn't save enough money.

Although the bill forbade hospitals to shift uncovered costs for Medicare and Medicaid patients to other payors, the administration warned that hospitals would do just that, avoiding any meaningful efforts to economize.

And the bill would save "only about $500 million over the next five years, or 100 times less than [the original administration plan] and 60 times less" than the latest compromise, according to Nelson.

The administration was also unhappy that the bill as reported omitted two important cost-saving features of earlier versions: a limit on payments to hospital-based physicians (anesthesiologists, radiologists, pathologists), and automatic phase-in of reimbursement limits for costly "ancillary" services like lab tests and drugs.

Unless the Senate accepted the Nelson amendment on the floor, HEW officials said, they would recommend to the president that he veto the bill.

Talmadge's bill had the qualified support of two leading opponents of the Carter plan, the Federation of American Hospitals and the American Hospital Association.

It was bitterly opposed by organized labor because, of all the alternatives pending, it was the least favorable to blue-collar hospital workers.

Nelson Amendment. The Nelson amendment adopted by the full Senate included several concessions to opponents. Like the compromise worked out earlier in the year by Rostenkowski, Nelson's plan endorsed the industry's voluntary effort to control hospital costs. It provided for standby mandatory controls on hospital revenues from all payors if the voluntary goals to cut hospital revenue increases to about 12 percent annually were not met.

There was a broad "pass-through" exemption to protect blue-collar hospital worker wages. And under mandatory revenue limits each hospital would have its own limit based on its expenses. The industry had objected that Carter's original across-the-board 9 percent revenue limit for all hospitals was a "meat-ax" approach that could force hospitals with unusual costs out of business.

The amendment applied the fixed-rate payment system to all hospital charges — those paid by private insurers and individuals as well as by Medicare and Medicaid. The system was similar to that in the Talmadge bill, but its version of incentives and penalties was less favorable to hospitals than Talmadge's.

Under the Nelson amendment, the hospitals' voluntary cost control effort and the new reimbursment system would run at the same time. Mandatory controls would go into effect if the voluntary effort failed to meet its goals, and they would apply to all revenues, not just routine costs. In addition to financial penalties (reduced reimbursement) for hospitals failing to comply, there would be tax penalties for both hospitals and other payors (insurance companies) for overcharges or overpayments.

A similar reimbursement system for ancillary costs would be developed by July 1981. Until then the voluntary effort would apply.

Several exemptions were added to the Nelson amendment to build support for it.

Senate Floor Action. After voting 42-47 against a motion to table the Nelson compromise, the Senate passed the bill by a 64-22 vote. Earlier it had tabled by a 69-18 vote the tougher, original administration cost containment bill as reported in 1977 by the Human Resources Committee. Passage of the bill was attributed to strenuous lobbying by organized labor, private insurance trade associations, and many groups that depended on federal "categorical" (targeted) health funds, as well as representatives of health maintenance organizations (HMOs); parliamentary ambush; and a pervasive belief that a "yea" on the controversial bill was "safe" because the House would not pass it before adjournment.

Inflation was the dominant theme of Senate debate, and after the vote sponsors credited their success to new congressional awareness of "the rising concern of Americans about rampant inflation in the health care industry," as Kennedy put it.

1979 Revised Plan Killed

The administration renewed its campaign to contain hospital costs on March 6, 1979, when it sent a new proposal to Congress (HR 2626, S 570). Again, however, the effort proved unsuccessful. The House Nov. 15 decisively rejected the bill and adopted instead a substitute that White House press secretary Jody Powell termed "a joke."

Administration Proposal

Like compromise bills of the 95th Congress, the president's 1979 proposal permitted voluntary cost-cutting efforts of the industry to continue as long as set goals were met. The legislation provided for mandatory revenue controls beginning in 1980, if the hospital industry as a whole failed during 1979 to hold revenues to a 9.7 percent rate of increase. The annual rate of increase would be adjusted for inflation in the cost of goods and services hospitals had to buy. An extra 1.8 percent increase would be allowed for increases in population or new hospital services.

Even if the mandatory program were triggered in, about 57 percent of U.S. hospitals could escape controls under a variety of exemptions in Carter's plan, according to Califano. Exemptions included hospitals in states with successful mandatory or voluntary cost control programs; small, non-urban hospitals; hospitals less than three years old; and HMO hospitals.

Revenue limits would be tuned to wage hikes for blue-collar hospital workers and to inflation in a "market-basket" of goods and services purchased by hospitals. There would also be adjustments for population increases and for changing patterns of medical care that would increase a hospital's "service intensity."

Hospitals judged "efficient" when compared with similar hospitals could get a "bonus" that would up their permitted rate of revenue growth, while "inefficient" hospitals would be penalized. For this part of the program, hospitals would be compared by case-mix, by location (city or rural) or by other characteristics.

The bill also authorized stiff tax penalties both for hospitals that overcharged and for anyone who paid the excess charges. It included an "anti-dumping" provision to keep hospitals from meeting the revenue limits by refusing to accept patients with very costly illnesses. And it provided up to $10 million for fiscal 1980 and funds "as needed" for three years thereafter to help states set up or continue operating their own hospital rate-setting programs.

The only major difference between the 1979 administration bill and the 1978 Senate bill was that the new proposal did not include the Medicare and Medicaid reimbursement changes proposed by Talmadge.

Intense Lobbying on Hospital Costs in 1979

The White House itself coordinated the lobbying for its hospital cost control bill in 1979, unlike 1977 and 1978 when it left that job to the Department of Health, Education and Welfare (HEW, now Health and Human Services) and was criticized for doing a poor selling job. While the White House failed to get involved in the hospital cost debate until late in the 1978 session, it began organizing and expanding its list of supporters early in 1979.

Under presidential assistant Anne Wexler, the White House put together a coalition of more than two dozen organizations representing the insurance industry, labor, the elderly and state and local government organizations to lobby on behalf of the administration bill. The coalition included the National League of Cities, the National Association of Counties and the National Association of State Legislators. They supported the Carter bill because it would cut down on their contributions to the health delivery system.

Some 1,200 county officials, meeting in Washington, D.C., the week of March 5, 1979, were dispatched to Capitol Hill to discuss the bill with their representatives and senators. And a meeting of about 250 coalition members held at the White House March 15 with Vice President Walter F. Mondale was followed by a lobbying foray to the Hill.

Many supporters of the bill saw it as a necessary first step in the fight for national health insurance. Richard E. Merritt, human resources director of the National Conference of State Legislatures, said the bill established an important precedent in assuring a state role in administration of hospital cost containment. "If the states are eliminated from the regulation of hospitals [costs] now, you've essentially eliminated them from a role in the future," Merritt said.

Wexler, along with HEW Assistant Secretary Richard D. Warden, also organized briefings for represen-tatives of business groups in an effort to broaden the administration's base of support beyond the insurance industry. However, the business community gave administration overtures a cold shoulder. Jan Ozga, health care director for the U.S. Chamber of Commerce, which opposed the administration bill, characterized it as "the first step toward price controls" for all goods and services, a view widely echoed among business groups.

The Business Roundtable, a group composed of the executives of major corporations, and the National Association of Manufacturers also opposed the administration bill.

Indeed, the insurance industry was the only major business group to support the Carter plan. During the 1978 debate, the Health Insurance Association of America, representing some 320 insurers, played a major role in winning Senate passage of the measure that eventually died in the House.

Industry Efforts

None of the White House efforts were lost on the hospital industry, which campaigned as aggressively against the bill in 1979 as it had in previous years.

In addition to the Federation of American Hospitals (FAH), which represented 780 of the nation's 986 investor-owned hospitals, the industry's principal spokesmen were the American Hospital Association (AHA), which included among its members most of the nation's hospitals, and the American Medical Association (AMA).

The industry argued that Carter's proposal would have only a minuscule effect on inflation, that it would be a regulatory nightmare, that it unfairly singled out the hospital industry for price controls, and that it was unnecessary because hospitals' voluntary efforts at controlling costs were working. It also argued that the bill would result in "rationing" of health care.

The 1979 bill also omitted a major feature of Carter's original 1977 bill, a $2.5 billion national cap on capital expenditures for hospital construction, major medical equipment or other improvements.

Despite the exemptions, the bill would save an estimated $1.4 billion in federal spending in the first year of mandatory controls, with most of the savings coming from "a small minority of hospitals who are . . . profligate" in spending, Califano said. Total federal savings for fiscal years 1980-84 would be $21.8 billion, and overall savings for both private and public payors for that period would be $53.4 billion, according to Califano.

The president challenged Congress to demonstrate its commitment to fighting inflation by acting quickly on the bill. With inflation threatening the "basic societal structure" of the nation, Congress should disregard special interest pressures and pass the legislation, Carter said. He blamed the hospital lobby for the defeat of the earlier bill, and said the industry lobby was "even more determined and equally well financed" in 1979.

Congressional Action

In the end, the industry lobby won out again. On Nov. 15, the House dumped cost controls entirely and by a 234-166 vote, with 99 Democrats voting against the president, adopted a substitute that simply created a national study commission on hospital costs and authorized some funds for state cost control programs. It was a major legislative defeat for the president, who had called the bill his top-priority anti-inflation measure of the year.

The substitute was sponsored on the floor by a respected young Democrat and Carter supporter, Richard A. Gephardt, Mo., although it had been pushed in committee by Republicans. After opting for the study commission and rejecting a move to kill even that legislative gesture by recommitting it to committee, the House voted 321-75 to pass the bill.

Republican members wanted to recommit the bill for fear that if Democratic supporters had anything at all entitled "cost control" to take to conference with the Senate, the House could still face a strong cost control bill in 1980. But Henry A. Waxman, D-Calif., chairman of the House Commerce Subcommittee on Health, a co-sponsor of the administration bill, said the very large House vote against Carter's plan meant that it was "most likely" dead.

House leaders had warned Carter he did not have the votes to win, but he insisted the bill be brought to the floor before Congress left for its Thanksgiving recess. Despite ominous vote counts, the White House apparently believed the inflation issue would bring members around at the last minute.

The president's initial reaction to the vote was "unprintable," according to Powell. Powell later characterized the House action as a "victory for the highly financed special interest [hospital] lobby and a defeat for the common good."

When it came to the floor, HR 2626 was a considerably weaker version than the 1977 bill, which itself had been substantially scaled down by the president.

Of the four congressional committees with jurisdiction over the bill, only the Senate Labor and Human Resources Committee reported it relatively intact in 1979. The Senate Finance Committee rejected Carter's plan, approving instead a revision of Medicare and Medicaid hospital payments only (HR 934).

The administration did not press for a Senate vote on mandatory controls in 1979, reportedly because it did not have the votes to win. Several conservative senators had threatened to filibuster any cost control measure that came to the floor.

The future of hospital cost control legislation remained cloudy as of mid-1980, although the administration indicated it would attempt to make mandatory controls part of any national health insurance plan Congress passed. ∎

Troubled Hospitals Seek Congressional Aid

Although their timing could not have been worse, a coalition of hospital, labor, county and city officials banded together in late 1979 and early 1980 to ask Congress for a sizable bailout for financially troubled hospitals — a bailout that could cost hundreds of millions of dollars.

Washington's preoccupation with budget-cutting in 1980 did not give them much hope of massive federal aid. But without a quick infusion of funds, health experts warned, many of the hospitals which had functioned for decades as a de facto "national health system" — providing medical treatment for the poor and near-poor — could be forced to shut down critical services, or even close their doors.

The numbers were not firm, but health analysts said at least 200 U.S. hospitals had piled up deficits totaling hundreds of millions of dollars a year.

Concerned members of Congress, such as New York's Rep. Charles B. Rangel, D, and Sen. Jacob K. Javits, R, were especially worried about public and certain private hospitals in medically underserved, poor communities. By law or by custom, these hospitals admitted patients regardless of ability to pay. Rangel and Javits warned that other cities also would soon feel the problem.

In Feb. 29, 1979, testimony before Rangel's Ways and Means Health Subcommittee, Carol Bellamy, city council president of New York City, warned that cities were "losing the fight" to finance the public "hospitals of the last resort" that served an estimated 11 million to 25 million Americans who had no insurance coverage. Such medical landmarks as Cook County Hospital in Chicago, Jackson Memorial Hospital in Miami and Grady Memorial in Atlanta were in deep financial trouble, in large part because more and more of their patients were unable to pay their bills. In 1978, Grady Memorial in effect gave away $29 million worth of uncompensated services, as much as it received from Medicaid for care provided to low-income beneficiaries of that program. Tiny rural hospitals complained they were suffering as well.

The number of non-paying patients had grown as states pared down Medicaid, the state-federal program for the poor. The cost of care for illegal immigrants also had become a serious financial problem for hospitals in New York, Chicago, Los Angeles and many Southwestern states. Inflation, shrinking local tax bases and certain cost control efforts magnified the impact on hospital budgets of non-paying patients, according to hospital officials.

Although their plight appeared alarming, it would not be easy for the hospitals to extract additional federal aid from Washington in 1980. The Carter administration believed that in most cases the "major responsibility" for hospitals "rests with state and local governments," according to Health, Education and Welfare (HEW, now Health and Human Services) Under Secretary Nathan J. Stark in testimony before Rangel's subcommittee. And the hospitals' constituents, the poor, "are not a very popular commodity," Rangel observed.

Powerful Support

But the poor had some powerful allies lined up on their side in the fight, including the hospital lobby and the American Federation of State, County and Municipal Employees (AFSCME). Some 300,000 AFSCME members worked in health facilities. And hospital officials developed impressive access on Capitol Hill during their three-year campaign against hospital cost control legislation. *(Story, p. 19)*

Members who opposed aid to hospitals risked charges that they had abandoned important community institutions. Nevertheless, it was expected that when debate began, skeptics undoubtedly would blame the hospitals' problems on inept management, obsolete physical plants and excess capacity. Some critics even suggested that seriously troubled hospitals should be allowed to fail, sending patients to more successful neighboring institutions. In several states, public officials were already turning over public hospitals to private management.

But that was no solution, warned Dr. Quentin Young, chairman of Cook County Hospital's Department of Medicine and chairman of the Coalition for the Public General Hospital. Young said private hospitals routinely turned away uninsured patients and often rejected Medicaid beneficiaries as well. Public general hospitals were "a precious and irreplaceable national resource," and allowing them to close, Young said, was "the Marie Antoinette solution."

Reasons for Deficits

The developing fiscal crisis among hospitals had almost as many causes as there were hospitals in trouble, according to federal and hospital officials studying the

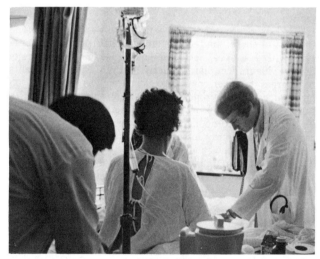

Hospitals have become the only source of health care for millions of Americans, especially the poor and uninsured. Closing one not only means loss of a health facility for neighborhood residents but loss of many jobs.

problem. Inflation, poor planning, inadequate Medicaid payments and local conditions such as physician shortages or large numbers of illegal aliens all contributed to the deficits of many hospitals.

Hospital officials said widespread health insurance coverage and a new stress on controlling costs had all but ended the traditional "Robin Hood" method of financing medical care for the poor by overcharging the "rich." Nine out of 10 Americans in 1980 had some sort of health insurance, although coverage for many workers, such as retail clerks and clerical workers, was scanty. What had occurred was that doctors had taken their insured patients to sleek suburban hospitals and high-powered medical centers. The exodus of paying patients left large public general hospitals and charitable private institutions with a growing pool of non-paying patients.

Public and private charity hospitals were also burdened by "dumping" — transfers from private hospitals of patients who were uninsured or whose health insurance

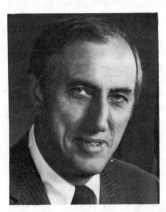

"The assumption should not be made that all hospitals in financial trouble should necessarily be saved ... with their present missions, modes of operation and governance."
—Nathan J. Stark, under secretary of health, education and welfare

benefits had expired. Rep. Henry A. Waxman, D-Calif., told Rangel's subcommittee that Los Angeles County Hospital received 2,000 such "involuntary transfers" each month.

Hospital administrators said they wanted to spread the cost of these "bad debts" among their paying patients. But, with few exceptions, Medicare, Medicaid and major private insurance plans strictly limited their payments to charges for their own beneficiaries. The emphasis on hospital cost containment in the latter part of the 1970s further constrained such hospital practices as using "profits" from well-to-do departments — radiology or laboratories — to defray losses of less lucrative departments, such as emergency rooms.

Most of the financially distressed hospitals suffered from one or more of the following problems:

Inflation

As prices of basic hospital supplies soared, so did interest rates for capital, which was critically important in the high-technology health care industry. Medical care was becoming increasingly expensive, in part because doctors had the capability to do more for patients than they were able to do previously. Sophisticated medical machines revolutionized diagnosis and treatment; and, as a result, many more specialized technicians were put on hospital payrolls. "Medicine is the only industry that

is both labor intensive and technology intensive," a Federal Trade Commission attorney observed.

Public general hospitals have traditionally relied heavily on financing from city and county revenues. But by 1980, inflationary pressures were stiffening local taxpayers' resistance to increased spending for these institutions. For example, Georgia's Fulton County routinely spent one-fourth of its annual tax revenues on Grady Memorial, according to the hospital's executive director, J. S. Pinkston Jr. But in 1979, when the county printed individual tax bills with the amount each taxpayer was "contributing" to the hospital, reaction was quick and angry. Irate citizens complained that "they could not afford such a price for services they generally did not use — services ... for the poor," he said.

Medicare, Medicaid Inadequate

Many Americans have not been able to pay for much medical care but, on the other hand, they have not been able to qualify for medical assistance. For example, the National Health Law Program, a consulting organization that advises lawyers working in the health field, found that less than a third of Southern families with incomes below the poverty level qualified for Medicaid.

Some states let inflation strip the working poor from their Medicaid rolls by the simple expedient of not raising income eligibility levels. Another state tactic that enlarged the pool of non-paying patients was tightening up on Medicaid eligibility determinations, or deliberately delaying this "certification" process until long after the patient had checked out of the hospital.

In Illinois, for example, the certification rate for Cook County Hospital patients dropped from about 62 percent in 1973 to 22 percent in 1979. Cook County Commissioner John H. Stroger Jr. blamed this steep decline in certification for most of the hospital's $84.8 million deficit in 1979.

Hospital administrators complained that Medicare and Medicaid reimbursement formulas crunched them in several ways. "Reasonable cost" reimbursements for inpatient services did not appear to be a major problem, but states could and had set fees for procedures on outpatients that were well below real cost. For example, three Pennsylvania children's hospitals were required to "accept $12 for each clinic visit as payment in full [from Medicaid] ... even though the real cost is ... $35 to $40" or more for non-routine care, according to Albert Wareikis, vice president of Children's Hospital of Philadelphia.

These lower outpatient rates posed a particularly severe problem in medically underserved communities, where many people relied on hospital clinics and emergency rooms for basic medical care. Many private insurers also set low reimbursement rates for outpatient services, contributing further to the problem. In 1978, New York hospitals lost $235 million in unreimbursed outpatient care.

Hospital administrators also said Medicare and Medicaid had not factored in an adequate amount for depreciation allowances to enable them to replace old equipment with the next, more sophisticated generation of medical machinery. And public hospital officials were irritated by the fact that for-profit hospitals could charge Medicare and Medicaid for a "return on investment" allowance, but public hospitals received no comparable reimbursement.

Illegal Immigrants

An estimated three million to six million foreign-born persons were living illegally in the United States in 1980, and a large number of them depended on local hospitals and clinics for what health care they received. Reluctant to risk detection by immigration officials, they were also difficult for hospital bill collectors to track down. These "undocumented persons" were a major drain on hospitals that served them, said Rep. Tony Coelho, D-Calif. One tiny hospital in Coelho's district almost bankrupted itself and the county government that supported it when it spent more than $75,000 in one year treating an injured, "undocumented" farmworker. More and more illegal immigrants had been routinely using public clinics for non-emergency care, according to Coelho.

Hospital officials said either that they were unable to distinguish between U.S. citizens and undocumented persons, or that they could not ethically refuse to care for them.

Court decisions during the late 1970s discouraged Immigration and Naturalization Service "sweeps" for illegal immigrants. Coelho complained that this trend — in effect a national decision to relax immigration laws — left local governments staggering under the costs of providing services, including medical care, to illegal aliens.

Other statutes, including anti-discrimination laws, that could distribute non-paying patients more evenly among hospitals, also were not being enforced, according to Rangel. As an example, he cited the fact that no New York state hospitals were in compliance with Hill-Burton charity care requirements.

The 1946 Hill-Burton act required medical facilities receiving federal construction funds to make services available to all persons residing in their area and to provide a "reasonable volume" of free care for the indigent. The obligation was to continue "for all time," and most of the nation's hospitals were so obligated, according to HEW spokesman Frank Sis. But enforcement has been "non-existent," Sis said. The original law and the title of the health planning act that replaced it provided no sanctions against violators.

Spokesmen for the National Health Law Program said federal and state tax laws also contributed to the problem, because they allowed private nonprofit hospitals to receive tax-deductible charitable contributions without requiring them to provide charity or reduced cost care to needy patients.

Management Problems

Hospitals were extremely sensitive to charges that they created their own fiscal problems by failing to set up proper record-keeping and billing procedures, by inefficient purchasing procedures and other management problems. Although few administrators would say so publicly, many public hospitals never developed the business expertise of some of the for-profit hospitals, because their mission had never been to make money. As Robert B. Marvin, administrator of a small hospital in north Florida, told Rangel's subcommittee in early 1980, because of its "philosophical approach," a public hospital, "which is there only to provide a place to treat the sick, does not develop the extent of expertise necessary to expand its profitability."

Dorothy Lang, a staff attorney with the National Health Law Program, testified before the subcommittee that Los Angeles County Hospital's "inadequate" billing system cost the county "millions of dollars of Medicaid revenue" that was not collected. But even that inadequate system cost more than $10 million a year, and "given a choice of spending scarce resources on patient care or on billing mechanisms," many public hospitals opted for patient care, Long said. Marvin added that the "less sophisticated" public sector had been less effective than the private sector in winning concessions from state and federal governments.

Outlook

Early in 1980, Rangel launched a series of field hearings on the fiscal problems of hospitals and persuaded the Ways and Means Committee to ask the House Budget Committee for $100 million for aid to distressed hospitals in fiscal 1981. Waxman, chairman of the Commerce Subcommittee on Health also was pushing a hospital aid budget request. The major options being considered were:

● Adding allowances for "bad debts" to Medicare and Medicaid reimbursement formulas.

● New distress grants targeted on hospitals meeting certain criteria, such as number of uninsured and Medicaid patients.

● Revisions of existing programs, such as waivers in federal programs to reimburse for costs of caring for illegal immigrants, or stationing National Health Service Corps doctors at hospitals in medically underserved areas.

All of the above measures were generally regarded as temporary relief for a chronic problem. Any long-term

---

Public general hospitals have been "a precious and irreplaceable national resource," and allowing them to close would be "the Marie Antoinette solution."
—Dr. Quentin Young, chairman, Coalition for the Public General Hospital

---

solution appeared to be unlikely as of 1980, not only because of budget problems but because of serious flaws in existing data on hospitals. No one involved in the problem could definitively say just how many hospitals were endangered, which should be helped, or how much it would cost.

In his testimony, Stark suggested that there might be a "few" badly needed hospitals that merited federal aid. HEW had already stretched existing authorities to bail out Brooklyn-Jewish Hospital and two smaller New York institutions. The image of "fat" and "bloated" hospitals pushed by former HEW Secretary Joseph A. Califano Jr. was absent from the department's policy pronouncements in 1980.

But Stark was quite cool to the idea of Medicare and Medicaid payments to hospitals to cover reimbursement for bad debts. That could cost the federal government as much as $500 million a year, he estimated. It would also put each hospital in the position of determining eligibility and benefits for a national medical assistance program, he suggested.

Stark also implied that state and local governments and private payors should be compelled to share any responsibility for bad debts, but the idea was controversial and the administration in 1980 was taking a "hard look" at it.

Some sort of distress grant seemed to be the most likely outcome, but Stark, Rangel and others said they wanted to make certain that the aid was targeted on hospitals that needed it most. "While many of our nation's hospitals might consider themselves financially hard-pressed ... we are concerned with ... relatively few," Stark said.

Existing data was not fine-tuned enough for such targeting, officials said. Comparisons between institutions would be basic to deciding which hospitals should be helped, but the many different styles of hospital accounting in effect in 1980 virtually ruled out such comparisons on a national scale. "Words mean different things to different accountants. One hospital's 'bad debts' become 'charity work' at another. A county hospital might gather every imaginable charge into its 'deficit' column so it can ask for more money from the county," a hospital finance officer explained.

These accounting differences might be reduced under regulations set by HHS to require hospitals to report their costs for Medicare and Medicaid under a uniform system. But as of mid-1980, the regulations had compounded basic problems with the two major data sources, the American Hospital Association's (AHA) annual voluntary reporting system and Medicare cost reports. AHA officials privately called their data "soft," because under their voluntary system, many hospitals either did not report at all or did not fill in all information requested. HHS officials said they had very good numbers for what

hospitals spent annually, but that they did not have enough information to analyze hospital deficits. A deficit could be caused by bad management, by failure to bill Medicare or Medicaid, by illegal aliens or by any combination of these and other factors, but "these are much more subtle comparisons than we can make now," said Suzanne Stoiber, a member of the HHS Task Force on Financially Troubled Hospitals.

Stark and Rangel appeared to agree that once adequate data became available, aid should go first to hospitals whose problems stemmed from their commitment to caring for the uninsured or poorly insured. They also agreed that priority should be given to aid to hospitals in medically underserved areas.

A third major cause of fiscal troubles — management problems — raised the most painful political questions. No one wanted to pour money into wasteful systems, and Rangel was clearly distressed by the deficiencies of several endangered hospitals in his Harlem district. But some of the most poorly managed hospitals were also perceived in their communities to be the most needed. If they were to fold, Rangel feared, jobs would be lost and black staff doctors would be unable to obtain admitting privileges at nearby white hospitals. Dealing with this dilemma could result in new controls for hospitals, such as outside audits or management reviews, as a condition for federal assistance.

"The assumption should not be made that all hospitals in financial trouble should necessarily be saved, or even supported, with their present missions, modes of operation and governance," cautioned Stark. To Rangel, the best long-term solution would be comprehensive national health insurance. "But," he noted wryly, "You could have a convention in a telephone booth of folks who want that." ∎

Would More Competition Cut Health Costs?

A stiff shot of competition is the best cure for the nation's feverishly inflated medical industry, according to a controversial economic theory that has been gaining ground in Congress.

Although it conjures up visions of cut-rate appendectomies and medical price wars, the theory actually involves a series of changes in the nation's tax and health regulation laws.

These changes would create powerful financial pressures on the nation's medical system, forcing doctors, hospitals and health insurers to organize themselves into competing units that would strive to keep prices down and quality up, according to proponents of the theory. Americans also would have to pay more of their own health care costs instead of relying on insurance to cover them; that would make them more cost-conscious and more likely to question the necessity, quantity and cost of their medical services, the theory goes. The nation was spending an estimated $218 billion on health care in fiscal 1979.

The leading advocates of the competition theory were economists Alain C. Enthoven of Stanford University, Martin Feldstein of Harvard, and Clark C. Havighurst, an antitrust attorney specializing in medical economics, who was teaching at Duke University. On Capitol Hill, the economists' recommendations were shaping up as a highly visible alternative to national health insurance and federal health regulation.

The theory — sometimes referred to as the competition model, or the free market model — appeared to offer Congress a solution to some vexing problems in health care without either new regulations or new spending.

Two groups with considerable clout in Washington — the insurance industry and hospitals — found the concept an effective argument against government intervention. Another visible advocate was the influential Minnesota consulting firm, InterStudy, which was deeply involved with health maintenance organization (HMO) development. The segment of the medical marketplace that could gain the most from a congressional tilt toward the competition model was the HMO, or prepaid health plan.

Competition advocates liked the prepaid plans both for their internal economies and for their competitive impact on the traditional fee-for-service U.S. medical system. The plans provide medical care for a fixed fee and thus must hold their costs within their budget. The changes competition advocates proposed for HMOs would merely put the plans on an equal footing with the fee-for-service sector.

Benjamin W. Heineman Jr., assistant secretary for health, education and welfare (HEW, now Health and Human Services), and other prominent health professionals warned in 1979 that competition alone would not cure the ills of America's high-technology, psychologically complex style of medicine. "I don't think medicine works like a fruit and vegetable market," said Robert M. Ball,

senior scholar at the Institute of Medicine, a branch of the National Academy of Sciences which conducts major science policy studies. Or, as two contributors to the respected *New England Journal of Medicine* put it: "It is difficult to envision the operation of 'smoothly working market forces' in the American medical exchange, where quality is very hard to define, necessity is in the eye of the beholder, and the public is hostile to the queue and willing to pay to avoid it."

Economist Alice M. Rivlin, head of the Congressional Budget Office (CBO), testified that any savings from putting the competition theory into practice would take years to show up. In addition, the changes envisioned by Enthoven, Feldstein and Havighurst had potentially explosive political implications. Any promotion of prepaid health plans would be on a collision course with one of the most firmly defended principles of the American medical establishment — what American Medical Association officials have referred to as "the sacred doctor-patient relationship" based on fee for service.

And, to bring about the competitive marketplace envisioned by the economists, Americans would have to pay many medical bills that have been covered by their health insurance, or new taxes on the insurance itself. These changes would not be popular with Americans accustomed to having their health bills covered by insurance, and they were opposed by organized labor, which bitterly denounced any suggestion that it yield all-expenses-paid health plans for its members.

Nevertheless, while President Carter and Sens. Edward M. Kennedy, D-Mass., and Russell B. Long, D-La., sparred over how much more health insurance the nation could afford, Enthoven, Havighurst and Feldstein were, with some success, urging Congress to go their very different route and opt for less. They also called for less government interference in the health care system.

House members James R. Jones, D-Okla., Dave Stockman, R-Mich., Bill Gradison, R-Ohio, and Phil Gramm, D-Texas, a former economics professor, were pushing competition as an alternative to hospital cost control legislation. Stockman and Gramm, in the name of competition, also led efforts to weaken an extension of the controversial health planning system.

Pieces of the competition theory also emerged in alternatives to national health insurance introduced by House Ways and Means Committee Chairman Al Ullman, D-Ore., and Republican Sens. Richard S. Schweiker, Pa., and David Durenberger, Minn. Even Carter's and Kennedy's rival national health plans boasted elements designed to promote competition. *(Major competition proposals, box, p. 38)*

The Theory

Nine out of 10 Americans in 1979 had some form of health insurance — either private or Medicare or Medicaid. Many economists believed that this extensive coverage — despite its many gaps — had expanded the variety of medical services and treatments available to Americans far beyond the real health needs of individuals.

Insurance shields individuals from the true cost of treatment and protects doctors and hospitals from bad debts. And fee-for-service reimbursements, which most health plans provide, reward doctors for prescribing more and more care. There is no incentive for thrift, according to the advocates of competition. Claimed Schweiker: "Our health insurance system now resembles a free lunch arrangement for doctors and hospitals." Rivlin observed: "Patients want the best of care, and doctors feel free to provide it."

Health insurance paid for an individual by an employer or the government — so-called third-party insurance — "is a totally inappropriate way to finance medical care," said Enthoven. "People need to realize that medical care is scarce and costly," added Stockman.

Government regulations such as health planning and HMO standards have compounded the effect of such third-party payments, protecting inefficient medical care providers from going out of business and holding back innovative ones, competition advocates claimed. The federal tax subsidy for private health insurance plans — worth $10.8 billion a year — also has contributed to the problem, the economists said, because it gives employers tax relief for their employee health plan costs (the higher the costs, the more the relief) and encourages workers to take raises in the form of more health insurance rather than taxable dollars.

Existing law permitted employers to exclude from their taxable income all contributions to employee health and accident plans. Employees paid no income taxes on the health insurance coverage they received from employers, and individuals who itemized their deductions could deduct part of their insurance premiums. "Our federal tax system invites almost limitless health care spending," said Ullman.

By contrast, according to competition advocates, creating financial pressure on individuals would force them to question whether they really needed another test or another doctor visit, and to insist on health plans offering the best benefits for the least money. The resulting consumer pressures would ultimately produce a competitive marketplace, they said — if Congress also minimized regulations. As bulk buyers of health services, insurers and others organizing health care plans could exert downward pressure on costs. The need to attract members would prompt reinvestment of profits in better benefit packages, and excessive treatment would have to be eliminated in order to keep prices competitive and still make a profit, competition supporters said.

As discussed in congressional committees during 1979, the competition model brought together the work of several theorists. Enthoven stressed encouragement of HMOs. Feldstein focused on the impact of federal tax subsidies on health insurance and on consumer cost-consciousness. Havighurst, who had been a consultant to the Federal Trade Commission (FTC), was most interested in identifying elements in the existing medical system that had anti-competitive effects.

Enthoven put many of these ideas into a "Consumer Choice Health Plan" which he drafted in 1977 for his longtime friend, then-HEW Secretary Joseph A. Califano Jr. The plan was rejected as a Carter administration

national health plan, although elements of it did show up in the administration proposal.

Enthoven proposed a mixed system of tax credits and vouchers for the poor, to give all Americans a basic, minimum purchasing power in a competitive health care market. To produce that "system of fair market competition," Enthoven told the Senate Finance Committee June 21, 1979, four principles would have to be implemented:

Multiple Choice. Each year a consumer would be allowed to enroll in any qualified health plan operating in his area. Under the existing system, many employees had no choice, or no incentive to choose a cost-saving plan such as an HMO because their employer paid for whatever type of coverage they chose. (The same was true for Medicare beneficiaries.) "Employers are saying to the most costly fee-for-service doctors, 'It doesn't matter what your costs are, we'll pay the whole thing'," Enthoven said.

Fixed-Dollar Subsidy. Each consumer would get the same amount of financial help toward the purchase of his health plan membership — from Medicare, Medicaid, employer or tax laws — no matter what plan he chose. Those choosing more expensive forms of coverage, such as high-option plans with little or no cost-sharing, would have to pay the difference themselves.

Uniform Rules. A uniform set of rules would be needed for all types of plans to keep insurers or others from profiting by such practices as preferred risk selection or deceptive, inadequate coverage.

Doctors In Competitive Economic Units. Enthoven predicted that doctors feeling economic pressures would organize themselves into groups to provide care. These groups would have to control costs to keep premiums low enough to attract consumers. To achieve these ends, Enthoven proposed new limits in federal tax law. He said favorable tax treatment should be allowed only for plans that offered:

● Basic benefits, as defined for federally qualified HMOs. A minimum standard package of benefits "would standardize a lot of fine print, make plans easier to compare." The basic HMO package included inpatient and outpatient hospitalization, physician care including consultation and referrals, limited mental health benefits, testing, X-rays and preventive services such as childhood immunizations, well-baby clinics and adult checkups.

● Catastrophic expense protection, limiting the maximum amount a family would spend out of pocket each year to $1,500 or $2,500.

● Continuity of coverage, such as automatic coverage of newborns and the right of unemployed persons, divorcees and surviving spouses to convert to individual coverage at group rates.

Problems in the Theory

Health professionals interviewed by Congressional Quarterly in 1979 uniformly agreed that a dose of competition might improve the health care market — but that the theory did not provide answers to some of the hardest questions about the health care industry:

● **Desire for Insurance**. Will Americans accept less health insurance? The extent of existing coverage, plus the longevity of national health insurance as a political issue, suggested that Americans deeply feared medical bills and preferred paying predictable, fixed amounts even if they did not use the benefits.

The experience of the nation's 23 million elderly with a major cost-sharing insurance program, Medicare, illustrated this point. In 1978, 15 million aged Americans spent nearly $4 billion for 19 million policies to supplement their Medicare coverage, according to the House Committee on Aging. The average cost of each policy was about $200 a year, committee staff calculated — a substantial bite into the reduced income of many of the nation's aged, but an amount they were willing to pay to protect themselves against costs Medicare did not cover, such as drugs, part of hospitalization costs, chronic nursing home care, eyeglasses and dentures.

Experience with a group of federal employees suggested that many younger people, too, would rather pay high premiums for high-option health coverage than pay medical costs out of their own pockets. Mary Giannola, a counselor for HEW employees on their health plans, said a majority chose high-option coverage even though it can cost a young family as much as $600 a year in extra premium payments. High-option pays for more services and has lower deductibles than comparable low-option plans costing perhaps $100 a year in premiums. Because the federal employees' health program offered

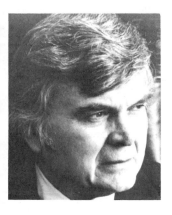

"Our federal tax system invites almost limitless health care spending."

—Rep. Al Ullman, D-Ore.

a wide range of choices and required employees to contribute to the costs of more expensive types of coverage, the economists said it showed how a truly competitive medical market would work.

But in one respect the federal program did not yet bear out economists' expectations: that HMOs or similar prepaid arrangements would compete effectively. Office of Personnel Management statistics showed that in the past 10 years, as medical bills soared, enrollment in HMOs and similar comprehensive plans grew slowly. In 1968, 8 percent of federal employees chose the prepaid plans; in 1978 only 9 percent picked this option. The economists blamed the slow growth of HMOs on strict regulations mandating an expensive range of services and requiring plans to base premiums on the health characteristics of their community ("community rating") rather than on the actual group covered ("experience rating"), which private insurers could do.

● **'Shopping' for Care.** Can consumers effectively "shop" for health care? Probably not, said Ball of the Institute of Medicine, who has written extensively on national health insurance. "It is very difficult for any but the most sophisticated purchaser to find [good medical care] or to recognize it when he does," he said.

Studies have attributed about 70 percent of health spending to decisions by doctors. Few patients feel qualified to challenge doctors' opinions, at least on major illnesses. And how are consumers to make informed choices when doctors themselves disagree on exactly what constitutes good care and what is excessive? Ball asked. "A physician in good conscience can say, 'I could do a little more,' and not necessarily be motivated by greed," he added.

Shopping for health insurance can be as confusing as shopping for a doctor or hospital. Nearly $1 billion of the $4 billion Medicare beneficiaries spent on supplementary coverage in 1978 went for overlapping coverage, with the elderly purchasing double or triple coverage for some things while omitting others completely, according to the Committee on Aging. Even health professionals can have trouble comparing insurance plans.

But advocates of competition claimed consumers could make reasonably good choices without mastering all the complexities of plans, because "at the end of the year, all you really care about is, did it work? If it didn't, you'd choose another plan," suggested Stockman aide Donald W. Moran.

● **Fraud.** Can market forces control fraud? One longtime congressional health aide offered this succinct view of a regulation-free market: "First you have fraud. Then you have regulation. That's *why* we have regulation — because individuals can't know enough to protect themselves from people who cheat them out of services they need, or sell them treatments they don't need."

Health professionals concerned about fraud often cite a California scandal involving prepaid health plans (PHPs), private entities that promise to provide comprehensive medical services to patients for a fixed fee. The PHPs proliferated after 1972 when the state began promoting Medicaid enrollments in them. Abuses included administrators siphoning off enrollment funds into for-profit subsidiaries they owned and withholding medical care needed by members. "Instead of performing surgeries, pain-killing drugs were given to patients. Children were not immunized. Sick patients were placed in clinic holding rooms instead of hospitals where they belonged," Sen. Sam Nunn, D-Ga., told a 1978 Senate Finance Committee hearing. Nunn headed a subcommittee that investigated the plans.

One result of the scandal was new regulation — among other things, a 1976 decision by Congress to require HMOs to meet federal standards as a condition for receiving a state Medicaid contract. And the California Legislature in 1977 barred certain conflicts of interest for plan officials and some marketing practices that had been used by some of the plans.

A more recent problem, reported to the Senate Finance Committee by its chief health staff aide, Jay Constantine, involved "competition" among Manhattan hospitals to fill empty beds with Medicaid- and Medicare-eligible alcoholics and drug addicts. The hospitals paid cab drivers to sweep the streets for these public patients, who were checked into expensive acute-care beds instead of being enrolled in far less costly outpatient treatment programs, Constantine said. This pattern of abuse, he said, was detected by a PSRO (professional standards review organization), a component of federal regulatory apparatus that had often come under fire from free-market advocates.

But proponents of more competition said such scandals only strengthened their arguments that the government cannot police the market as effectively as price-conscious

Major Bills to Promote Competition . . .

A number of bills to promote competition in the health care industry were introduced in the 96th Congress.

The three most ambitious plans were those of Republican Sens. Richard S. Schweiker, Pa., and David Durenberger, Minn., and House Ways and Means Committee Chairman Al Ullman, D-Ore.

The three plans had certain basic features in common. All required employers to offer their employees a choice of more than one type of health insurance coverage. They required employers to contribute the same amount for each employee, regardless of the type of coverage an individual chose. Employees choosing plans costing less than the basic contribution — such as those with a high deductible — would get a cash rebate from their employer for the difference.

These changes would be enforced through federal tax law. The existing law permitted employers to write off contributions to all types of health coverage as a business expense and permitted employees to receive those benefits as tax-free "income." Under the competition proposals, only plans meeting certain criteria would be eligible for this special tax treatment.

One House bill (HR 3943) introduced by Ways and Means Committee member James R. Jones, D-Okla., would permit the special tax treatment only for health insurance plans requiring a 25 percent annual hospitalization deductible, up to $2,000 or 15 percent of gross income.

Medicare Reimbursement

Durenberger, Ullman and the Carter administration also wanted to change existing Medicare reimbursement policy to promote enrollment of Medicare beneficiaries in health maintenance organizations (HMOs). The basic legislative proposal would authorize Medicare to pay an HMO 95 percent of what comparable services would cost for a Medicare beneficiary in the fee-for-service system. (Under existing law, HMOs had to use less favorable and more cumbersome methods of determining Medicare charges.)

The effect of the changes would be to permit HMOs to keep more of their "savings" (compared to fee-for-service charges) than they could under existing law. They would also be paid on a prospective basis rather than after services are delivered (retrospectively) — the basic federal reimbursement method which was administratively difficult for HMOs.

Carter and Durenberger would require that these savings be spent to lower the cost of Medicare premiums or improve benefit packages.

Details of 1979 Plans

Following are key details of the major plans:

Schweiker Health Care Reform Plan (S 1590)

Employer Plans. Requires employers with 200 or more employees to offer at least three distinct health plans. Requires all employers to offer at least one health plan with a 25 percent deductible (beneficiaries pay 25 percent of hospitalization costs, up to 20 percent of their income, before benefits begin).

● Mandates fixed employer contributions for health benefits, and provides for a tax-free rebate to employees choosing low-cost coverage.

● Designates collective bargaining agents as administrators for the choice of health plans.

Catastrophic Insurance. Requires employers with 50 or more employees to provide health insurance for workers' medical expenses exceeding 20 percent of income in any given year. Requires this coverage to continue for six months after an individual leaves a job. Employers and or employees would pay for this coverage, as negotiated.

● Permits (but does not require) states to assign to private insurers high-risk "uninsurable" individuals, the self-employed and others without health insurance. In states with such programs, insurance companies could not receive any federal money (for Medicare and other federal programs) unless they provided "assigned individuals" at least catastrophic coverage and a package of preventive health benefits at a fixed premium, set slightly above what they would charge for large-group coverage.

Medicare. Eliminates a 150-day limitation on hospitalization. Requires instead that individuals pay up to 20 percent of their hospital costs each year, but limits combined hospitalization and physician payments by an individual each year to 20 percent of annual income.

consumers. "These abuses have risen in our current 'heavily regulated' system. We put a little more faith in the people themselves," said Michael Pollard of the FTC's Office of Policy and Planning. "We have some faith in the integrity of professionals to provide services that should be provided," Pollard added. "I can't imagine that there are that many doctors whose values are going to change overnight" if regulations are loosened up.

And InterStudy's Walter McClure testified that the market offers a more efficient cure for excess hospital beds than does regulation: failure. "Markets are very good at shrinking industry," McClure said.

● **Requirements.** Would new regulations be needed to promote competition? Yes, said Washington, D.C., health consultant Stanley B. Jones. Without some basic rules, doctors, hospitals, insurers or other organizers of health plans might compete by deceiving consumers instead of improving the product, warned Jones, who critiqued the Enthoven plan for a 1977 HEW conference. Jones, who was a member of a firm drafting Kennedy's national health bill, postulated certain goals for any national health system: access, quality, comprehensive care and reasonable cost. For a competitive market to produce these results, Jones said, the government should do the following (some of these features were included in Enthoven's plan):

● Standardize insurance options, so that consumers could compare different products and avoid being misled about defective plans.

...In Health Care Industry Introduced

Preventive Health. Requires all health insurance plans, as a condition for special tax treatment, to cover a basic package of preventive health benefits including maternal and infant care, childhood immunizations and adult checkups.

Durenberger Health Incentives Reform (S 1485)

Employer Plans. Requires employers with 25 or more employees to offer at least three different health plans, including at least two health maintenance organizations (HMOs) that meet federal or state standards.

To qualify as non-taxable fringe benefits and employer tax exclusions, plans would have to provide a basic benefit package, limit the maximum expenditure per family to $3,500 a year, prohibit any exclusions for prior medical conditions, prohibit cancellation of coverage for any reason other than failure to pay premiums, cover dependents and provide continuity of coverage for unemployed persons, divorced or widowed spouses.

• Requires equal employer contributions to health plans and cash rebates to employees choosing low-cost coverage.

• Limits the amount of a tax-free employer contribution to the average national premium cost for a federally qualified HMO.

Medicare. Authorizes the prospective payment, 95 percent formula for Medicare beneficiaries enrolling in qualified HMOs or other prepaid plans.

Ullman Health Plan

Employer Plans. Limits tax-free employer contributions for health benefits to the cost of the least expensive federally qualified HMO, if that option is available. Where no federally qualified HMO is available, limits the tax-free employer contribution to the national median cost of such plans.

• Requires employers with 25 or more employees to offer a qualified prepaid health plan if requested to do so by such a plan.

• Requires employers not offering an HMO to provide a low-cost plan, that is, one not costing more than half the median cost of federally qualified HMOs.

• Requires equal employer contributions to all types of health plans, and taxable cash rebates for employees choosing low-cost plans.

Medicare. Authorizes the prospective payment, 95 percent formula for Medicare.

Medicaid. Requires Medicaid to establish a statewide demonstration project like Project Health in Portland, Ore. In that program, a public agency serves as a broker for competing health insurance plans, and eligible low-income people pay for benefits on a sliding scale reflecting both their income and level of benefits chosen.

Other Proposals

Carter Administration. The president's national health plan, which relied heavily on employer-based, mandatory catastrophic coverage, would promote more informed consumer "shopping," according to Health, Education and Welfare (HEW, now Health and Human Services) officials. Employers and employees would have information on qualified plans. The administration plan also required disclosure of physician fees for the public program (Healthcare) covering the aged and poor. *(Carter health plan, p. 15)*

Carter's plan would restrict favorable tax treatment of private health insurance plans. The personal income tax deduction for insurance premiums and medical expenses would be permitted only when combined expenses exceeded 10 percent of adjusted gross income, not 3 percent as in existing law. However, the plan would also permit employees to take mandated new benefits as tax-free additions to income, if employers substituted these benefits for part of wages.

Kennedy Health Plan. Sen. Edward M. Kennedy's, D-Mass., Health Care For All Americans Act was the only proposal to place an annual dollar limit on total national health spending. This feature was critical, to force hard bargaining over costs and services, according to Kennedy aide Richard Froh. Without it, a competitive market could drive up total spending as providers tried to attract customers by offering more generous coverage.

Like Carter's proposal, Kennedy's plan relied heavily on the private insurance industry, and assumed competition among carriers for customers. But the industry would be limited by more stringent regulations — not what competition advocates had in mind. *(Kennedy health plan, p. 14)*

• Require doctors and other providers to publish their prices.

• Put a ceiling on payments to providers, to force "hard bargaining" over prices.

• Prevent insurers from "reacting to the new pressure by organizing poorer quality care."

• Keep insurers from excluding high-risk individuals from plans by "experience rating," now a standard method of keeping premium costs down. However, Jones pointed out, if regulations made risks for insurers too high, they might simply stop writing health policies.

• **Transition Problems.** One of the strongest arguments against relying on competition in the health industry was that it could take a long time to work.

Employers who used their bulk insurance purchasing power to bargain on prices and services, and those which self-insure, could find the mandated "freedom of choice" extremely disruptive, according to the Finance Committee health staff. Permitting employees to opt out of a plan reduces the bargaining power of an employer, and could undermine self-insurance schemes. Healthy, low-risk persons might choose less costly plans, leaving a pool of high-risk, expensive employees wanting the most lavish coverage.

Another problem, Heineman noted, was that "the resources just aren't there" to support tough competition in many parts of the country. And Ball questioned whether it would be useful to have "two inadequate hospitals competing in a small community." Relying on market forces to distribute health services could exacerbate the very difficult problem of maldistribution of doctors and other health professionals. "Competition won't do anything for 50 million Americans" who now live in rural and inner-city areas, Heineman insisted.

Economists were impressed with the competitive medical market of Minneapolis-St. Paul, where seven HMOs enroll about 12 percent of the population. Not only did the prepaid plans keep costs in bounds for members, they also exerted price-lowering pressures on other providers, admirers said.

But with only 217 HMOs nationwide enrolling about 6 percent of the population, there was not enough "market penetration" to make a significant difference. The experience of Minneapolis and California, where the Kaiser HMO was a major competitor for patients, could stem from unique historical or demographic factors that could not be reproduced uniformly across the nation, according to Irving Wolkstein, a former HEW official associated with Jones.

Nevertheless, Havighurst insisted, "The real problem is to get the first olive out of the bottle in this industry. Once that happens, competition will force changes very fast."

Outlook

Most observers expected continuing debate on the competition theory as Congress struggled with hospital cost control and national health plans.

One half of the economists' equation — peeling away regulation — could meet with some success in the increasingly anti-regulatory atmosphere of Capitol Hill. But changes in the tax laws or other major alterations of the existing system faced formidable political problems.

The health insurance industry could provide a critical boost — or setback — to the competition concept. But as of 1980, the theory, with its hard scrutiny of medical choices by doctors and "lean" benefit packages, had not proved popular with the industry because those ideas made beneficiaries unhappy, and unhappy beneficiaries tended to switch to more generous plans.

In addition, the existing tax subsidy had stimulated the insurance business. And health care inflation "basically benefits the industry because it means more money to flush through their investments. They'd have to become convinced that prepaid plans could be profitable for them" for the idea to win industry support, said a congressional source.

But perhaps the biggest problem with the competition model was that it would require a major shift in national attitudes toward health insurance. "The perceived need is for insurance — protection before one becomes poor — and that perception is just about universal," Ball wrote. For elected representatives, dealing with that attitude raised political problems.

What it all came down to, according to Sen. John C. Danforth, R-Mo., was "visibility." The advocates of competition hoped to reverse medical inflation by making health care spending a painfully visible part of every family's budget. ∎

Manpower Policy Hits Aid to Med Schools

The day is coming when a medical education could cost as much as a four-bedroom house.

Deep slashes in federal aid to medical schools, under congressional consideration in mid-1980, could mean that in the future, to finance four years in medical school, a would-be doctor would have to:

- Have rich parents, or,
- Accept mandatory service in the military or in a remote rural area or urban ghetto to "pay back" government scholarships, or,
- Borrow heavily. Loans of $7,500 a year, for four years, for tuition alone, might not be unusual. At prevailing interest rates, such a loan could balloon to more than $140,000 as the young doctor paid it back during the first years of his practice.

Budget-cutters in the administration and Congress, citing an expected doctor surplus, have taken a bead on the multimillion-dollar array of federal grants and contracts for medical and other health professions schools that were up for renewal in 1980.

Authorizations were tumbling. Between January and March 1980, President Carter sliced about 15 percent off the funding levels in his health manpower reauthorization proposal — levels that the affected interest groups already considered too austere. The House Commerce Committee, however, approved a bill (HR 7203) authorizing funds well above Carter's request, and the Senate Labor and Human Resources Subcommittee on Health in May 1980 approved a bill authorizing $1.4 billion for manpower programs for fiscal 1982-84, about 40 percent higher than existing levels.

End to 'Free Ride'

Despite these actions, the mood of many in Congress was summed up by retiring Sen. Richard S. Schweiker, R-Pa., who said his alternative manpower bill (S 2144), signaled "an end to the free ride."

Some members seemed irritated at doctors' high incomes. "Working people are taxed to finance the education of . . . people who are going to be rich," grumbled Rep. Phil Gramm, D-Texas.

With reduced federal support to the schools, the burden of financing their professional education was expected to fall more heavily on students and their families. Medical school tuition in 1980 was averaging $5,000 a year — ranging from under $2,000 at some state schools to as much as $14,000 at one western school. Taxpayers' money provided about 60 percent of the cost of educating doctors, according to Edward M. Kennedy, D-Mass., chairman of the Senate Human Resources Subcommittee on Health. Tuition was sure to jump as federal aid shrank, said the Association of American Medical Colleges (AAMC).

Although the magnitude of educational debts could provoke anxiety in even a well-to-do family, a House aide suggested, "Can you think of a better investment? The return is guaranteed, and at a very high rate." One economist estimated that the 1980 freshman medical student could expect an average income of $123,000 a year (in 1988 dollars) when he began practicing eight years hence.

Nevertheless, the austerity drive by Congress and the administration worried some people, including Rep. Tim Lee Carter, R-Ky., a physician and ranking minority member of the House subcommittee. He warned that the prospect of starting practice with such a large debt would drive all but children of the rich out of medicine. And Jay B. Cutler, chairman of the Coalition for Health Funding, warned that the proposed changes could result in higher doctors' fees and less "idealism" in the medical profession, less willingness to locate in underserved areas where fees are lower. "There's no miracle that's going to make the docs move from Park Avenue if medical school costs them an arm and a leg and another arm," he said.

Meanwhile, nurses, public health officials and other non-M.D.s worried that their professions were in for the same sort of cuts as the doctors, despite their lesser earning power.

Other Problems

Another major issue in the health manpower debate was how to provide medical services in the remote country areas and impoverished city neighborhoods that doctors have generally avoided. In 1980, the effectiveness of the National Health Service Corps (NHSC), which had been a major component of federal efforts to spread doctors more evenly, was being questioned as Congress reviewed its scholarship program. *(See chapter on rural health care, p. 56)*

Other concerns were continuing shortages of active nurses, a dropoff in the number of minority students choosing medical careers, and new demands for experts in such fields as environmental and occupational health, cost control and management of health care systems.

Federal Aid to Medical Schools

Since 1956, when it authorized the first federal aid for schools of public health, Congress has established loan, grant and aid programs for schools and students of medicine, osteopathy, dentistry, veterinary medicine, ophthalmology, podiatriaty and pharmacy (informally known as MOD-VOPPs, for their initials) and for training nurses, public health experts, emergency medical workers and other health professionals. Fiscal 1980 authorizations for these programs totaled $1.3 billion, although appropriations were less than half that amount — $542 million.

Aid to health professions schools generally falls into three broad categories:

- Capitation grants to schools. Calculated according to the number of students enrolled, the grants originally were intended to induce schools to increase class sizes. In 1976, eligibility for these grants was tied to a requirement that a substantial number of advanced training (residency) positions in hospitals connected with medical schools be devoted to general pediatrics, general internal medicine or other primary care specialties. The aim was to produce more general practitioners at a time of increasing specialization of doctors.

● Grants and loans for construction and special projects, to start up new schools or new educational programs, such as family practice residencies, or to bail out existing schools in "financial distress."

● Aid to students, such as traineeships, scholarships and subsidized loans. Aid often was designed to promote certain priorities, such as increased enrollment of disadvantaged or minority students, or service to manpower

---

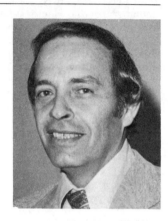

"There's no miracle that's going to make the docs move from Park Avenue if medical school costs them an arm and a leg and another arm."

—Jay B. Cutler,
Coalition for Health
Funding

---

shortage areas. Holders of Public Health Service scholarships of the 1960s could qualify for "loan forgiveness" if they served in shortage areas. In 1972 Congress authorized NHSC scholarships, which require recipients to pay back each year of support with a year of service.

Development of Manpower Policy

The supply of doctors in the United States was deliberately limited for the first six decades of this century, until 1963, when Congress authorized the first direct federal aid to medical education.

Between 1925 and 1965, medical enrollments grew from about 6,500 to 8,500, while the nation's population climbed from 106 million in 1920 to 179 million in 1960.

A pivotal 1910 report by Abraham Flexner for the Carnegie Commission fostered early moves to shrink medical education programs. Flexner found that many "medical schools" were little more than organized apprenticeships, run by local practitioners for students who had barely finished high school. Students trailed their mentors on daily rounds and rarely saw the inside of a laboratory or an anatomy theater. His report and public concern with the uneven quality of medical education prompted the closing or absorption of many substandard programs.

The prime mover was the American Medical Association (AMA), which denied accreditation to unsatisfactory schools and thereby assured that their poorly trained graduates were ineligible for state licensure. Accredited schools were pressured to limit class sizes to ensure adequate teaching and use of facilities. By 1915, the number of medical students was down to about half the number that had been in training a decade earlier.

Initially, the AMA's goal was to assure the quality of medical care. But as the Depression cut into patient

incomes and, accordingly, into demand for medical services, AMA control of medical education helped maintain doctors' earning power, according to a 1978 study by the Council on Wage and Price Stability (COWPS). The study cited evidence that the AMA "sought to limit the supply of new physicians to prevent erosion of income."

Until the late 1950s, the AMA objected strenuously and successfully to any major expansion of medical education, particularly with federal subsidies, although there was some indirect federal funding through research grants.

First Federal Aid

By 1963, the AMA had come to support limited federal aid to medical education, and Congress enacted the first Health Professions Education Assistance Act (PL 88-129). That law and subsequent amendments provided federal loans and scholarships for students of medicine, dentistry, osteopathy, optometry, podiatry, pharmacy and veterinary medicine, along with construction funds for medical and nursing schools.

During the 1960s, Congress extended and expanded this act and also authorized aid for training nurses and allied health professionals. The concept of using specially trained nurses, physician assistants and other mid-level practitioners to deliver babies, handle routine complaints and provide basic medical services received considerable attention.

The 1963 act did not alleviate the shortage problem immediately. Several studies, including those of two presidential commissions, recommended that the number of physicians in the United States be substantially increased. In 1967, according to statistics compiled by the World Health Organization in Geneva, nine countries had a higher ratio of physicians to population than did the United States.

Behind the legislation of the 1960s was a growing sense of concern that the nation's need for medical care was rapidly outstripping the capacity of available health personnel. Warnings of a doctor shortage began shortly after World War II. They resulted partly from the fact that medical examinations of draftees had revealed "untreated, undiagnosed disease" on a scale not previously suspected, according to Dr. Thomas Kennedy of the AAMC.

In the 1950s, the baby boom and extended life expectancies suggested that more medical care would be needed, both at the beginning and toward the end of life. Medicare and Medicaid, enacted in 1965, increased pressures on the health system as the elderly and the poor began to use their new access to medical treatment. At the same time, private health insurance plans were expanding rapidly, encouraging more people to seek medical care. And because of medical advances, doctors could do more for patients. The combination of public and private third-party payers tended to protect physician incomes, and this apparently further softened AMA resistance to growth of the profession, according to the COWPS study.

Health Manpower Act

By 1970, the Carnegie Commission and others were predicting critical shortages of as many as 50,000 doctors. Congress responded with the Comprehensive Health Manpower Training Act of 1971 (PL 92-157). A new feature was capitation grants, which amounted to "bonus" per-student payments to medical schools, to encourage expansion. These funds also became a source of needed income for the schools, theoretically more stable than occasional injections of grant money for construction or special projects. The 1971 act also continued funding for construction and subsidized loans, as well as special help for schools with severe financial problems, one-time grants for new schools and financial aid for U.S. students studying in foreign medical schools.

The 1971 act showed some awareness that the sheer numbers of doctors might be less important than what kind of doctors they were and where they practiced. Loan-forgiveness and scholarship provisions were included to promote service in shortage areas, and there were funds for a new "generalist" specialty, family medicine.

In 1972, Congress authorized the National Health Service Corps (NHSC), which had already been established administratively.

Problems

Between 1971 and 1974, when the Health Manpower Act came up for renewal, it became apparent that simply increasing the total number of doctors was not curing maldistribution and overspecialization.

Between the late 1960s and 1979, the number of medical schools grew from around 80 to 125, and the annual number of U.S. medical school graduates nearly doubled, from 8,000 in 1963 to 15,000 in 1978. But the percentage of primary care doctors went in the opposite direction. By 1975, only 38 percent of practicing physicians were involved full-time in primary care, Health, Education and Welfare (now Health and Human Services, HHS) Department figures showed. Concentration of doctors showed up on both coasts and in urban centers, while the South and Plains states continued to suffer chronic shortages. *(Health care shortage map, p. 45; physician distribution table, p. 44)*

One study cited by the General Accounting Office (GAO) showed that the city of Chicago lost a third of its private doctors between 1950 and 1979, while its suburbs gained nearly the same number of new practitioners.

In medically underserved areas, the percentage of private doctors in practice actually declined in the decade following 1963, according to the HHS Department. However, although the number of shortage areas had increased since federal aid to medical education began, that growth might simply show that the ways of defining shortages had become more sophisticated.

The low percentage of physicians in primary care practice in 1975 compared dramatically with 1931, when more than 90 percent of practicing doctors were in general or primary care practice. It was also well below the standard set by the AAMC of 50 percent primary care doctors.

Remedies

Between 1974 and 1976, the House and Senate separately approved stiff mandatory measures to try to correct maldistribution and overspecialization. But they failed to agree on a bill until members opted for an incentive approach instead.

A 1974 House bill would have required students to repay capitation support paid on their behalf to medical schools if they did not practice in underserved areas. The Senate bill required medical schools receiving federal aid to allot 25 percent of the positions in their incoming classes to students who agreed to practice in underserved areas for a minimum period of time.

The 1976 bill was finally written in conference, and its provisions were considered a victory for medical schools and organized medicine.

Conferees rejected both the student "payback" and scholarship "quota" schemes. Instead, they agreed to boost funds for the scholarships requiring service later, in the belief that students would join an expanded program. They adopted a modified version of the residency training "quota" for primary care, dropping a stiff Senate plan for national allocation of residencies. Under the bill, schools could get capitation funds only if they ensured that an increasing percentage of first-year residencies in hospitals affiliated with medical schools were in primary care.

A controversial condition for capitation grants added by Congress was that schools expand their third-year classes by accepting American students then studying at foreign medical schools. The bill also severely restricted the entry of doctors trained abroad who were not U.S. citizens.

The 1976 bill included a new federally guaranteed loan program, but not at low, subsidized interest rates. Loans were at high market-level rates, to make the service-related ways of financing a medical education more attractive by comparison. The bill expanded the National

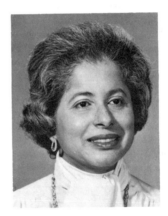

"We can't keep dumping funds into nurse education to train people to be administrative assistants and secretaries."

—Health and Human Services Secretary Patricia Roberts Harris

Health Service Corps and authorized other scholarships only for persons with exceptional financial need. *(Provisions, appendix p. 41-A)*

In 1977 Congress took another step to try to remedy shortages of medical services in rural areas. It authorized Medicare and Medicaid payments for services of nurse practitioners and physician assistants in rural clinics and in certain medically underserved urban areas. Existing law had allowed reimbursement only for services performed under supervising physicians, but the mid-level practitioners were often the only source of medical attention in shortage areas. *(Appendix, p. 59-A)*

1980 Manpower Issues

Changing estimates of the number of future doctors was a major factor in the 1980 drive to cut federal aid to medical schools. But America's 126 medical schools were deeply dismayed by the prospect of funding cuts which, according to AAMC's Dr. John Sherman, could hurt an important national resource — the sophisticated medical centers which group schools with hospitals and research facilities.

U.S. Physician Distribution, 1978

State	Civilian Population	Private Physicians	Per 100,000 Population
Alabama	3,719,000	4,554	122
Alaska	379,000	460	121
Arizona	2,327,000	4,918	211
Arkansas	2,176,000	2,610	120
California	22,021,000	52,194	237
Colorado	2,626,000	5,600	213
Connecticut	3,084,000	7,705	250
Delaware	577,000	972	168
D.C.	666,000	3,491	524
Florida	8,499,000	18,353	216
Georgia	5,024,000	7,259	144
Hawaii	838,000	1,808	216
Idaho	872,000	1,010	116
Illinois	11,205,000	20,628	184
Indiana	5,368,000	6,993	130
Iowa	2,895,000	3,635	126
Kansas	2,323,000	3,618	156
Kentucky	3,464,000	4,699	136
Louisiana	3,934,000	5,955	151
Maine	1,081,000	1,752	162
Maryland	4,100,000	10,390	253
Massachusetts	5,761,000	14,985	260
Michigan	9,178,000	14,290	156
Minnesota	4,006,000	7,676	192
Mississippi	2,383,000	2,571	108
Missouri	4,840,000	7,839	162
Montana	779,000	1,024	131
Nebraska	1,553,000	2,338	151
Nevada	651,000	925	142
New Hampshire	867,000	1,542	178
New Jersey	7,303,000	13,820	189
New Mexico	1,196,000	1,869	156
New York	17,722,000	47,021	265
North Carolina	5,478,000	8,428	154
North Dakota	640,000	825	129
Ohio	10,736,000	17,325	161
Oklahoma	2,852,000	3,650	128
Oregon	2,440,000	4,546	186
Pennsylvania	11,740,000	22,149	189
Rhode Island	931,000	1,967	211
South Carolina	2,852,000	3,873	136
South Dakota	683,000	723	106
Tennessee	4,336,000	6,808	157
Texas	12,869,000	20,143	157
Utah	1,302,000	2,225	171
Vermont	487,000	1,075	221
Virginia	4,994,000	8,653	173
Washington	3,722,000	6,981	188
West Virginia	1,859,000	2,565	138
Wisconsin	4,677,000	7,271	155
Wyoming	420,000	479	114
TOTAL (50 States and D.C.)	216,432,000	404,190	187

Source: American Medical Association, *Physician Distribution and Licensure in the U.S., 1978*

Perhaps what disturbed Sherman most was the feeling that the schools were being abandoned after gearing up a decade earlier to meet Congress' demand for more doctors. The educational system, which takes seven years or more to produce a doctor, was only just beginning to show the impact of policy changes adopted in the early 1970s. "We made good-faith efforts," Sherman said. "We can't turn on a dime."

The schools felt particularly squeezed in 1980 because they faced not only congressional thrift in the health professions programs, but also HHS regulations that could crunch teaching hospitals. Among other things, HHS planned to limit Medicare and Medicaid reimbursement and special allowances for nursing and malpractice insurance.

The Numbers

By 1990, America will have almost 600,000 physicians, compared with 379,000 in 1979, and that could constitute a slight "excess," according to an HHS study. The congressional Office of Technology Assessment (OTA) foresaw a surplus as well, but noted that the total might not be considered a surplus if there were a change in national priorities. For instance, 600,000 might be an appropriate number of doctors, an OTA report suggested, "if it is considered desirable for use to rise, for physicians to spend a few extra minutes with each patient, or for physicians to have shorter workweeks."

Minority enrollments in medical schools have peaked at 6 percent of students — half of the target set by the AAMC. The decline in these enrollments could be accelerated by increased stress on student borrowing, according to AAMC's Sherman, who noted that many "black families and poor families just aren't easy with debts."

Nursing organizations and the Carter administration have been bitterly at odds on whether there are enough nurses. The National League for Nursing and the American Hospital Association said there was a critical shortage — as much as 100,000 nurses nationwide. Hospitals in Tennessee had shut down beds for lack of nurses. The unemployment rate for nurses was only 2 percent, indicating a high demand.

Yet President Carter and, before him, President Ford, tried, largely without success, to shut off most federal aid to nurse training. They argued that there were enough trained, licensed nurses and that the shortages simply reflected a high dropout rate. About a third of the estimated one million trained nurses were not practicing. *(See Rural Health chapter, p. 57)*

The Office of Management and Budget (OMB) calculated that over the past decade, some $1.3 billion in federal funds had been invested in nursing education programs. "We can't keep dumping funds into nurse education to train people to be administrative assistants and secretaries," said HHS Secretary Patricia Roberts Harris.

New Specialists Needed

Another "numbers" issue was raised at hearings in the spring of 1980 by the Association of Schools of Public Health, whose spokesmen warned that the schools were not producing enough graduates to carry out congressional mandates on environmental and occupational health and health planning, or to pursue such national priorities as cost containment.

Sen. Jacob K. Javits, R-N.Y., deeply concerned about actual and threatened hospital failures in New York,

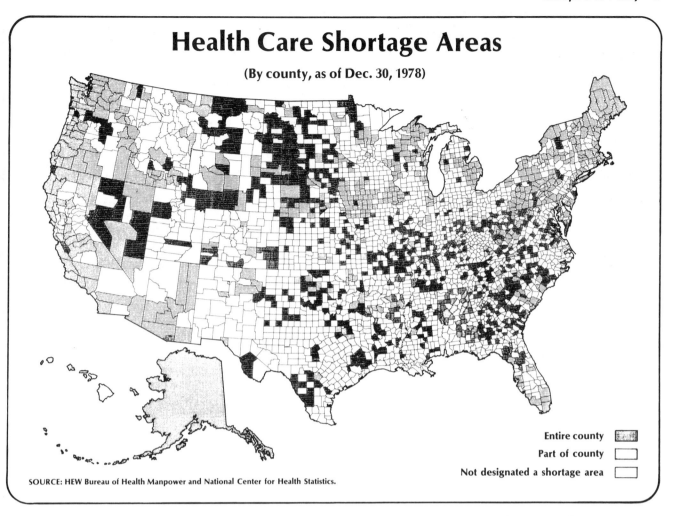

Health Care Shortage Areas

(By county, as of Dec. 30, 1978)

Entire county

Part of county

Not designated a shortage area

SOURCE: HEW Bureau of Health Manpower and National Center for Health Statistics.

warned that health care systems were "undermanaged, ill managed, . . . not managed at all." By 1985, according to Labor Department statistics cited by Javits, the nation would need 230,000 health administrators, compared to the 160,000 employed in 1976. Yet only 1,500 trained administrators were graduating each year, Javits said.

The 1979 Surgeon General's report, *Healthy People,* also warned that efforts to improve the nation's health through disease prevention programs would suffer unless more trained personnel were available.

The nation's 21 schools of public health had a combined enrollment of 7,000 students. More than 80 percent of their graduates worked for government, nonprofit agencies or universities; their mid-career earnings averaged $30,000 a year.

Maldistribution

Although the number of first-year medical school enrollees had doubled in the last decade, as of December 1979 some 50 million Americans still lived in medically underserved areas, according to an HHS report.

However, researchers had begun finding some evidence that both geographical and specialty maldistribution could be lessening. One research team predicted that by 1985, about 85 percent of Americans would have access to primary care — the sort of continuing medical attention provided by general practitioners. In 1980, one out of five Americans apparently received primary care from

physicians trained as specialists, according to a controversial study published in 1979 by the *New England Journal of Medicine.* This finding appeared to reverse a common assumption that the availability of primary care was declining.

A second research group, at the RAND Corporation in Santa Monica, Calif., found that highly qualified ("board certified") physicians, nudged by growing competition, were "diffusing" to small and medium-size towns. Work by the RAND group indicated that between 1970 and 1977, there was a 15 percent growth in the number of doctors practicing outside urban areas.

The growth in numbers of doctors and the possibility that increased competition would promote better distribution prompted Rep. Dave Stockman, R-Mich., to support vigorously an attempt in the House subcommittee to phase out the NHSC program. Rep. David E. Satterfield III, D-Va., sponsor of the proposal to phase out the scholarships, appeared less interested in the competition theory. Satterfield said he was disturbed by House Appropriations subcommittee findings that NHSC doctors "worked shorter hours and fewer days" than private practitioners.

Carter Policy and Response

President Carter wanted to prod more health professionals into entering general and family practices in poor city neighborhoods and remote rural counties. To

U.S. Military Faces Serious Doctor Shortage . . .

While American medical schools were churning out new doctors in record numbers, the U.S. military was facing serious disruptions in its medical services because of acute and increasing shortages in medical personnel.

Congress hoped to alleviate the situation by sweetening the financial incentives for doctors to serve in the armed forces, and in February 1980 cleared a bill (HR 5235) to boost special pay bonuses and provide other financial incentives for them to join and remain in the military services.

However, the bill fell victim to President Carter's budget-cutting campaign, and he vetoed it March 11. While acknowledging the shortage of physicians in the armed forces that the bill was designed to cure, Carter said the legislation was a "good example . . . of the type of unjustified federal largess that we must stop if the budget is to be balanced." *(Vetoed bill, appendix p. 78-A)*

Ignoring the threat of a second presidential veto, the House Armed Services Committee approved a new military pay bill (HR 6982) April 1. Although administration officials told the panel they had no objection to the pay provisions for doctors, they said a veto would be recommended if Congress also insisted on increasing the pay of dentists and other health care providers.

Nonetheless, the House committee approved an amendment requiring that the existing bonus for dentists — which was discretionary — be guaranteed. The new bill contained the same extra pay for military doctors — up to $29,500 a year above officers in the same grade — as that in the vetoed version. However, the pay provisions in the original bill for military dentists, optometrists, podiatrists, veterinarians and Public Health Service doctors were eliminated in favor of an extension of existing bonuses for those specialists.

In drafting the legislation, the House committee hoped to attract more doctors into the military and retain them for longer periods by increasing the extra pay for younger doctors. The bill provided higher pay for doctors who were certified by medical specialty boards and those who were in great demand by the armed services. Some medical specialists were in such short supply that the services had to contract with civilian doctors to provide care.

In addition to the maximum $29,500 bonus for doctors (most bonuses would be about $20,000), the bill would continue existing bonuses of up to $16,250 for dentists and $1,200 annually for optometrists and veterinarians.

The Senate Armed Services Committee reported a similar bill on May 13 (S Rept 96-749).

The Doctor Shortage

Since the end of the draft, with its automatic replacement of needed personnel, the services had been hurting for doctors, dentists and other health professionals. In fiscal 1979, the Army, Navy and Air Force together needed about 1,500 more doctors than they had on active duty, according to Defense Department testimony before the Senate Armed Services Committee in 1979.

Defense officials warned that the shortage threatened the military's preparedness for war, the quality of peacetime medical care for members of the armed forces, retirees and their families, and recruiting efforts for the all-volunteer army.

In 1979, military M.D.s made $20,000 to $59,000 a year in basic pay plus bonuses. That compared with an average civilian doctor's annual income, after expenses but before taxes, of $70,000, according to Defense Department officials.

The service obligations of more than 3,000 of the military's 10,000 doctors were due to expire in the summer of 1980. Pentagon officials were concerned that many physicians who might stay if their pay were increased would get out unless they were assured Congress would act soon.

The shortage of doctors in the armed services began developing when the "doctor draft" ended in 1973. Young doctors were not automatically joining the services, and many of those who were in left when they had repaid their scholarship obligations or when they reached a stage in their training where, in private practice, income soared.

The doctor shortages could be costly. For instance, military specialists in the highly paid field of radiology were so rare that the Defense Department was running ads in medical journals, offering civilian doctors as much as $100,000 a year to take military patients on contract. Surgeons and orthopedic specialists — considered critical to defense preparedness — were also in particularly short supply.

Defense officials were not looking to the glut of doctors predicted by the Department of Health and Human Services (HHS) to swell their ranks. "We've been hearing about doctor surpluses since the Fifties. We've been waiting for them. Doctors *could* join" the military if they began to feel crowded, "but we don't expect it," said Col. Jack Murphy, an aide to the assistant secretary of defense for health affairs. "The people we have aren't in it for the money anyway. They want to serve," he added.

Murphy's comment notwithstanding, disparities between military salaries and the higher earnings of civilian practitioners have always lured many doctors into private practice once they had completed their military obligation.

Doctors leaving the service complained that the existing salary structure was unfair; a $30,000-a-year military radiologist performed the same duties as his $100,000 civilian colleague on contract. Military doctors also complained that shortages of equipment and support staff hampered their work, that military life in general could be unsettling and, ironically, that military medical care for their families was sometimes unsatisfactory.

Congressional Efforts

During the 1970s, Congress took several steps to try to ensure adequately staffed medical corps for the armed forces:

• In 1972 it created medical school scholarships that must be "paid back" with active duty.

... Congress Revives Vetoed Incentives Legislation

• In 1974 it authorized bonuses — in addition to basic military pay — of up to $13,500 a year for doctors opting to stay in active duty.

• In 1977 it funded a new military medical school (created in 1972), over the strenuous objections of the Carter administration.

• In 1979 it agreed to raise the military medical scholarship stipend to the same level as similar civilian health manpower scholarships, index the scholarships for inflation and provide new bonuses for active-duty doctors who had gone to medical school on military scholarships. It also told the Defense Department to supply more "ancillary personnel" — nurses, clerks and aides — to assist doctors.

Services Curtailed

As a result of the doctor shortages, defense officials, the General Accounting Office (GAO) and congressional committees agreed, the military health system was experiencing the same sorts of dislocations that accompanied uneven distribution of medical resources in civilian health care.

Of 123 military hospitals studied by the GAO, 60 percent had "either closed some medical services or curtailed them for up to six months," according to the agency's August 1979 report. Because of this, some spouses and children of active-duty personnel were being turned away — or were refusing care — from military hospitals, as were military retirees.

"People are herded into crowded waiting rooms where they must stew for over an hour ... before seeing an overworked, tired and angry physician," reported one anonymous respondent to a GAO survey on military medical care. Others complained that military doctors were "surly" or uninterested in their problems; physician assistants, rather than fully trained doctors, saw patients; months-long waits for routine appointments were common; and emergency medical conditions were not always diagnosed and treated promptly.

Even active-duty personnel had chosen or been forced to go to civilian doctors and hospitals, where the cost to the government was substantially above that of in-house care, according to the GAO. Fully one-fifth of the armed forces active-duty personnel who responded to a GAO survey said they were unable to obtain care they needed at military facilities, or that they preferred to go off base.

Many respondents said they preferred to use the Civilian Health and Medical Program of the Uniformed Services (CHAMPUS) rather than on-base care. But that program was not without problems — the largest one being its cost. In fiscal 1978, CHAMPUS reimbursement per patient day for hospitalization was $283.93 (including some payments by patients themselves), while the average per-day cost at an Army hospital was $171.75, according to Lt. Gen. C. C. Pixley, U.S. Army surgeon general.

While on-base treatment was free, CHAMPUS required those who used the plan to pay a portion of their civilian medical bills themselves. This could be a severe hardship for enlisted men, although higher ranks did not seem to find these payments a problem, according to GAO.

CHAMPUS has also been plagued with administrative problems, such as the bankruptcy of one regional carrier that was supposed to pay hospital and doctor claims. In some communities doctors refused to see CHAMPUS patients because they disliked the program's payment rates and red tape. And when military bases were located in medically underserved regions, it was difficult for personnel to even find any off-base medical facilities.

'Misleading' Statements

The GAO report ascribed some of the dissatisfaction with military medicine to misleading statements by military recruiters, by a 1974 House Armed Services Committee report and by military retirement manuals. These materials suggested that active-duty members of the armed forces, their families and military retirees were entitled to complete medical treatment at military facilities. In fact, federal law has "only guaranteed medical care in military facilities to active-duty members," according to the GAO. Others could use military facilities, but only if space were available, and in a priority system that placed retirees last.

Almost half the individuals responding to a GAO questionnaire "believed they were receiving only part of the care to which they were entitled," according to the report.

GAO investigators suggested that military medical resources were spread too thin, and proposed several options for congressional consideration, including some that would involve major upheavals in the existing system.

Defense Department's Defense

Defense officials and their congressional supporters said they felt the GAO overstated some of the system's problems and overlooked the basic reasons a fully staffed direct care system was needed.

A department response to the report suggested that it had inappropriately focused on peacetime military medicine, ignoring "in large part the relationship between the wartime/contingency readiness mission of the military health services system and the health benefit mission. One interfaces with and impacts the other," said Assistant Defense Secretary Vernon McKenzie.

Basically, the Defense Department argued that it needed a fully staffed direct care system for two reasons: to guarantee a benefit that was important in recruiting volunteers, and to make sure that adequate medical resources were in place for any military action. Also, without a large and varied medical practice like that provided by the direct care system, it would be even more difficult to retain doctors, it was thought.

On June 26, 1980, by voice vote and without debate, the Senate agreed to substantial increases in pay bonuses for Veterans Administration doctors and dentists. The bill (S 2534), which had passed the House June 23, was signed by Carter June 28, ending the fight over how generous the measure ought to be.

further the dual goal of promoting primary care and putting it where it was needed, the president wanted to eliminate general support (capitation) for training health professionals and increase spending for programs training primary care and family practitioners, for new urban and rural clinics and for the National Health Service Corps. As expressed in the budget that Carter proposed in 1979 for fiscal 1980: "Financial aid to learn a lucrative profession should only be extended in exchange for a commitment to work in an underserved area."

The administration's 1980 legislative proposal (HR 6800) would authorize $361 million for health professions education and the National Health Service Corps in fiscal 1981 and "such sums as needed" for the following two years. It would repeal capitation aid and construction and start-up grants for the MOD-VOPP schools, with similar repeals for schools of nursing. Nursing schools also would lose funds for advanced training programs designed to produce teachers and administrators, a training program for nurse-anesthetists, and nursing student loans.

A subsidized loan program for particularly needy health professions students would be phased out, while a second program providing funds at commercial rates of interest would be continued, with its 12 percent interest ceiling eliminated.

The bill proposed new grants to states for reducing geographical maldistribution of health personnel, and extended the NHSC scholarship program and funding for family medicine and other generalist training programs.

Objections to Carter Plan

While drying up federal aid to health care training might delight fiscal conservatives, it raised sharp objections from educators, students, health practitioners and members of Congress from states where health professionals were scarce.

Medical school officials argued that it was unfair to expect them to solve the maldistribution problem. Both the AMA and AAMC maintained that professional training could not carry the burden of redistributing health personnel. "Doctors are not going to places where they're needed," said AMA official Dr. Leonard Fenninger, who was the first chief of manpower at HEW in 1967. "But neither are other people, like teachers and lawyers and accountants, going where they're needed." Like other highly trained professionals, most doctors preferred to work near colleagues and near clinical and cultural resources of major cities. Many also liked the shorter hours and greater prestige of specialty practice, as well as the higher fees. Medical schools and residencies could not effectively redirect these motivations, Fenninger suggested.

The schools also complained that flip-flopping federal policy disrupted the long process of training doctors. When Congress first demanded more doctors, the schools doubled the capacity of the medical education system. In 1980, they said, they were being left to pay for new tenured faculty, new buildings and other costs of expansion. Without federal help, some could go under, they said. Particularly painful would be the termination of the general purposes capitation grants. The schools needed this sort of "flexible money" to develop new ways of training medical students, to recruit minorities and to make other improvements, it was argued.

Others, including backers of comprehensive national health insurance, opposed cutting health manpower funds. Like President Carter, they also wanted to target funds on shortage areas, but they saw a growing need for more doctors and other health professions if broad universal health care coverage were adopted.

Proposed Solutions

In sum, it appeared that dealing with manpower shortages was enormously complicated. Problems of maldistribution and overspecialization were so difficult that even socialist nations, with considerably more control over health personnel, were having trouble resolving them, according to Dr. Julius B. Richmond, Health and Human Services assistant secretary for health.

Manpower decisions were difficult because there were several potentially conflicting types of demands.

There were demands to:
● Improve access to health care in shortage areas.
● Hold down medical costs by promoting primary care, which was less expensive than specialty medicine.
● Increase the number of black, Indian, Spanish-speaking and other practitioners that were underrepresented in the health care professions.
● Maintain the research and patient-care functions of academic medical centers.

The complex psychology of career choice cast doubt on the effectiveness of the most popular proposed solutions for manpower problems: education subsidies with "strings attached," and reform of reimbursement systems.

Some experts suggested that subsidies for training programs did not really change hearts and minds — that dollar incentives were wasted on dedicated individuals who would seek out shortage areas anyway, and the extra pay would not persuade many others to serve.

The requirement that half a medical school's first-year residencies be in primary care was not working, the New England Journal of Medicine said in 1978, because decisions to specialize came after the first year. Two-thirds of students who began general internal medicine residencies later chose "further subspecialty training," researchers reported.

But there were some promising trends. HEW figures showed that three out of four medical schools in 1979 had family practice departments, which were non-existent before 1969. Another HEW report, published in August 1978, showed that the number of primary care doctors had grown at a faster rate than the overall population.

The importance of non-dollar motivations made Fenninger and others skeptical of another dollar-based strategy popular with economists writing about health policy: reimbursement reform.

In 1978, the Institute of Medicine recommended eliminating the powerful fee incentives that encouraged doctors to choose an urban specialty practice. It said Medicare, Medicaid and private insurers should pay the same fee for a given procedure, regardless of where it was performed. City-based doctors were earning more per procedure than rural doctors. In one of its most controversial recommendations, the Institute also suggested that the fee be the same "regardless of whether the services are provided by physicians, nurse-practitioners or physician assistants."

A massive overhaul of reimbursement would run into the same stiff resistance doctors have always shown to efforts to tinker with their fees. On the other hand, it would have to be a major component of any national health insurance plan, according to former HEW Under Secretary Hale Champion.

A third strategy for dealing with medical service shortages was to subsidize specific health care centers. Relying on this approach, however, still would not ensure uniform availability of health care. "Poor families living in a neighborhood without a governmentally funded health project may receive no benefits, while needy families in a more fortunate community may receive comprehensive care," noted Karen Davis and Cathy Schoen in a 1978 Brookings Institution study, *Health and the War on Poverty.*

Carter's budget for fiscal 1980 had boosted funds for urban and rural clinics, but slashed spending for Area Health Education Centers, medical school training and clinical centers located in remote areas. A GAO report had praised this program, suggesting that it had "considerable long-term potential ... to overcome some of the important professional objections to shortage-area practice."

Other proposed solutions included promoting the use of non-M.D. health care providers and allowing uncontrolled growth in the supply of doctors, to create a competitive marketplace.

Mid-level professionals, sometimes called "physician extenders," could perform more than half the procedures usually performed by doctors, and both physicians and consumers appeared satisfied with the quality of their services, according to a Congressional Budget Office (CBO) study. They also tended to "settle in rural and urban areas not frequented by physicians, and could therefore improve access to health care, the study said.

Services provided by non-M.D.s could be dramatically lower in cost. For instance, salaried nurse anesthetists earned about $19,000 a year, while their M.D. counterparts earned $75,000 a year or more in fees. Their training also cost less — $10,000 to $12,000, compared with more than $60,000 to train a physician, according to CBO estimates.

In sum, "the multiplicity of objectives and the strengths and weaknesses of alternative approaches make it unlikely that any single strategy for meeting the health care needs of the poor [and underserved] will be adequate or effective," according to Davis and Schoen. "A mixed approach, modified to meet the unique needs of different population groups, is required."

House, Senate Committee Action

Two congressional committees called for a retooling of federal aid programs for schools of medicine and other health professions, placing more of the financial burden for their education on students themselves.

But despite reduced federal spending levels in bills approved by the House Commerce and Senate Labor and Human Resources committees, they still greatly exceeded the levels set by the president, thereby risking a veto.

The bills (HR 7203, S 2375) also flew in the face of President Carter's repeated attempts to end most federal support for schools of nursing and to eliminate general-purpose "capitation" grants to schools of medicine and other health professions.

While the Senate committee eliminated these controversial grants, it would give schools a similar type of institutional support contingent on their meeting certain "national goals," such as steering graduates into general practice careers. The House bill continued capitation grants, but phased down authorization levels sharply.

Service Corps Questioned

Both committees called for changes in the National Health Service Corps (NHSC), indicating skepticism about the way the Department of Health and Human Services (HHS) had developed that program.

The House bill continued the corps, but with new stress on members setting up private practices in underserved areas. Only three scholarship recipients chose that option in 1978, according to the committee.

The Senate bill cut corps scholarships sharply and created a second mandatory service program to provide subsidized federal loans to students who would be subject after graduation to a sort of "draft" by lottery.

Funding Levels

As reported May 15 (H Rept 96-978), the House bill authorized $684 million for fiscal 1981, including spending for NHSC, and provided a three-year total authorization of $2.4 billion, according to Congressional Budget Office (CBO) estimates. (House committee figures for the authorizations were lower because CBO added in actual dollar estimates for certain items which the committee carried as "sums as necessary.")

The Senate committee assumed programs would operate at existing levels in fiscal 1981 under a continuing resolution, and began authorizations in fiscal 1982 at $443 million. The three-year total for the Senate bill would be $1.5 billion. These figures did not include the NHSC service program.

Health Service Corps

The House committee authorized the payment of corps doctors by the private or non-profit public institutions at which they were serving their obligated time, rather than only by the federal government. It also broadened the definition of shortage areas in which corps members could use the private practice option.

The committee authorized local health planning agencies (Health Systems Agencies, HSAs) to approve or disapprove designations of shortage areas, although the secretary of HHS could override these decisions, and permitted local medical societies to comment on these designations also. Some local doctors and health officials had sought a greater say in whether NHSC personnel were sent into their area.

Another change, designed to help financially pressed city and county hospitals, directed HHS not to require publicly funded hospitals to share the cost of salaries for corps members stationed there.

The House bill authorized $92 million for NHSC scholarships in fiscal 1981, $101 million in fiscal 1982 and $109 million in 1983. The three-year total for the corps service program, including salaries and other expenses of corps members working off their obligations, was $444 million.

The Senate committee set NHSC scholarship authorizations at about half the House figure ($55 million for fiscal 1982, $48 million a year in fiscal 1983 and 1984) and did not fund the service component of the program.

State Service Scholarship Program. The Senate bill created a new program of federal matching grants for states wishing to operate service-contingent scholarship programs similar to the corps. Authorizations for these grants were set at $6 million, $13.5 million and $15 million in fiscal years 1982-1984.

Student Aid

The House bill continued federal loan guarantees for health professions students — a program known as HEAL — but raised the maximum permissible interest rate for these loans from the existing 12 percent ceiling to the cost of money to the government plus a 2 percent allowance for administrative costs.

Limits for individual loans were raised to $20,000 a year, from $15,000, for all students except nursing, pharmacy, public health and health administration students. Their new ceiling would be $12,500 a year.

The House bill also continued a second student loan program with subsidized interest rates, for needy students. S 2375 would phase that program out by fiscal 1982.

The Senate bill would replace both loan programs with a new "service-contingent" loan program that could require most borrowers to repay their loans with federal service.

Students could borrow directly from the government, but must agree to be available after graduation for mandatory federal service in manpower-shortage areas. Interest on their loans would be held at a 7 percent, subsidized rate (3 percent for nurses, public health students and certain others) while students were being trained; after they graduated, the interest rate would rise to the cost of money to the government plus 1.5 percent.

Graduates who had received these loans would be liable for one year after graduation or completion of post-graduate training to be called for service, but only if Congress in that year appropriated funds to pay them. Borrowers could either volunteer or be given an assignment by the secretary of HHS. Those called for the mandatory service program would serve a year for each year they had a loan, and their indebtedness would be repaid by either the federal government or by states participating in the service portion of the program.

The interest subsidy could continue after graduation in certain cases. Among those who could qualify for interest subsidies would be doctors in residency or advanced training programs, practitioners in primary care, preventive medicine or physical/rehabilitative medicine, psychiatrists, and individuals who pursued careers in research, teaching or government service or practiced in underserved areas.

The Senate bill authorized $13 million, $20 million and $40 million for this program in fiscal 1982-1984.

First-year scholarships for students with exceptional financial need were continued by both bills, with the House measure permitting second-year scholarships if enough money was appropriated.

Aid to Schools

The House bill continued capitation funding but, for all schools except public health and nursing, phased down authorizations levels as follows: The fiscal 1981 authorization for these grants would be 75 percent of the fiscal 1980 appropriations level; for fiscal 1982, 50 percent, and for fiscal 1983, 25 percent.

Public health and nursing schools would receive capitation grants at slightly increasing levels.

The Senate bill ended capitation grants, substituting instead a new system of "national priority incentive grants." Like capitation funds, the new grants would be based on the number of students enrolled. To qualify, however, schools of medicine, osteopathy, dentistry, veterinary medicine, optometry, podiatry, pharmacy, nursing and public health would have to meet at least two of the following conditions:

● Courses in health care economics, nutrition, physical medicine and rehabilitation, geriatrics, nutrition or occupational and environmental health would have to be offered.

● Schools would have to maintain 65 percent of their first-year residencies in primary care or ensure that 20 percent of their graduates entered family practice.

● Schools could also qualify if they offered community preventive health programs, increased the number of graduates entering research careers or maintained minority enrollment at 15 percent of the student body.

Both the House and Senate bills continued federal grants for departments of family and general internal medicine and dentistry, for area health education centers and for programs to encourage minority students to enter health professions. The House bill permitted funds to be used for programs to identify promising minority students and provide special education projects for them.

Grants for starting new schools of medicine, osteopathy and dentistry were ended by both House and Senate committees.

Both bills continued almost the full range of existing aid programs for nursing schools and their students.

The other major difference between the bills was in student aid. The House measure continued nursing student loans and scholarships, while the Senate version cut them back sharply. Nursing students would be eligible for the new service-contingent subsidized loan program, however.

Foreign Medical Graduates

The House Commerce Committee also reported a separate bill (HR 7204 — H Rept 96-943, Part I) revising certain immigration rules for graduates of foreign medical schools working in the United States, particularly in residency or other advanced training programs.

Both the House bill and provisions of S 2375 would waive certain requirements for foreign medical graduates (FMGs) who had entered the United States on temporary visas, if enforcement of the requirements would keep these individuals from practicing medicine and if this loss would "substantially disrupt" health services at hospitals or other facilities. ∎

Rural Health Care: A Continuing Problem

Living in the country can be hazardous to your health. That has been the conclusion of those who have examined the relationship between where Americans lived and the kind of health care they received. Doctors have tended to live and work in affluent areas close to large cities, leaving rural areas, as well as the inner cities, inadequately served. "The need for decent, affordable and accessible health care," Vice President Walter F. Mondale said in 1978, "is one of the most pressing unmet needs in rural America today." Health care "is simply another vital service the system has decreed 'off limits' to rural people — a striking example of 'placeism,' or discrimination against persons because of where they live," wrote Richard J. Margolis in the June 20, 1977, *New Leader.*

While 30 percent of all Americans lived in rural areas, these areas had only 17 percent of the nation's primary care physicians in 1979. (Primary care physicians are those in family practice, internal medicine, pediatrics, and obstetrics and gynecology — medical specialties related to general practice.) Shortages of medical personnel have not been confined to physicians. There were 30 percent fewer dentists and 30 percent fewer nurses per 100,000 population in rural areas than in metropolitan areas. Many rural communities lacked the financial resources to build and maintain health care facilities. Even when health professionals and facilities were available, rural patients might not have access to such preventive services as nutrition counseling and health education. Furthermore, rural residents often faced special environmental health hazards, including substandard housing, inadequate sewage disposal facilities and impure water supplies.

All of these factors have had a harmful effect on the health of rural residents. They suffer from higher rates of chronic disease than do urban dwellers; they are over 40 percent more likely to be afflicted with emphysema, for instance. Infant mortality rates in rural America, according to statistics for 1969-73 from the Department of Health, Education and Welfare (HEW, now Health and Human Services), ran to 21.4 deaths per 1,000 live births, in contrast to 19.3 in metropolitan areas.

The geographic variation in infant mortality rates reflected the "uneven distribution of medical resources," according to a report published by HEW in 1978. In 1973, the latest year for which complete statistics were available, there were 48 obstetricians and gynecologists for every 100,000 women of child-bearing age in metropolitan areas and only 18 elsewhere. The pediatrician-child ratios were even wider — 11 (rural) and 35 (metropolitan) per 100,000 children under age 15.

Physician-Population Ratios

In 1977, according to the American Medical Association (AMA), there were an average of 180 private physicians per 100,000 persons in this country — or one physician for every 555 persons. The ratio ranged from 228 in New England and 220 on the West Coast to 129 in the central Southern states of Alabama, Mississippi,

Tennessee and Kentucky. At one extreme, there were only 100 physicians for every 100,000 South Dakotans but 252 for every 100,000 New Yorkers. (In 1980, the administration estimated that the ratio had risen to 200 physicians per 100,000 population for the entire United States.)

According to the AMA, 139 counties in the United States had no active physicians as of Dec. 31, 1977. These counties made up about 3.9 percent of the U.S. land area and about 0.2 percent of the population (521,700). HEW's Health Resources Administration, which keeps tabs on the adequacy of health care by geographic region, identified about 1,100 areas with a total population of about 16 million, as having a "critical shortage" of primary care physicians. About four-fifths of these areas were rural.

Even when physicians are available, rural residents may find it difficult to get to them, especially where public transportation is in short supply. Community organizations that provide rural patients with transportation to hospitals and clinics have been hard hit by rising gasoline prices. "In the first five months of this year [1979], we spent 53 percent of our annual budget for gasoline and maintenance for vans," said Lorraine Ruday, transportation coordinator for a community action group in predominantly rural Greene County, Pa. "That was before gas prices really started to go up fast, and now I can't see that it's going to ever get any better. We can't risk overspending our budget so we've just got to economize more." The Greene County community action group owned five 12-seat vans which, among other things, were used to take poor people for routine physical examinations in Pittsburgh, some 50 miles away, according to the Aug. 17, 1979, *Wall Street Journal.*

What do people do when they are sick and there is no doctor or hospital nearby and they cannot afford transportation? "The absence of nearby facilities usually means putting off care until an illness is so severe that it can no longer be ignored," said Nancy Lane, a health program analyst for the Appalachian Regional Commission, a federal-state partnership that plans and provides technical and financial assistance for economic development in Appalachia. "Their kids get hospitalized because they've waited too long. Their babies die." Office visits and medication are "luxuries" for people barred by geography and low income from reaching doctors or clinics, Lane said. More accident-related deaths occur because of the distance from health care. "Nobody knows what to do with them [the victims], and they throw them in the back seat and drive," Lane explained.

The federal government classified almost the entire Appalachian region as medically underserved. The area's physician-to-population ratio in 1976 was 158, significantly lower than the national average. In mountainous, isolated southern and central Appalachia, the infant mortality rate in 1976 was 1.5 times the national average, according to statistics compiled by the Appalachian Regional Commission.

State Programs to Alleviate Shortages

Problems in rural health care were by no means limited to Appalachia. Health care was inadequate or non-existent in other rural areas of the country — especially in the West. In Wyoming, for example, about 40 percent of the doctors practiced in the two largest cities, Cheyenne and Casper, according to Robert G. Smith, executive director of the state medical society, in the March 11, 1979, *New York Times*. Of the approximately 1,000 physicians practicing in Idaho, some 200 lived in the Boise area, and 400 others lived in or near the cities of Twin Falls, Idaho Falls, Pocatello and Coeur d'Alene, according to Donald Sower, president of the Idaho Medical Association. "Rural physicians earn less than their urban colleagues," said Dr. Neil Swissman, president of the Nevada State Medical Association. "They must be available 24 hours a day, have fewer opportunities for continuing medical education, and have less frequent contact with their colleagues for consultation."

Some states have set up programs to encourage doctors to practice in rural areas. Nevada's Rural Health Project, for example, runs a program in which physicians from large communities spend time working with doctors in rural areas. This gives the rural physician the opportunity to share professional knowledge or to take time off. Several states have programs in their state medical colleges to encourage students to settle in small towns and communities. The states either partially or fully forgive student loans if the student decides to practice in a rural, underserved area.

Some medical colleges offer students the choice of studying part-time in rural locations. Other schools encourage students to choose the field of family medicine or admit a selected number of students who live in rural areas. "If a person is from a rural, low-income area," said Dr. Louis W. Sullivan, dean of the Morehouse College Medical School in Atlanta, in a *New York Times* news service story of Aug. 30, 1978, "we think there's more likelihood he'll go back there to practice." Some state agencies, as well as those run by private organizations, have set up programs to train "non-physician providers" (nurses and physician's assistants) to work in underserved areas. These programs — characterized by a U.S. General Accounting Office (GAO) report of August 1978 as "alternative type" health care programs — have "increased the number of primary care providers and improved access to the medical delivery system for substantial numbers of people."

One such program, the North Carolina Rural Health Centers, was administered by the state Office of Rural Health Services. The program, which began in 1973, operated health care centers in small communities across North Carolina. The centers were operated mostly by nurse practitioners under the supervision of physicians in nearby communities. In the 12-month period that ended June 30, 1979, the North Carolina Rural Health Centers served some 35,000 patients.

Kentucky runs a Frontier Nursing Service in the southeastern or Appalachian part of the state. The service operated a 40-bed community hospital and mobile care clinic, satellite nursing clinics and a family nurse and midwifery school. About 85 miles northwest of Albuquerque, N.M., in Cuba, is a large outpatient clinic run by the Presbyterian Medical Services' Checkerboard Area Health System. Open since 1971, it provided health care to some 10,000 residents scattered over 4,000 square miles of northwestern New Mexico. Satellite centers provided medical care in outlying areas.

Reasons Doctors Choose Urban Areas

Two faculty members from the University of Rochester School of Medicine and Dentistry surveyed physicians who practiced and some who had left practices in two rural New York counties. The survey indicated that both groups of doctors were concerned with maintaining contact with their professional colleagues and gaining access to advanced medical treatment facilities. Doctors who had left most frequently cited their wish to change their type of practice and problems with the limited opportunities for professional growth. Factors such as long working hours and low income were not as important, according to the survey, which was published in the February 1978 issue of *Medical Care*.

One physician in the survey commented: "There is too much to do in a small town and because of the type of training programs not given in medical school and internships, no one is going into general practice. We in the country saw no relief in sight for our increasing burden. I am one physician who loved general practice, the people, the community, the intellectual atmosphere, etc., but was forced by the lack of new medical manpower to give up general practice."

The responses from physicians deciding to settle in small communities generally emphasized personal and medical considerations. The factor named most often was that "small community living appealed to me." Other reasons frequently cited were the desire to locate near a good community hospital or to have a medical center in a nearby city. Another frequent answer was that the doctors felt there was a need for physicians in a particular community and decided to meet it.

Doctors in other states expressed similar sentiments. "The country pace is more my style than the city," said Dr. Janne Olson of Fawn Grove, Pa., in the Oct. 17, 1979, *Baltimore Sun.* "I have enough confidence in my abilities to be able to fly by the seat of my pants [without backup support from city specialists]. The most important thing here is to be able to recognize your limitations, to know when something is too much for you to handle and refer it on to someone else."

Cultural, educational and recreational opportunities and climate also played a part in doctors' thinking about where they would practice. "In sum," Joel D. Bobula and Louis J. Goodman wrote in a 1979 AMA publication ("Physician Distribution and Licensure in the U.S., 1977") "professional and social amenities as well as prior exposure to urban life are major factors underlying the current geographic distribution of physicians. Economic factors, which may have played an important role in the past, no longer appear to be of primary importance."

Not all analysts agreed with that assessment. Richard J. Margolis maintained that economic considerations were the primary factors involved in doctors' choices of location. Margolis wrote that both rural health care and the national health care system suffer because of "an obsolete fee-for-service system that makes entrepreneurs out of healers, encouraging them to practice among the affluent; a tendency to embrace specialties or subspecialties and eschew the responsibilities of primary care; and an overreliance on technology that drives up prices and reduces the patient to little more than a broken machine needing repair."

Distribution of Doctors and Hospitals, 1978

	Total (100.0%)	Metropolitan Number	Percent	Non-Metropolitan Number	Percent
Total Physicians (12-31-78)	407,953	354,690	86.9	53,263	13.1
Total Patient Care	325,783	281,984	86.6	43,799	13.4
Office Based Practice					
General Practice	45,148	30,952	68.6	14,196	31.4
Medical Specialties	64,624	57,794	89.4	6,830	10.6
Surgical Specialties	73,540	62,979	85.6	10,561	14.4
Other Specialties	55,631	49,436	88.9	6,195	11.1
Hospital Based Practice	86,840	80,823	93.1	6,017	6.9
Other Professional Activity*	29,786	28,031	94.1	1,755	5.9
Inactive	26,831	21,752	81.1	5,079	18.9
Not Classified	25,553	22,923	89.7	2,630	10.3
Hospitals (1978)	6,074	3,209	52.8	2,865	47.2
Hospital Beds (1978)	991,189	757,762	76.4	233,427	23.6
Resident Population (1978)	219,768,500	164,797,900	75.0	54,970,600	25.0
Income (1978)					
Per Capita	$ 6,552	$ 6,995		$ 5,277	
Per Household	$18,722	$19,854		$15,263	

* Includes 6,495 Medical Teaching, 10,359 Administration, 10,366 Research, and 2,566 Other.

SOURCE: American Medical Association, *Physician Distribution and Medical Licensure in the U.S., 1978*

Legislation to Influence Doctor Location

At the heart of the rural health care problem was the decision by a majority of doctors to specialize in fields that frequently required them to locate near major medical centers. According to 1977 AMA figures, only 55,149 — or 13.1 percent — of the nation's physicians were classified as general practitioners or in family practice. That small percentage translated into fewer physicians and lower quality health care for rural areas.

Although by the early 1970s the doctor shortage had been nearly eliminated statistically, there remained a problem of geographical and specialty distribution. In 1976 Congress passed a bill that reflected health manpower analysts' worries less about the overall physician supply than about getting enough doctors in the right places and right medical fields. The bill guaranteed continuation of basic federal support for medical, dental and other health professional schools through September 1980. For students, the bill offered a new federally guaranteed loan program as well as a big expansion in scholarships requiring practice in doctor shortage areas as a member of the National Health Service Corps.

The bill's chief sponsor, Rep. Paul G. Rogers, D-Fla., said it was one of the most important measures Congress passed that year. "It is designed to continue . . . financial assistance to schools and students of health professions," Rogers said. "More importantly, it is designed to reverse several critical trends in the American health care system today and will chart the course for health care delivery through the next decade." President Ford, who signed the bill into law on Oct. 12, 1976, said the measure addressed the major problems of geographic and specialty maldistribution and was "a definite step toward improving health care delivery." *(Appendix, p. 40-A)*

Medical Student Interest in the Family

There was some evidence that more medical students were turning to careers in primary care — family practice, internal medicine, pediatrics, and obstetrics and gynecology — medical specialties that are needed in many areas of the country. According to the American Academy of Family Physicians, about 55,000 American doctors practiced family medicine and 2,360 new doctors started training in family practice in 1979. According to the Association of American Medical Colleges, 95 of the nation's 125 medical schools in 1979 had either family practice or family and community medicine departments. In addition to that, some 400 hospitals and health centers nationwide offered training programs in family practice. AAMC figures indicated that 62 percent of the 1979 medical school graduating class chose either family practice, pediatrics, internal medicine, or obstetrics and gynecology.

Some believed that the growing interest in family practice was part of the holistic health movement, which is based on "the concept of the human body and mind as a fully unified biological system capable under most circumstances of warding off disease or overcoming it." According to this philosophy, the primary function of the physician is to engage to the fullest the ability of the body to right itself. In so doing, the physician is expected to take into account all the interacting factors that may figure in breakdown — emotional strains, job or family pressures, faulty nutrition, environmental hazards such as noise, overcrowding, smoke, etc. Dr. Edward J. Kowalewski, chairman of the Department of Family Medicine at the University of Maryland in Baltimore, quoted in the *Baltimore Sun*, Oct. 17, 1979, characterized the practice of family medicine as meaning "total responsibility for you and your family. We are responsible

Indian Health: Better Than It Was...

"We're keeping Indian babies alive these days — but how well they are when they grow up is another story."

That assessment of the status of Indian health — the good news and the bad news — was made by David Chavkin, a Washington attorney with the National Health Law Program. It was the view Congress was getting, too, as it began taking stock of the programs authorized by the 1976 Indian Health Care Improvement Act (PL 94-437), which was due to expire in 1980. The Senate passed a four-year reauthorization June 2, 1980 (S 2728); the House had not yet acted on its version (HR 6629) as of mid-1980.

Federal investments in medical services and improved water and sewage systems have brought some impressive gains in the health of native Americans over the past 25 years, including dramatic improvements in infant mortality rates and longer life expectancy. But American Indians and Alaska natives as a group were still significantly less healthy than Americans in general. (The term "Indians," as used in this story, refers to both groups.)

And because of official Washington's preoccupation with a balanced budget, the chronic underfunding of Indian Health Service (IHS) programs was not expected to end in 1980.

Success — Compared to What?

Recent statistics showed that Indian infant mortality and deaths from certain childhood illnesses have dropped more than 70 percent since 1955. Death rates from childbirth, tuberculosis, pneumonia and many other treatable or preventable conditions have also fallen significantly for Indians. "Success.... Some programs work," proclaimed a recent *Washington Post* editorial on the IHS.

But the statistics obscured how much catching up Indians had to do from the dismal record of illness and early death of 25 years ago, when the Department of Health, Education and Welfare (HEW, now the Department of Health and Human Services, HHS) took on the Indian medical program previously run by the Interior Department's Bureau of Indian Affairs.

"The health status of American Indians and Alaskan natives ... still lags 15 to 20 years behind that of the general population," HEW concluded in a 1979 review of the nation's health.

Indians still had a shorter life expectancy than other Americans, said IHS project officer Dr. Robert C. Birch. Indian rates of infant and childhood deaths, fatalities from flu, pneumonia and tuberculosis, and disabilities such as hearing loss from ear infections still exceeded national norms.

Alcoholism, accidents and depression — medical problems deeply rooted in social conditions — were growing in Indian communities plagued by poverty and unemployment. Cirrhosis of the liver, often associated with alcoholism, was the fourth largest killer of Indians in 1980. Suicides among native American groups rose 47 percent between 1970 and 1977.

An emerging health issue was the exposure of certain Indian communities in the Southwest to radiation. About half the nation's uranium was located on Indian reservations. The Senate-passed bill would require uranium mine and mill operators to compensate the IHS for diagnosis and treatment of cancer or other diseases related to radiation exposure. *(Radiation story, box, p. 108)*

High Expectations Unmet

To attack these health problems, Indians estimated they would need about $2.8 billion over the period 1980-84. Their expectations seemed drawn from the glowing promise of the 1976 act to provide "the highest possible health status to Indians."

But HHS Secretary Patricia Roberts Harris passed this cost estimate on to Congress earlier in 1980 with the chilly comment that the figure reflected "the need for some optimal health care services which are well beyond ... services normally provided." (Just preparing the plan on which that estimate was based, Harris observed, cost nearly half a million dollars.)

The Carter administration requested $72.2 million in fiscal 1981 and "such sums as needed" for the three following years for the so-called "PL 437 programs" — recruitment and training support for Indian health professionals, water and sewage systems for Indian homes and reservations, health services for "urban" Indians living off reservations, other health services and construction of facilities.

The administration request fell well below the fiscal 1980 authorization of $234 million — of which $115 million was appropriated. (Total spending for federal native American health programs was running about $600 million a year, under authorizations of the 1976 act and the 1921 Snyder Act establishing federal responsibility for Indian health.)

Congress was also far from approaching the Indians' ideal figure in 1980. The Senate bill passed June 2, 1980, was a four-year, $524.6 million reauthorization (S 2728) which allotted $105.6 million in fiscal 1981 for PL 437 programs. A less generous House version reported May 15 by the House Interior Committee (HR 6629 — H Rept 96-975, Part I) authorized $87.5 million for fiscal 1981, and a four-year total of $435.3 million.

Early Indian Programs

Indian health became a federal line item in 1911 when Congress appropriated $40,000 for services, after decades in which first military and then civilian physicians on federal salary provided some sporadic treatment.

The 1921 Snyder Act authorized, somewhat vaguely, spending for "relief of distress and conservation of the health of Indians." But programs were never well funded or fully staffed, and Indian health suffered from the combined effects of this neglect, plus poverty and other social problems.

Congress' decision in 1954 to transfer Indian health programs to HEW's Public Health Service brought some progress, but even in 1976 "Indian communities and Native villages were plagued with concerns other Ameri-

. . . But Much Improvement Still Needed

can communities had forgotten 25 years previously," according to the Senate Select Committee on Indian Affairs' May 15 report on S 2728 (S Rept 96-758).

The 1976 act and an earlier measure, the 1974 Indian Self-Determination Act (PL 93-638), mandated a less paternalistic approach to Indian health problems, with more control of health programs by native Americans themselves. The 1974 act provided authority for tribes and groups to contract with the federal government to run their own programs, and, by 1980, there were three tribal hospitals and about 210 Indian-run health clinics. The Indian Health Service administered an additional 44 hospitals and more than 400 clinics providing full-time or part-time professional staff.

The 1976 act was intended to enhance Indian control by mandating federal consultation with tribes and villages on their needs, and by providing scholarships and other programs to increase the number of Indian health professionals. It was also meant to improve substantially the health services themselves. Major features of that act:

● Spelled out the federal commitment to Indian health in some detail, unlike the 1921 act.

● Made Indians eligible for Medicaid and Medicare, under certain circumstances.

● Authorized new health programs for "urban" Indians living away from reservations. It had been IHS policy to locate health services on reservations, but some estimates suggested that as many as half of the nation's 900,000 to one million Indians did not live on reservations. (Population figures for Indians were in dispute; Indian officials usually maintained there were more Indians than federal figures showed.)

● Continued authorizations for federal programs to create or improve water and sewage systems for Indian reservations and individual homes.

Indian Health Problems

HHS Secretary Harris sent Congress the administration's reauthorization proposal in April 1980, along with an ambitious national health plan for native Americans that had been compiled from more than 200 tribal health plans. A 1979 HEW report derived from those plans recorded many of the statistics on improved native American health, but it also offered some bleak glimpses of continuing problems.

Perhaps the biggest problem after lack of funds was the sizable gap between Indian expectations for IHS and what the federal government considered adequate. For example, Indians tended to expect IHS to provide comprehensive medical care directly or pay for it on contract from private doctors and other providers. But the administration insisted Indians should seek care from non-IHS sources as much as possible, and that the contract funds should only be used as a last resort. Other problems noted by the report:

● The doctor-to-population ratio for native Americans was half the overall rate for the nation, while 71 percent of IHS nursing positions were unfilled, although the IHS said up to 80 percent of basic health problems could be treated by nurse practitioners and other non-MDs.

● "Rural Indians" — those living off reservations but far from city-based Indian programs — might be virtually without services because of their distance from IHS facilities. Those who could qualify for Medicare often could not pay the mandatory premiums and other fees for the program. For some Indians, cultural and language differences were barriers to joining the programs. Poor Indians eligible for Medicaid faced the same problems as other rural poor — scarcity of practitioners, refusal by local doctors to accept Medicaid patients, and state restrictions on eligibility or covered services. One state with a large Indian population, Arizona, had no Medicaid program.

● While a "significant majority" of Indians appeared to live no more than 30 minutes from an outpatient facility and 90 minutes from hospital care, lack of a car or public transportation made these facilities inaccessible for many. Other "barriers" included language and reluctance to abandon traditional healing systems.

● Dissatisfaction with IHS services. Howard Bad Hand of the National Indian Health Board in Denver said, "We're very impressed by what they [the IHS] accomplish with what little they have." But the report said many non-Indian IHS professionals suffered from "culture shock" and turnover was high. Record-keeping and "other forms of communication are . . . fragmented so that providers do not know who is doing what to whom." Some native patients suspected that the inexperienced or foreign-trained doctors they encountered at IHS facilities were "just here to practice on us," the report noted.

Legislation

The Senate-passed Indian health bill authorized $89.3 million more for PL 437 programs over the four-year life of the bill than the House version. The extra dollars in S 2728 would go for new scholarships to prepare Indian students for health careers, bigger boosts in alcoholism treatment programs, and new health programs for Indians distant from both reservation and urban Indian health facilities.

The Senate bill also mandated that IHS provide contract health services for Arizona Indians, and contained provisions dealing with the potential new problem of radiation exposure among Indians. The House bill contained none of these program changes.

Radiation Provisions. The Senate bill mandated a study and some compensation for the costs of illnesses caused by radiation exposure. The narrowly drawn provision would require mine or mill operators to pay IHS for diagnosing and treating illnesses caused by workplace exposure to radiation. These payments would only be for individuals eligible for IHS services who were also, "by reason of . . . employment, entitled to medical care at the expense of [the] employer," according to the committee report.

The compensation provision was intended to prod companies into more actively protecting the health of their workers.

not only for medical care but for the continuation of good health, for preventive medicine. What has happened is that the patient has been cut to pieces, and we sometimes forget that each piece is part of the whole. Our job is to take care of the whole. This is the oldest tradition in medicine."

HEW's National Health Service Corps

One federal program that would fare well under Carter's health manpower plan was the National Health Service Corps (NHSC), which was set up in 1970 to improve the delivery of health services to areas of urban and rural poverty.

The agency, within the U.S. Public Health Service, pays the salaries of physicians and other health personnel, including nurses and physician's assistants. The corps, whose fiscal 1980 budget was $82 million, also provides scholarships to students who promise to join the corps upon completion of their medical training. The administration requested $230 million in 1981 funding for NHSC services and scholarships. At this level, funding for the program would increase 260 percent over 1977.

The corps works with scholarship recipients while they are in school. Meetings and seminars are arranged to keep the students informed about new Health Service Corps programs. The corps encourages students to take courses in different fields, but emphasizes primary care areas. Scholarship recipients get credit for working in rural clinics where they receive on-the-job training from National Health Service Corps doctors or other health professionals.

In 1979 there were some 4,500 medical school students holding National Health Service Corps scholarships. Some 2,500 other National Health Service Corps doctors were completing residency programs. They are deferred from their service commitment until they complete residency training. For each year of government scholarship support, the recipient "owes" a year of service either in a health manpower shortage area or in a medically underserved one. HEW officials generally were pleased with the program's progress. "It's going very well and developing rapidly," said Dr. Fitzhugh Mullan, the National Health Service Corps director. "Of the roughly 1,850 people we have on board right now, about 1,000 are physicians. The rest are physician's assistants, dentists and other health practitioners." In the 12-month period that ended Oct. 1, 1978, the corps placed 1,289 individuals at 668 sites across the nation, including 694 physicians, 210 dentists and 385 other health personnel such as nutritionists and medical social workers. In 1978, 89 percent of the people in the National Health Service Corps were in rural areas.

What effect has the program had on medically underserved areas? "As far as we can tell it is the most tangible and predictable vehicle to move manpower into shortage areas," said Dr. Mullan. "Many of our people are in places where doctors have never been before or places where doctors have retired 20 years ago and the community has not been able to get a replacement." Dr. Mullan said that many of the health workers — both scholarship recipients and those who have volunteered to work for the National Health Service Corps in underserved areas — were remaining in rural areas. "For volunteers," he said, "we are showing a retention rate annually of about 40 percent of those finishing their basic tours and remaining at their placement, and another 10

percent converting to private practice in that area. That's about 50 percent of the people who get out there sticking beyond their tour of duty."

Observers said that the full impact of the program would not be felt until more students receiving scholarships completed their medical training and went to work in medically underserved areas.

Mullan's assessment appeared to be contradicted by an uncomplimentary 1978 GAO report which noted that only 42 physicians, out of the 800 who had served in the corps, had decided to settle permanently in the underserved areas where they had worked. Corps doctors were not as productive as private-practice counterparts and, as a short-term method of providing medical care, the corps was extremely expensive, the report added.

In addition, a 1980 report by the House Appropriations Subcommittee on Health found that NHSC doctors "worked shorter hours and fewer days" than private practitioners. The critical report concluded that the corps was an expensive and questionable long-term solution to maldistribution because:

● Corps doctors saw fewer patients per year than private practitioners.

● The corps "retained" only 50 percent of its physicians in underserved areas past their period of obligated service.

● The choice of location for corps personnel and the federally funded facilities in which they worked was occasionally unsatisfactory, and the site-selection process was becoming unfairly skewed away from rural areas.

AMA Executive Vice President James H. Sammons, in a letter to the Appropriations panel, concurred with the findings, and added that the "AMA has received many complaints" about placement of corps doctors where the need was "marginal." He said private physicians could provide less expensive care. "It is our belief that if these individuals and families [in shortage areas] could obtain health insurance through the private sector, many of the problems of access to care would be eliminated," Sammons wrote. He also urged improved transportation for underserved areas.

An HEW response questioned some of the study's figures and sampling processes, and observed that the subcommittee investigators did not comment on the quality of care, except to note that preventive services were considered effective. HEW also suggested that low productivity and relatively low retention rates of NHSC physicians could reflect both their inexperience and the difficulty of their mission. Their patients often are individuals unaccustomed to medical care and so may consume more time. And, as Rep. Barbara A. Mikulski, D-Md., pointed out, "Poor people's medicine is hard medicine. It burns you out."

Rural Health Clinics

There are other federal programs designed to get more doctors and other health personnel into rural areas. HEW's Community Health Center Program was set up in 1975 to support ambulatory health care projects in areas with scarce or non-existent health services. The center awards grants to qualified public or nonprofit health organizations located in medically underserved rural or inner-city areas. The program, which helps plan, develop and operate clinics, had a budget of $25 million in 1979. *(Appendix, p. 27-A)*

The Rural Health Clinic Services Act (PL 95-210), passed by Congress in 1977, was designed to extend Medicare and Medicaid reimbursement to services provided by nurse practitioners and physician's assistants in rural health clinics. These nurses and paraprofessionals often were the only sources of medical care in doctor-short areas. Until the law was passed, only medical services provided by physicians could, in most cases, be reimbursed by federal health programs for the elderly and the poor. The bill was designed to encourage the development and use of rural health clinics and to keep some of the existing clinics from going broke. Without Medicare or Medicaid coverage of their services, many rural residents either did not get adequate care, had to pay for it themselves despite financial hardship or had to be treated as bad debts by the clinics. Financial problems had forced some clinics to close and threatened the existence of others. When the bill was signed into law by President Carter Dec. 13, 1977, about 550 rural health clinics were in operation. *(Appendix, p. 59-A)*

To be eligible for Medicare or Medicaid reimbursement a clinic must be directed by a physician or have an arrangement with one or more doctors to review periodically the services furnished by the paraprofessionals. The clinic also must be located in an area that is designated by HHS as having a medically underserved population or a shortage of primary care specialists. As of Oct. 1, 1979, about 440 clinics had been certified by the government. One hundred other clinics would be joining the list shortly, according to Dr. Michael E. Samuels of HHS's Bureau of Community Health Services. "One of the things we're finding out is that these are fairly low-cost operations especially when compared with billings from major hospitals. The average billing from one of the clinics is about $10-$15 per encounter. That won't even handle lunch at a hospital," he said.

Other federal efforts to improve rural health care include the Migrant Health Centers program, which supports the delivery of health care services to migrants, seasonal farm workers and their families. The migrant program, in effect since 1962, was reorganized in 1976. The centers serve some 557,000 persons, providing diagnostic services, treatment and preventive services as well as dental care, nutrition counseling and other services. The administration requested $45 million for the program in fiscal 1981.

A program called the Health Underserved Rural Areas was established in 1974 to provide funds to public and private health or dental services. The objective is to attract health personnel to rural areas. The Rural Health Initiative is administered by HHS's Bureau of Community Health Services, and oversees several other programs, including the Community Health Centers Program, the National Health Service Corps, the Health Underserved Rural Areas, the Migrant Health Program and the Appalachian Health Program.

There were a number of other federal projects to help rural areas attract medical personnel. Under one HHS program the government repaid 60 percent of educational loans when registered nurses, and doctors of medicine, dentistry, optometry, pharmacy, podiatry, osteopathy or veterinary medicine signed a contract to practice in an underserved area for two years. A program run by the Departments of Labor and HHS trains migrant and seasonal farm workers as medical paraprofessionals. The federal Job Corps operates a program to encourage trainees to work in rural health care centers. The Farmers Home Administration of the U.S. Department of Agriculture sponsors a program that encourages construction or improvement of community medical facilities, including hospitals, clinics and nursing homes.

Vice President Mondale announced in 1978 that the Farmers Home Administration had signed an agreement with HEW's Health Services Administration to set aside a portion of funds from the Community Facility Loan Program to be used for loans to nonprofit or government applicants who want to build or remodel rural clinics or health centers for migrant workers. The White House estimated that by 1982 some 300 clinics serving 1.3 million persons would be built using government money for construction, renovation or equipment.

Nurses' Education

Congress has legislated federal support for nursing education since 1956. The first comprehensive nurse training act (PL 88-581) in 1964 established construction grants for new schools, project grants to upgrade training and financial aid for students, with loan forgiveness for nurses working in health-care-shortage areas. In 1971 Congress authorized federal repayment of all but 15 percent of education loans for nurses working in underserved areas (PL 92-158).

President Carter in 1978 vetoed a two-year, $206 million-a-year reauthorization of the federal nursing education support program. Any future federal assistance, Carter said, "should be limited to geographic and specialty areas that need nurses most." *(Appendix, p. 68-A)*

Carter said the veto would not disrupt existing nursing programs since they could continue to receive funds through fiscal 1979 under a continuing resolution. However, early in 1979, the president sought cuts in general support funds already appropriated for 1979, leaving money only for nurse practitioner and other advanced types of training. The proposal brought angry complaints from nurses and some legislators. But Congress finally gave Carter a partial victory on the cuts, authorizing only a one-year, $103 million extension of federal aid for nursing education. The nurses' training measure, which was signed into law on Sept. 29, 1979 (PL 96-76), was intended to continue aid long enough to permit a general congressional review of federal aid to all health professions training. The bill directed HEW to conduct a study of the nation's nursing needs. *(Appendix, p. 77-A)*

The federal government's recognition of rural health problems and the enactment of programs to meet these special needs have been "positive" developments, concluded a July 1979 report published by the Department of Agriculture. "However, even with this federal commitment," the report went on to say, "the rural health system is not on par with that in urban areas." Further improvements to the rural health care system, the report said, would require an imaginative use of available resources by local communities. "More community colleges could be training students for health service careers," the report stated. "Communities can also be active in training residents to serve as emergency medical coordinators to deliver basic first aid until more specialized emergency services are available. Local residents who have a commitment to the community can also be involved in health education and promotion activities." ∎

Health Planning System Comes Under Fire

The controversial federal health planning system, which had been living on borrowed time since legislation reauthorizing it went down to defeat in the House in 1978, got a reprieve in 1979, when Congress cleared a three-year, $987 million extension of the embattled legislation (PL 96-79).

Its friends, recognizing that the very mention of federal health planning was raising hackles around the country, soft-pedaled the legislation. They just wanted the system reauthorized, and were willing to go with minor changes, rather than try to put stronger teeth into the law.

Some of its logical enemies — conservatives who had attacked the system in the past as unwarranted federal intrusion into the private health sector — had suddenly hopped on board as cosponsors of the legislation. Although the law had been a perennial target of arguments against excessive federal regulation, several Republicans began to promote it as an alternative to President Carter's hospital cost control bill.

As Congress debated continuing the network of state and local planning agencies, this inadvertent coalition of liberal and conservative support appeared to guarantee renewal. It also seemed to guarantee no very dramatic changes in the system, since liberal members did not want to load it with more controversy, and conservatives did not necessarily want to strengthen it. Potentially troublesome provisions were cleared in advance with the American Medical Association (AMA), among others.

Overall, the 1979 bill did not add any new regulatory authority. While officials at the Department of Health, Education and Welfare (HEW, now Health and Human Services) were not entirely happy with some of the features of the legislation, they said they were pleased that the bill survived without a significant weakening of the law. What resulted, according to HEW lobbyist Gerald Connor, was "a courageous decision by Congress to continue a difficult program — and take some of the bugs out of it — in a year when regulation isn't very popular."

Background

The health planning system was established in 1974, when Congress passed legislation (PL 93-641) creating a national network of local planning agencies to improve health services and cut health costs by preventing unnecessary development of health facilities and by establishing priorities to determine which facilities and services were necessary.

These responsibilities were to be carried out by local health systems agencies (HSAs), which covered health service areas of 500,000 to three million residents. Statewide health planning and development agencies were also established to coordinate the long-range health planning activities of the local agencies.

The 1974 legislation also replaced the 28-year-old Hill-Burton hospital construction program with a program that emphasized modernization of existing hospitals and new construction mainly of outpatient facilities. Construction of new inpatient facilities was restricted to areas with recent rapid population growth. *(Appendix, p. 13-A)*

In 1977, Congress extended the act for one year only, to give the Carter administration time to review the program and recommend changes. In its report on the legislation (HR 4974 — H Rept 95-116), the House Interstate and Foreign Commerce Committee said that although 196 HSAs had been designated (approved by HEW), other sections of the program had not been moving as rapidly. National health planning policy guidelines were to have been completed within 18 months of enactment of the bill, and work on them was "seriously behind schedule," the committee said. So was creation of the new National Council on Health Planning and Development.

1978 Debate on the Bill

Although the Senate in 1978 passed a three-year extension of the program, the House killed the measure; subsequently, the program received a simple one-year extension. As reported by the House Commerce and Senate Human Resources committees, the legislation would have made many minor changes in the complex multi-level planning system — amounting to a "tune-up, not an overhaul," according to one committee aide.

A storm of protest had erupted when the Department of Health, Education and Welfare issued guidelines in 1977 that appeared to mandate hospital closings, particularly in rural areas. *(Appendix, p. 61-A)*

What the 1977 dispute told members of the health panels was that "people want state and local control" of decisions about health care delivery, said Commerce Committee aide Robert Crane. The reported similarity of many letters to members of Congress suggested a second lesson — that the health care industry had lost none of its ability to mount a powerful lobbying effort on Capitol Hill.

The committees responded by increasing the role of governors and local elected officials in state and regional planning processes and instructing the secretary of HEW to make sure the planning panels were "broadly representative" of community interests. Many of the planning agencies had been accused of catering to the local medical establishment and neglecting the health needs of the poor and minority groups.

Major Issues

The strongest supporters of the planning system went to some pains to ensure that the reauthorization would move through the 96th Congress.

For instance, officially, the administration continued to support a tough prohibition on physicians' purchases of very expensive medical equipment, which the Senate narrowly approved in 1978. The provision's sponsor, Sen.

Edward M. Kennedy, D-Mass., backed off from the curb, however, picking up instead a weaker version from the 1978 House Commerce Committee bill. Kennedy's move reflected a behind-the-scenes agreement with the AMA, so that the association would not work actively against new provisions designed to promote health maintenance organization (HMO) development. HEW officials said privately they would not push for the stronger version.

Another example of reluctance to overload planning with difficult issues was the question of "decertification" — phasing out of existing facilities if "appropriateness reviews" showed them to be underused. In 1974 and again in 1978 there was some talk of mandatory decertification, but the 1979 bill opted instead for financial incentives to pay off the cost of closing or consolidating these facilities, on a voluntary basis only.

HEW officials as well as congressional supporters downplayed the planning system in 1979 for several reasons. HEW Secretary Joseph A. Califano Jr. told members of Congress that the complex network of state and local planning agencies was still too weak to carry out the major burden of containing health care costs. Henry A. Waxman, D-Calif, chairman of the House Commerce Subcommittee on Health, said that despite enormous efforts by planners, "health planning is far from mature in many parts of our country [and] some HSAs have performed miserably."

Another issue was control: planning priorities have flowed upward from community-based agencies (HSAs), not down from HEW. Any ambiguity over who was to make planning decisions seemed to have been settled by the 1977 fracas over HEW planning guidelines for hospital beds and special services. In the aftermath, Congress told HEW to make allowances for regional differences, particularly those of rural areas. The 1979 bill deleted a statutory requirement that state health plans be consistent with national guidelines. "We [HEW] do not have the ability to control health planning through [the planning] legislation," said Califano.

Probably the most important factor in Califano's soft sell of health planning was a desire not to divert attention from the administration's embattled hospital cost control proposal. Republican opponents of that plan were asking why Congress should enact new health regulations when the existing planning system was designed to save money.

Finally, the most enthusiastic supporters of planning said that 1979 was the year to protect the troubled system, not load it down with new controversy.

How the System Is Working

It was not clear that, even under the best of circumstances, the planning system could succeed at both of its congressionally mandated tasks: to assure "equal access to quality health care" while keeping down the costs. The decades-long debate over national health insurance had not produced a universally accepted answer on how to achieve both of these goals simultaneously.

And conditions under which the planning systems worked were far from ideal. Local and state units were being created and setting their agendas during the stormy 1977 struggle and many faced stiff resistance from local medical establishments. HEW had been slow to issue guidelines, leaving agencies without any very clear idea of what they were supposed to do. The absence of guidelines

and standards also made agency decisions more vulnerable in litigation.

However, the record was not all dark. Individual HSAs had earned high marks for effectiveness. The system had led to "extensive participation by citizen volunteers in the local health planning process," according to Dr. Julius B. Richmond, assistant HEW secretary for health. Richmond said 203 HSAs were functioning in 1979 with 80 percent of them fully designated (approved by HEW). Most of the states had completed state health plans by mid-1979. Richmond also cited HSA efforts to attract dentists to rural Alabama and to combat high infant mortality in a California ghetto as examples of HSA success in improving access to health care.

Nevertheless, since its creation in 1974 the system has been caught in a cross-fire of complaints that it did both too much and too little.

HSAs that took tough stands against popular projects could find themselves overridden by elected officials or tied up in lawsuits.

Physician groups and hospitals frequently evaded agency denials of very expensive equipment, such as computerized X-ray machines (CAT scanners). The federal law required states to administer programs certifying the need for very expensive equipment in hospitals, but some physician groups had bought the machines after a hospital had been denied certification and operated them in rented hospital space.

An American Enterprise Institute (AEI) study found that state certificate-of-need laws probably slowed the construction of unneeded hospital space, but had done little to curb capital investment in very expensive equipment or costly special services like coronary care units.

Some agencies simply were not making tough decisions because they were dominated by hospital administrators and other health establishment members, or because they feared that legal challenges would drain their resources.

The planning system also was vulnerable to chronic objections that it was anti-competitive and in violation of federal antitrust law.

Despite these problems, the planning system was viewed as useful, for different reasons, by a broad range of supporters. Backers like Sen. Kennedy said the system was beginning to save substantial amounts of money. Kennedy claimed that every dollar spent on the planning process kept $8 from being spent on unneeded projects.

To the extent that the planning system protected the established fee-for-service medical practices and hospitals from competition, it also had the qualified support of organized medicine. The AEI study found that the system often kept competing new services, like prepaid group practices (health maintenance organizations or HMOs) from entering the medical marketplace.

1979 Senate Action

While a House subcommittee was busy watering down the health planning program, the Senate quietly passed a reauthorization of the act.

On May 1 by voice vote the Senate passed a three-year, $997 million reauthorization (S 544) of the Health Planning and Resource Development Act. There was no debate. Kennedy, sponsor of the measure, simply inserted a statement of support in the *Congressional Record*. The bill retained two provisions from the 1978 bill designed to encourage HMOs and to curb doctors' buying of very expensive medical equipment, but both were weaker than versions approved by the Senate in 1978, reflecting a private compromise between HMO interest groups and the AMA, in which each agreed not to object to the other side's amendments to the statute.

In its April 26 report on S 544 (S Rept 96-96), the Senate Labor and Human Resources Committee said the health planning system had made an "excellent beginning" despite slow implementation of the 1974 law and much litigation challenging planners' decisions and the validity of the law itself.

But the planning process has been "full of turmoil," and these problems had been pointed out in testimony:

● Domination of the boards of local planning agencies by providers, with inadequate representation of poor and medically underserved groups.

● Negative impact on the development of health maintenance organizations. "There appears to exist a misunderstanding of the HMO concept and discrimination against HMO applications at both the HSA and the state level," the report said.

● Continuing excesses of hospital beds. This indicated to the committee that the law had yet to fulfill its potential for curbing duplicate services.

● Slowness of states in adopting acceptable "certificate-of-need" laws. These laws, which required state-level approval of new major investments in health services, based on local (HSA) findings of need, were a critical element of the planning law. Only eight states had such laws in effect.

● A major loophole in the 1974 law that permitted physicians to purchase very expensive medical equipment even if local and state planners decided that it was not needed. In some instances, doctors were buying the equipment after hospitals, which were required to seek approval for the purchases, had been turned down.

Committee changes in existing law were intended to respond to some of these problems. But differences between the 1978 and 1979 bills reflected an anti-spending and anti-regulatory mood. There were the weakened HMO and medical equipment provisions and a new emphasis on "competition." And the 1979 authorizations were more than $600 million under the amount approved by the Senate in 1978.

In a separate view, Gordon J. Humphrey, R-N.H., said the health planning act unnecessarily delayed projects and that it hadn't saved much money. Coordination of health services "would best be effected by informal arrangements among them and the attention of local government," Humphrey said.

In his floor statement, Kennedy called the planning process "one of the most impressive cost containment programs in the health field." He cited a survey showing that between 1976 and 1978, planners had blocked $1.8 billion of "unneeded capital investment expenditures" of a total $7 billion worth of proposals.

1979 House Action

The House passed its version of the health planning bill July 19 by a 374-45 vote, after the bill had been reported by the House Commerce Committee May 15 (HR 3917 — H Rept 96-190).

House Health Panel Moves To the Right

In a development that spelled trouble for high-priority health bills of the Carter administration, the moderate House Commerce Subcommittee on Health, formerly chaired by Rep. Paul G. Rogers, D-Fla., moved sharply to the right in the 96th Congress.

A prime victim of this movement was the 1979 reauthorization of the health planning systems program. A powerful new coalition of conservative Democrats and Republicans, led by David E. Satterfield III, D-Va., and Dave Stockman, R-Mich., rewrote the bill extending the program, adding amendments that went to the basic assumptions of the 1974 laws.

The initial success of the coalition upset arrangements among interest groups, members of Congress and the Carter administration that were intended to smooth the way for extension of the controversial planning system. Before markup began, committee and administration staffs and lobbyists were not predicting major amendments.

But once Satterfield and Stockman "realized they'd reached criticial mass in the subcommittee, that they had the votes, they decided to rewrite the whole act," as one lobbyist for the American Medical Association (AMA) put it.

Another explanation for the surprise attack on the planning law came from Eliot Stern of the American Health Planning Association: "We underestimated the extent to which enemies of hospital cost control legislation would try to use the planning act as a foil — after first drawing out all its teeth." Administration witnesses had been asked repeatedly in hearings why Congress should regulate hospital costs when the planning law already in existence was supposed to do the job.

Satterfield and Stockman clearly did not buy the basic assumption of the hospital cost containment bill, that federal regulation was the answer to inflation in health care costs. And, said Stockman, "this is just the beginning."

Stockman and others on the committee enthusiastically promoted the concept of a "free market" medical system in which providers compete for patient dollars, going out of business if their prices were too high or their services unsatisfactory. Stockman said frankly that he would like to dump the planning law, but not in 1979, "because you can't go cold turkey."

"My concerns run to control and power," he said. "The more you centralize a system, the weaker it is." Another Satterfield priority, according to an aide, was ensuring "due process protection to the players in the planning game — including, of course, hospitals." Critics of Satterfield's amendments to the planning act said they strengthened the hand of hospitals and other health care providers in the planning process by further constricting the Department of Health, Education and Welfare's (HEW, now Health and Human Services) limited control over the system and by requiring procedures that consume much extra time.

The measure was drafted by the newly conservative and independent-minded Health Subcommittee, where a powerful coalition of conservative Democrats and Republicans, led by David E. Satterfield III, D-Va., and Dave Stockman, R-Mich., added amendments that challenged the foundations of the 1974 law.

What finally emerged after extensive subcommittee debate — and sporadic veto threats by HEW representatives — was a bill that would further loosen HEW's tenuous control over the national network of local and state health planning agencies. It also watered down provisions designed to protect the planning process from domination by hospitals and other local health providers.

As reported by the full committee, HR 3917 retained many features of the subcommittee bill, including an exemption for prepaid health services so broad that opponents said it could promote fraud and seriously weaken health planning. But the measure also strengthened the planning process in several important respects.

The only major amendment added on the House floor to the committee bill severely limited a "trade-off" procedure that opponents said was critical to the health planning process.

Arguing that some state agencies had been improperly setting conditions for proposed new medical services that had nothing to do with the medical need for a specific service, Satterfield offered an amendment, adopted by voice vote, that limited certificate-of-need decisions to questions directly related to medical need for the proposed service.

The House rejected 203-211 a Richardson Preyer, D-N.C., amendment that would have permitted the agencies to set broader trade-off conditions, as long as the criteria for the decisions were published and subject to public comment.

In other action, the House rejected 135-274 a Robert L. Livingston, R-La., amendment that would have converted local planning agencies to public units. Most were private corporations.

It refused on a standing vote to require local plans to explain what effect, if any, they would have on the medical ethics embodied in the Hippocratic oath. The House then defeated 55-364 a motion by the amendment's sponsor, Ron Paul, R-Texas, to recommit the bill to committee with instructions to add the ethics amendment.

House, Senate Bills Compared

The broad outline of the House bill was similar to that of the Senate-passed bill. It authorized funds for fiscal 1980-82 for local and state planning agencies and a national advisory commission, continued federal loans and project grants for some hospital modernization and construction, and discontinued state allotments of federal money for hospital construction.

Both bills also included the new limit on doctors' purchasing of major medical equipment, similar to the 1978 House version, which was weaker than the Senate provision. Both required integration of state mental health and drug- and alcohol-abuse plans with health planning, and excluded health planners from decisions affecting hospitals or other institutions with which they were associated. They also included the new program of incentive payments to encourage hospitals to close excess acute-care beds voluntarily or to covert them to other needs.

Major differences included authorization levels and standards for state certificate-of-need programs.

Conference Action

House and Senate conferees meeting Aug. 1 were each reluctant to cede ground on two major certificate-of-need questions: whether federal law should bar states from passing broader certification requirements and what sort of special treatment prepaid group health plans should receive.

Pre-emption

The pre-emption discussion was complicated by a deep disagreement between Waxman and Tim Lee Carter, R-Ky., chairman and ranking minority member of the House Commerce Health Subcommittee respectively, over the meaning of language in the bill.

"I never thought that the House language pre-empted the states. It was never even discussed" in committee, said Waxman. But Carter and the American Medical Association, whose lobbyist hovered near him throughout the conference, contended that the language in question did indeed prevent states from passing tougher certification laws. Their concern was that states would require certificates for major medical equipment located in doctors' offices, while many HMOs were going to become exempt from these requirements. Carter said young doctors shouldn't face unrealistic bars to establishing their practices.

The 1978 Senate bill had included the stiffer requirement that all major equipment purchases gain certification. The 1979 House and Senate versions required certification only for major medical equipment that would be used on inpatients — to mollify the doctors, according to Sen. Kennedy.

Conferees returned to the issue repeatedly without resolution, while Carter held firm. Finally, Waxman conceded that "Dr. Carter has very strong feelings [on the issue] and I believe the House ought to go along." Kennedy accepted the pre-emption, but insisted on a delayed effective date. Conferees settled on a date close to the next reauthorization of the planning law.

Other Issues

Conferees also worked out a complicated compromise that somewhat tightened the House exemption from certificate-of-need for HMOs and other prepaid health arrangements. Kennedy insisted on more closely defining what sort of prepaid schemes could qualify. House opponents of the HMO exemption had warned that this would encourage fraudulent plans.

A third difficult issue was what sort of conditions a state agency could put on its approval of a certificate-of-need application. Existing law did not limit these conditions, and advocates said planners needed to be able to make trade-offs — such as approving a new piece of diagnostic equipment only if a hospital promised to let all doctors in a community use it.

Satterfield's amendment to the House bill limited allowable conditions to questions of medical need alone. Satterfield was disturbed by reports that planning agencies had tried to force changes in hospital boards and enforce other conditions he thought were inappropriate. The conference compromise permitted only such conditions as were authorized in either federal or state laws — a plan that met Satterfield's concern that decisions be made according to clear, legal ground rules.

Conferees dropped a Senate-passed provision requiring state or regional planning agencies to evaluate federal health projects, such as Veterans Administration or Defense Department hospitals, if requested to do so. Both Senate and House Veterans' Affairs committees had strenuously protested this provision as an infringement of their jurisdiction.

Numerous other compromises on House and Senate differences, worked out in staff discussions but not discussed by conferees, were detailed in the conference report (S Rept 96-309) filed Aug. 9. In general, conferees split the difference on authorizations, and kept most of what each house had agreed to in substantive changes. For example, the Senate barred HSA board members from selecting their successors; the House had no similar provision, so conferees barred self-selection for half the board members.

Provisions

As signed into law Oct. 4, 1979, S 544 (PL 96-79):

Health Planning System

Guidelines and Priorities. Required an annual Health, Education and Welfare Department (HEW) review of national guidelines and regional and state health plans. Required periodic reports on the impact of health planning goals on health care delivery systems.

● Added these goals to national priorities for health planning: identification and termination of unneeded services and facilities; adoption of policies to contain health care costs, ensure more appropriate use of services and promote greater efficiency in the health care delivery system; promotion of outpatient treatment for mental health problems, where appropriate, and elimination of inappropriate hospitalization of mental patients.

National Council. Expanded to 20 members, from 15, the National Council on Health Planning and Development; required that at least eight members be consumers, including representatives from medically underserved areas.

Competition. Stated as a congressional finding that extensive health insurance coverage and the traditional payment pattern that reimbursed for services after they were provided had lessened price-consciousness and competition in the health care industry. Directed regional and state planning agencies to foster competition where possible, and to allocate the market for institutional and other services not responsive to competitive pressures.

Designation of Planning Areas, Agencies. Authorized state governors to request changes ("redesignation") in boundaries of health service areas (the jurisdiction of a health systems agency, or HSA), and required the secretary of HEW to consult with governors, local officials and state health councils before any redesignation. Required HEW to consult with affected governors and other officials for redesignation of a multi-state area. Required public notice and comment period before any redesignation.

● Extended to three years, from one year, the period for which a state or regional planning agency (HSA) could be approved by HEW ("designated"); required state planning agency comment on the performance of an HSA before redesignation.

● Required HEW, before it could terminate the designation of a state or regional planning agency, to provide

Health Planning Authorizations

As cleared by Congress Sept. 21, 1979, S 544 authorized the following amounts in fiscal 1980-82 *(in millions of dollars):*

	Fiscal 1980	Fiscal 1981	Fiscal 1982
Planning grants to health systems agencies	$150	$165	$185
Grants to state health planning agencies	35	40	45
Grants to state rate regulation programs	6	6	6
Grants to regional health planning centers	6	8	10
Construction grants to hospitals to meet safety, accreditation standards	40	50	50
Construction grants to hospitals in underserved areas or for conversion to outpatient or long-term care uses	—	15	15
Grants to hospitals for discontinuation or conversion of unneeded services	30	50	75
Total	**$267**	**$334**	**$386**

notice and an administrative appeal, and to consult with the governor, the state health coordinating council and the national planning council.

● Authorized the secretary to return a state or regional planning agency to conditional designation (instead of terminating it immediately) for unsatisfactory performance. Required termination or full redesignation at the end of the year of conditional status, with the established procedures for termination.

● Raised the minimum planning grant to an HSA; also authorized special grants for extraordinary expenses, such as travel in an unusually large jurisdiction.

Planning Agencies. Revised language that appeared to require quotas for different population groups on HSA boards, but insisted that boards be "broadly representative" of economic, racial and ethnic groups served; the handicapped; geographic areas within the HSA; and major purchasers of health care, such as labor unions. Required HSAs to provide for "broad" public participation in the selection of at least half the new board members.

● Required representation on HSA boards of hospital administrators, general-purpose local government officials, mental health and drug abuse interests, and any Veterans Administration hospitals and health maintenance organizations in the HSA area.

● For provider members of HSA boards: eliminated the "indirect provider" category and revised the income test for direct providers, to those who made one-fifth, rather than one-third, of their income from health-related activities.

● Required consumer majorities on HSA subcommittees.

● Broadened protection for regional and state planning agency members and staff against personal liability suits, and extended liability protection to the HSA itself.

• Prohibited HSAs from using federal funds to pay for lobbying. This prohibition would not prevent HSA staff and members from lobbying, as long as that was not their primary responsibility.

• Permitted HSAs to close portions of public meetings and records relating to confidential personnel matters or to judicial proceedings.

• Eliminated a requirement that a public HSA delegate personnel and budget decisions to a separate governing body.

• Barred HSA and state agency members from voting on decisions affecting institutions where they worked or had other substantial interests — or had had such an interest within the past year. Required written disclosure from members of any such relationships.

• Required HSA staffs to have expertise in financial and economic analysis, public and preventive health and mental health.

Health Plans. Stipulated that regional health plans, developed by HSAs, should focus on health care equipment and institutional services and facilities. This language, however, was not intended to "prevent an HSA from involving itself in improving the environment which impacts on health," the conference report stated.

• Required coordination of regional and state health plans with planning by drug and alcohol abuse and mental health agencies.

• Required regional and state health plans to describe both existing and needed health facilities, and to identify institutions needing modernization, conversion to other uses or closure.

• Required approval by the governor of a state plan; permitted disapproval only if the plan failed to meet statewide health needs, and prohibited federal funding for state agencies without a state health plan in effect.

• Required review and amendment of regional and state health plans every three years, instead of annually as in the original law.

• Deleted a requirement that regional health plans conform to national planning guidelines. Required HSAs to report and explain any inconsistencies with national guidelines to state planning units and the secretary of HEW.

Certificates of Need. Required state agencies to act according to established procedures on applications for approval (certificate of need) of proposed new health facilities and services, and to base decisions solely on the administratively established record. Required on-the-record hearings for certificate-of-need applications, as well as on appropriationess reviews, if requested. Barred personnel contacts outside official procedures on certification decisions.

• Required state agencies to set a period of time for deciding on a certificate-of-need application, and authorized judicial action to require a decision on an application if the state agency exceeded its set period of time. Authorized appeals of state agency decisions.

• Added these criteria for evaluating certificate applications: availability of needed resources for the project, such as capital and manpower; clinical needs and access to the new service of medical and other health professions schools; access to all area residents; costs and charges, and quality of care provided in the past by the applicant. Authorized state agencies to "batch" applications — that is, to compare similar proposals, choosing the best.

• Prohibited state agencies from placing any conditions on certification approvals, unless the conditions related directly to criteria spelled out in federal or state law or in HEW regulations existing before enactment.

• Required certificate approvals to include a timetable for establishment of the approved service, and required periodic state reviews of progress by the applicant. Authorized states to withdraw a certificate from an applicant failing to meet the timetable or to make a good-faith effort to do so. This was intended to keep applicants from preventing competitors from offering a service by holding on to a certificate but not acting on it. Also required certificate approvals to specify the maximum expenditure permitted for a project, and authorized further review if the project required more money than specified.

• Expanded a requirement for certificate-of-need approval to cover all diagnostic and treatment equipment worth $150,000 or more, regardless of location, if it was to be used on hospital inpatients. Permitted states to enact broader requirements, such as coverage for major medical equipment in doctors' offices that was not used on hospital patients, if such laws were enacted before Sept. 30, 1982.

• Prohibited states from requiring certificates of need for new inpatient health services, major medical equipment or major capital expenditures by a health maintenance organization (HMO, or prepaid group health plan) or group of HMOs meeting certain conditions. To qualify for the exemption, the HMO or other entity had to offer a basic package of medical services on a prepaid basis to at least 50,000 members; the service had to be accessible to all members; and at least 75 percent of patients expected to use the service had to be prepaid enrollees. An inpatient facility controlled by an HMO or one leased (long term) by an HMO could also qualify.

• Prohibited the sale or lease of exempt facilities, except to another entity qualifying for the exemption. For other purchasers, a certificate of need would be required.

• For HMOs failing to qualify for the exemption, required state agencies to approve certificate applications for services needed by enrollees that the HMO could not provide through existing institutions.

• Required state agencies to grant certificates of need for projects to repair safety hazards (as specified by fire and safety codes), or to comply with licensure or accreditation standards — but only for expenditures needed to meet these requirements.

• Required the General Accounting Office to report to congressional committees on the impact of the HMO exemption by Feb. 1, 1982.

Appropriateness Review. Added these criteria for state agency reviews ("appropriateness reviews") of existing institutional health services: need for the service, accessibility, financial stability of the institution, cost-effectiveness and quality of services provided. State agencies could decide whether to conduct reviews on a general, "regional" basis or institution by institution; eventually, however, the agencies were expected to produce specific information about specific institutions, to "provide the consumer with better information," according to the conference report.

Other Provisions. Required state review of applications for federal drug abuse, alcohol abuse or public health funds to be spent in more than one health service area. Required the secretary of HEW to disapprove applications rejected by the state for non-compliance with state plans. Authorized HSA reviews of state grants from federal funds. Permitted governors to override HSA dis-approvals of these grants.

● Barred HSA review of public health research or train-ing proposals, unless these projects would affect availability of health services for non-participants.

● Required states to collect annually price information on the 25 most-used health services, including hospital room rates, and required HSAs to make this information available to the public.

Funding. Provided for phased reductions in federal public health, mental health and drug and alcohol abuse funds to states failing to establish certificate-of-need programs meeting federal standards. This provision re-placed a provision cutting off all these federal funds for states failing to establish programs by Sept. 30, 1980. Authorized the secretary to cut the funds by 50 percent the first year, 70 percent the second year and 100 percent the third year, with the cuts to begin after a state leg-islature had had a full 12 months to enact the law.

● Authorized funds for fiscal 1980-82 for planning grants to HSAs and grants to state health planning agencies, state rate regulation programs and regional health planning centers.

Facilities Development, Termination

● Ended authorization for allotments to states for medi-cal facilities construction, and requirements for a state medical facilities plan.

● Authorized, through fiscal 1982, federal loans as needed, and loan guarantees. Expanded eligibility for both to nonprofit private hospitals meeting certain conditions, as well as public hospitals. Set these priorities for projects: discontinuation or conversion to other health uses of un-needed services or facilities; renovation and modernization of facilities, especially to meet fire, safety, licensure or accreditation standards; construction of outpatient medical facilities, or inpatient facilities in areas with rapid pop-ulation growth.

● Authorized federal loan subsidies for projects in urban or rural poverty areas.

● Authorized funds for project grants to hospitals to eliminate safety hazards or meet accreditation standards. ∎

HMOs: A Wave of the Future in Health Care?

In 1970, Americans spent about $70 billion for health care. By the end of the decade, the nation's annual health expenditures had soared to more than $230 billion. This enormous and steadily increasing health care bill led to widespread complaints that the public was not getting its money's worth and that the U.S. health care system was in drastic need of overhaul. Much of the criticism focused on the health insurance industry. Nine of every 10 Americans were protected by one or more forms of private or public health insurance, with yearly health insurance premiums averaging about $1,000 per person. However, it has been estimated that this insurance covered less than one-third of the total national health bill. Because most insurance plans paid much more for hospitalization than for outpatient care, doctors were encouraged to admit their patients to hospitals, thereby increasing medical costs. And since most plans paid only when the patient saw a doctor, after becoming ill, or entered a hospital, there has been relatively less emphasis on preventive care. *(Health insurance, p. 9)*

Many persons, in their search for an alternative to increasingly costly and fragmented medical care, focused their attention on health maintenance organizations. HMOs, as they are called *(see box, p. 68)*, typically provide comprehensive care for enrolled members on a prepaid basis. For a fixed sum paid at regular intervals the enrollee is entitled to any or all of the benefits offered without having to pay anything extra out of his own pocket.

In 1964, there were only 18 such organizations; by 1973, there were 42, with 4.3 million members. According to the Department of Health, Education and Welfare (HEW, now Health and Human Services), the total number of prepaid plans in the United States grew to 217 in 1979. The number of people enrolled in the plans was nearly 7.5 million, but this accounted for only about 6.3 percent of the population and about 3 percent of the nation's health expenditures. Among the best known of these group programs were the Kaiser-Permanente plan, with members in California, Oregon, Hawaii, Washington, Colorado and Ohio; the Health Insurance Plan in New York; the Group Health Cooperative of Puget Sound in Seattle; the Group Health Association of Washington, D.C.; and the Labor Health Center in St. Louis.

By the end of the 1970s, HMOs had been established in 36 states and the District of Columbia, with the preponderance of membership (three-fifths) in the West.

Of the prepaid plans operating in 1979, about one-half had received some federal aid, and 79 of them had been "officially designated," having met strict federal regulations. To qualify for federal aid, an HMO had to be public or nonprofit. The for-profit type of organization could receive loan guarantees of at least 10 percent if the projected membership was located in a medically underserved area. The Carter administration estimated that there would be 139 federally qualified HMOs by 1981.

There are basically three types of HMOs. More than half are group arrangements where the doctors and staff are salaried and work out of a single location. Another form is a practice in which doctors can be paid on a per-patient basis. A third form — one which has been growing — has been called an "HMO without walls." Under this arrangement, doctors form a group but retain their own offices, allowing patients to participate on a prepaid basis.

Pros and Cons of HMOs

HMOs have had many champions, and also detractors. The Group Health Association of America, the representative of prepaid group plans in the United States, cited advantages to the patient (relief from financial worry, health care in one location), to the physician, (normal work week at regular salary and no office overhead or need for costly malpractice insurance), and to the plan (less costly because of its emphasis on preventive medicine which reduces hospitalization). Strong opposition once came from the American Medical Association, which viewed HMOs as a step toward "socialized medicine." But this opposition had lessened considerably by the end of the 1970s (in 1978 the AMA began offering its employees in Chicago the option of joining an HMO instead of being covered under traditional hospitalization insurance). The official position of the association focused more on the quality of care that HMOs provided than on the socialized medicine aspects.

Some critics, including a number of persons enrolled in prepaid plans, complained that the care tended to be impersonal and that patients often had to wait several months for a medical appointment. But Dr. Gordon K. MacLeod and Jeffrey A. Prussin, co-authors of a March 1973 article in *The New England Journal of Medicine,* wrote that "the comparative studies that have been made strongly indicate that prepaid group practice plans help contain inflation in medical costs, lower the total cost . . . of medical and health care services to the individual enrollee and clearly reduce unnecessary hospitalization and elective surgery without sacrificing the quality of care."

In 1977, the average number of hospital days per 1,000 members for qualified HMOs was 425; for all prepaid plans, 519; for Blue Cross/Blue Shield (with about half of its 74 million members enrolled in health indemnity plans), 755. Studies have documented a 30 to 40 percent reduction in hospitalization costs for HMOs as compared with conventional plans.

By compensating doctors at the beginning, rather than the end, of their services, HMOs theoretically discouraged unnecessary tests and hospitalization. Because the income of doctors was dependent on the economic well-being of the organization, they had a strong incentive to avoid unnecessary costs. Group practice also provided an opportunity for the exchange of information and com-

Terms of Reference

Capitation. The amount of money required per person to provide covered services to a person for a specified time.

Community-wide plans. Plans in which membership is open to qualified groups or individuals in the community, rather than to members of specified unions or employees in specified industries.

Fee-for-service. The traditional practice of paying specific amounts for specific services received.

Foundation. An association of physicians who organize a management and fiscal structure that develops a fee schedule for individual physicians who join. The foundation usually markets the health plan to subscribers, makes claims payments and sets rates for subscribers.

Group health plan. Provides health services to persons covered by a prepayment program through a group of physicians usually working in a group clinic.

Group practice. A group of physicians who practice medicine together in one or more facilities and who share common overhead expenses, medical records, equipment and staff.

HMO. Health maintenance organization. As defined by the federal HMO act of 1973, it is a legal entity or organized system of health care that provides directly or arranges for a comprehensive range of basic and supplemental health care services to a voluntarily enrolled population in a geographic area, primarily on a prepaid or fixed periodic basis.

Prepaid group practice. Physicians and other health professionals who contract to provide a wide range of preventive, diagnostic and treatment services on a continuing basis for enrolled participants.

parison of services. In addition, a built-in control that discouraged undertreatment was regular review by participating physicians of one another's work.

"It has always been a paradox that doctors and hospitals are dedicated to keeping people well and healthy, yet generally derive most of their income from sickness," observed Dr. Cecil Cutting, former executive director of the Permanente Medical Group of Northern California. "By contrast, when prepayment is made directly to providers of care, both the hospitals and the doctors are better off if the patient remains well."

"The nicest thing . . . [about practicing in an HMO] is never to have to think about what this or that is going to cost a patient. I only have to decide what is appropriate," commented Dr. Jack Resnick, an internist with the Manhattan Health Plan. "For one thing, I don't have to put patients in the hospital just for tests or X-rays. We do them here. For another, if I come across something that's not in my field, all I have to do is walk down the hall and ask someone who knows. You can't get that kind of feedback in private practice."

"Because an HMO receives a fixed premium for all medical and hospital services, regardless of the amount of services utilized, it has an incentive to provide high quality, preventive care and not engage in excess hospitalization or to perform duplications or unnecessary tests," said Jack K. Shelton, a Ford Motor Company executive. Shelton's comment came during announcement in February 1979 of the establishment of a new HMO, the Health Alliance Plan of Michigan, by the three major automobile manufacturers and the United Automobile Workers.

"HMOs offer competition to a system badly in need of it," said former HEW Secretary Joseph A. Califano Jr. "They are demonstrating that they can compete — on a price and quality basis — with fee-for-service doctors and complex insurance policies that cover some fee-for-service medical and hospital care."

According to the HEW Office of Health Maintenance Organizations, the average monthly cost of belonging to an HMO in many areas in 1977 was below the cost of being insured just for hospitalization by carriers such as Blue Cross and Blue Shield. In addition, the monthly rates charged by many HMOs were rising more slowly than premiums charged by hospital insurers. However, in some locations the prepaid plans proved more expensive than conventional insurance, even after the more comprehensive benefits were taken into account. For example, in the Washington, D.C., area, the high option premium prices for prepaid plans tended to be somewhat higher than that of traditional insurance plans. But HMO spokesmen contended that their coverage was more comprehensive, records were more centralized, service was available 24 hours a day, and the total annual health costs to an individual or family might therefore actually be less expensive.

To many people, the idea of prepaid plans evoked an image of assembly-line medical franchises where patients saw a different or indifferent doctor each time they sought treatment. Actually, most health maintenance organizations have sought to provide the patient with a physician who would be consulted on each visit and was primarily responsible for the patient's care. And for many families, provision of unlimited pediactrics care was particularly attractive. According to Roger Birnbaum, director of the Rutgers Community Health Plan, HMOs helped offset the gap in primary health care caused by many physicians' abandoning family practices to take up more lucrative specialities. HMOs also could afford extensive coverage because relatively few members needed hospitalization, and the reduction in hospitalizations allowed the plans to spend more money on primary care.

On the other hand, there have also been widespread complaints that patients have experienced long delays in obtaining appointments, particularly for routine examinations. Although in emergencies they were likely to receive immediate service, they might not see the doctor they usually consulted, raising the possibility of inconsistent or insufficient diagnosis.

Government Backing for HMOs

In an effort to control rising health care costs and reduce hospitalizations, the federal government in 1973 began taking an active role in supporting HMOs, with passage of legislation authorizing financial support for the organizations.

Advocates of prepaid medical care denied that they were attempting to destroy the fee-for-service tradition. What they were trying to do, they insisted, was to give the consumer a choice. President Nixon, in signing the Health Maintenance Organization Act of 1973 into law on Dec. 29 of that year, stressed the element of choice.

Nixon had proposed federal assistance to HMOs in his 1971 health message to Congress as a means of increasing "the value of the services a consumer receives for each health dollar." In 1973, HEW set up a Health Maintenance Organization Service to distribute planning and development grants to prospective HMO sponsors. And late the following year, the president signed a bill which allowed Medicare and Medicaid beneficiaries to join prepaid group programs.

1973 HMO Law and 1976 Changes

The HMO law that finally emerged from Congress in 1973 was more limited than the one Nixon had proposed in 1971 but considerably broader than what the administration later wanted. A major reason for the retreat was seen as the AMA's opposition to a "federal subsidy" for HMOs. The law authorized $375 million in public funds in fiscal years 1974-78 to aid in the development of both nonprofit and profit-making health maintenance organizations, and it set forth a number of requirements for an HMO to qualify for federal assistance. Probably the most important requirement was that an extensive list of basic and supplemental services had to be offered. *(Provisions of act, appendix p. 4-A)*

That provision aroused considerable criticism. The full scope of services would be so costly, it was argued, that federally assisted HMOs would be at a competitive disadvantage with other prepaid plans and with fee-for-service arrangements.

Another provision of the law required that firms with more than 25 employees "include in any health benefits plan offered ... the option of membership in qualified health maintenance organizations which are engaged in the provision of ... services in the areas in which employees reside." But while employers were obliged to offer their workers an HMO option, if one was available, they were not required to pay any more of the cost than they already did toward the employees' existing coverage. If the employees opted for an HMO plan, they would have to pay any increased cost.

As a result of these complaints, Congress in 1976 passed legislation (PL 94-460) easing the HMO eligibility requirements. A coalition of private groups representing HMOs, insurers and labor, led by the Group Health Association of America, had begun working on proposed amendments to the act in late 1974. The administration also agreed that some provisions of the 1973 act were too strict. *(1976 revisions, p. 48-A)*

1978 Legislation

Two years later, HMOs got another boost when Congress cleared legislation (PL 95-559) providing a three-year, $164 million reauthorization for federal grants and loans for the prepaid group practices.

The final bill was considerably less ambitious than either the five-year extension originally sought by the Carter administration or the five-year, $415 million bill reported by the Senate Human Resources Committee. The measure was scaled down by both the Senate and the House.

The administration had proposed new financial incentives to encourage enrollment of Medicare and Medicaid beneficiaries in the health plans. And it wanted to exempt HMOs from certain restrictions of the federal health planning process.

It did not win these changes, but even the shorter reauthorization was considered a substantial reaffirmation of federal involvement in HMOs. In one important change, the bill added new financial support for HMO outpatient facilities, key to the plans' emphasis on reducing costly hospitalizations. The total amount of support for various stages of development and operation was raised, and certain requirements for staff and services offered were relaxed for the early, financially difficult years when an HMO builds membership. *(Provisions, appendix p. 67-A)*

But before either House or Senate committees reported the reauthorization legislation, the existing federal HMO program came under fire for slipshod management practices which included endorsing multimillion-dollar HMO loans without a fixed loan policy. And charges resurfaced that certain HMOs were defrauding their members and the federal government, or were so poorly managed that they would fail and default on federal loans. These charges, outlined in reports by the General Accounting Office (GAO) and the Senate Governmental Affairs Subcommittee on Investigations, figured prominently in debate on the HMO reauthorization. The doubts created by the reports, plus growing congressional resistance to expensive health programs, resulted in the more modest three-year reauthorization.

The proposed incentives to promote Medicare-Medicaid enrollments in HMOs never emerged from committee, in large part because some of the most memorable HMO abuses involved Medicaid HMO enrollments authorized by California in 1972. An administration proposal to exempt HMO ambulatory (outpatient) care facilities from federal planning review — thus putting them on an equal footing with outpatient services started by other entities like fee-for-service group practices — died with the health planning reauthorization (HR 11488).

In response to the criticisms of HMOs and the federal support program, the final bill included detailed HMO financial reporting requirements, with criminal penalties for false reporting. It also ordered the GAO to evaluate HEW efforts to improve its management of the program.

The bill that had originally been reported by the Senate Human Resources Committee reflected much of the president's program, except for Medicare and Medicaid amendments. It was the product of a collective effort involving the Washington Business Group on Health (a group representing about 150 major corporations), the AFL-CIO, health policy staff at HEW and the Consensus Group, a coalition that sprouted in the early 1970s to lobby for HMOs and helped shape the 1976 HMO amendments. Consensus Group members included HMO trade associations (the Group Health Association of America, the American Association of Foundations for Medical Care) and the insurance industry.

Thus, most of the interested parties — with the major exception of the AMA — had a hand in crafting the bill. Dan Hill, a spokesman for the AMA, said the association did not oppose HMOs *per se* but was concerned with what it viewed as unfair competition. If HMOs were to become a pervasive feature of the medical landscape instead of a limited experiment, they should not have the benefit of federal subsidies, Hill said.

Administration Efforts to Boost HMOs

In addition to legislative proposals, the Carter administration moved on a number of fronts to strengthen

Development of Prepaid Group Practices

Even before the Depression, there were HMO-type alternatives to conventional health insurance. It is believed that the first prepaid group practice was the Farmers' Union Cooperative Health Association, begun by Dr. Michael A. Shadid in Elk City, Okla., in 1927. To appeal to the farmers in the region, Shadid modeled his group plan on the cotton and supply cooperatives in the areas. Two years later, Dr. Donald Ross and Dr. Clifford Loos set up a private clinic in Los Angeles to provide better and cheaper medical care for employees of the Los Angeles Water and Supply Department.

The Los Angeles County Medical Society expelled Ross and Loos, but both were later reinstated after an appeal to the American Medical Association's (AMA) Judicial Council. The Elk City cooperative, according to a later account by Herman Miles Somers and Anne Ramsay Somers in their book, *Doctors, Patients and Health Insurance* (1971), "survived two decades of harassment from the local medical society and, in 1952, achieved a *modus vivendi* by agreeing to settle out of court a $300,000 'restraint of trade' suit against the society. The latter finally agreed to admit to membership the salaried physicians of the Elk City cooperative and the cooperative agreed to admit outside physicians and their patients to its hospital."

The first urban cooperative, Group Health Association of Washington, D.C., was started by employees of the Federal Home Owners Loan Corporation in 1937. It, too, was the target of strong AMA opposition. Two years after its establishment, the cooperative brought a lawsuit against the AMA and the D.C. Medical Society, charging them with restraint of trade under the Sherman Antitrust Act. In the 1943 case of *American Medical Association* v. *United States*, the Supreme Court upheld two lower court decisions which had found the AMA and its local affiliate guilty of violating the Sherman Act.

Despite a strong endorsement by the Committee on the Costs of Medical Care in 1932, the HMO prototypes attracted little public attention until the establishment of the Kaiser Medical Care Program in the 1940s. The founder of what later became the Kaiser-Permanente organization was Dr. Sidney R. Garfield who in the mid-1930s set up a prepaid group practice for construction workers in Southern California. In 1938 industrialist Henry J. Kaiser asked Garfield to organize hospital and medical facilities for construction workers at the Grand Coulee Dam in Washington state.

With the outbreak of World War II, Kaiser again invited Garfield to set up health care facilities for workers at his shipyards in California and Oregon. During the war, as many as 200,000 employees enrolled in the plan. When peace came in 1945, Kaiser decided to continue the plan and open it to all employed groups in the community. Kaiser-Permanente grew slowly until the 1950s. In 1950, there were only 150,000 members; ten years later there were over 800,000. Responding to Kaiser-Permanente's growth during that decade, California's San Joaquin Valley County Medical Society set up a Foundation for Medical Care in 1954 to counter the prepaid threat.

After conducting a study of the Kaiser plan, the National Advisory Commission on Health Manpower reported to President Johnson in November 1967 that the program "has achieved real economies, while maintaining high quality of care, through a delicate interplay of managerial and professional interests." The commission went on to say: "There has been created a cost consciousness among the health professionals and a health care consciousness among the administrators which enables them to work toward a common goal without either sacrificing or overemphasizing their own points of view.... The quality of care provided by Kaiser is equivalent to, if not superior to, that available in most communities."

By the end of the 1970s, the Kaiser plan, which was officially certified as an HMO in October 1977, was the world's largest nongovernmental supplier of health care in the nation, with more than three million members, 3,000 physicians, 26 hospitals with 5,700 beds, and 66 medical facilities. Its revenues exceeded $1 billion. One out of 10 Californians was a member of the plan.

the position of HMOs in the nation's health scheme. In March 1978, then-HEW Secretary Califano invited the chief executives of the "Fortune 500" (the nation's largest corporations), an additional 300 corporate representatives and more than 200 labor leaders to a day-long session on HMOs in Washington, D.C.

Also in 1978, the Federal Trade Commission took steps to curb discrimination by insurers or local practitioners against HMOs and combat other practices that might restrain their growth. The agency issued a consent order prohibiting a physicians' group and a Blue Shield plan in the state of Washington from boycotting or otherwise discriminating against HMO staff doctors. The FTC also launched "a nationwide investigation ... to identify other instances of anti-HMO conduct — said by many to be fairly widespread," said FTC Chairman Michael Pertschuk.

Steps were also taken to make internal improvements in the administration of the federal HMO program. And in 1979, the administration launched a 10-year development strategy focusing on 61 metropolitan areas with populations of 25,000 or more. These areas were distinguished by high growth rates, high health care costs or low enrollment percentages in HMOs.

In addition, in April 1980, the administration published interim regulations in the *Federal Register* that would permit HMOs to receive up to $2.5 million in direct loans or guaranteed loans to construct or buy facilities. This would be in addition to existing federal aid whereby HMOs could receive up to $4 million in loans and guarantees to defray expensive operating costs until sufficient membership was attained. "Because a new HMO generally operates at a deficit during its first five years, it may have difficulty raising private capital for construction of an ambulatory care facility," said Surgeon General Julius B. Richmond. "Yet, such a facility may be critical to handle the membership growth the plan needs to break even."

The administration's fiscal 1981 budget envisaged a growth in funding for the federal HMO program from $23 million in 1977 to more than $69 million in 1981. The administration again submitted legislation that would provide an incentive for Medicare beneficiaries to enroll in HMOs. The federal contribution to HMOs for enrolling Medicare recipients would be changed to 95 percent of the average Medicare expenditure, in return for HMOs providing broader benefits to Medicare recipients who chose this coverage.

Outlook

As the nation's health care system entered the 1980s, it appeared that HMOs might be capturing a larger share of the health care market. But they still faced numerous obstacles and problems, among them some continuing skepticism about the quality of health care they provided; cases of poor management and bankruptcy; difficulties in obtaining sufficient capital for huge start-up costs; and the reluctance of Congress and the administration to increase the budgets of any social service plan. Back in 1974, Dr. Richard H. Egdahl, writing in the May issue of *Prism*, an AMA magazine, predicted that it was "not likely that the Kaiser-type HMO will spread very rapidly in the next few decades because of the large initial capital investment requirements and the requirement of full-time salaries for participating physicians."

On the other hand, numerous studies and findings, including those by the Federal Trade Commission, have found that the growth of HMOs has encouraged competition in the health care industry by stimulating a new awareness of costs on the part of doctors and hospitals not participating in prepaid plans.

Both business and labor in general have come to support HMOs as a means to cut down on health insurance costs for union members and employers. As Douglas Fraser, president of the United Auto Workers, said in 1978, "When you're 'spending' 75 cents an hour [on health benefits] at the bargaining table, you're not spending it on wages, holidays or pensions."

Fraser predicted that management would perceive a common interest with labor in holding down medical inflation, and he cited as evidence a decision by the Labor-Management Group to turn its attention to health cost problems. The information group, chaired jointly by the presidents of the AFL-CIO and General Electric, was created to provide a forum for discussions between top labor and management officials on matters of mutual interest. On Jan. 19, 1978, the group issued a position paper stating that "labor and management should work to have legislative, regulatory, enrollment and other barriers to the development of HMOs which still exist removed."

While these recommendations were mild when stacked up against visions of a broadly available, comprehensive health care system advanced by some HMO proponents, they represented a significant shift to "less strong opposition" to HMOs on the part of business, in Fraser's view.

Although the venerable Kaiser-Permanente system was founded by an industrialist, many corporations have been uncomfortable with prepaid plans for general philosophical reasons and because they feel HMOs presented administrative complications, said Saul Kilstein of the Washington Business Group on Health. A particular complaint was the requirement that many employers must offer HMOs as an alternative to conventional health insurance; this made it difficult for multi-state companies to equate worker benefits, they said, since HMOs were not available in some regions.

Despite these reservations, however, Kilstein said business was beginning to regard at least large HMOs as appealingly cost-efficient. Many businessmen, he added, preferred a competitive "free market" HMO strategy for holding down health care costs to such alternatives as the regulation embodied in the administration's troubled hospital cost control proposals.

Unless a comprehensive national health insurance law were enacted with specific incentives for health maintenance organizations, their development was likely to depend almost solely on private business. Insurance company and corporation involvement has been increasing; Blue Cross has sponsored a number of pilot HMOs, and several large corporations have established prepaid programs, with varying degrees of success.

Whatever the future of prepaid plans, Arthur Weisman, senior vice president of the Kaiser Foundation, warned in August 1976, "Nothing said by me ... should lead any listener to the conclusion that appropriate medical care is inexpensive. It isn't. Moreover, it is erroneous to conclude ... that organized health-care systems will reverse the current trend of health-care cost escalation." But, he added, "what I have learned from experience is that organized systems can and do moderate health care costs." ∎

Medicare, Medicaid Plagued by Rising Costs

Fifteen years ago, on July 30, 1965, President Lyndon B. Johnson signed into law what has been generally considered to be the most important welfare legislation of his administration — the amendments to the Social Security Act of 1935 providing for the Medicare and Medicaid health programs. In signing the bill, the president said, "No longer will older Americans be denied the healing miracle of modern medicine. No longer will illness crush and destroy the savings that they have so carefully put away over a lifetime so that they might enjoy dignity in their later years."

Most observers agreed that the Medicare program has been largely successful in meeting the health care needs of the elderly. "Medicare has enabled old people without financial resources to get the health care they need," said Dr. Rashi Fein, professor of health economics at Harvard, in a 1975 assessment, "and it has prevented financial catastrophe for the rest of the elderly and their children. These were its main goals."

"Support for Medicare is related to the political influence of its aged constituency, but the esteem with which it is regarded is largely deserved," wrote Karen Davis and Cathy Schoen in their 1978 Brookings Institution study, *Health and the War on Poverty*. (Davis was later appointed a deputy assistant secretary of health, education and welfare in 1977.) "It has enabled many elderly people to receive health services in increasing amounts and quality. At least partially as a consequence of the improved access to medical care afforded by Medicare, the health of the aged has improved noticeably since the program began. Perhaps even more important, Medicare has helped protect the elderly and their children from the financial burden of large medical bills. It has also played a role in establishing minimal quality standards for hospitals and nursing homes, and it has enforced nondiscriminatory provision of services in hospitals."

However, both the Medicare and Medicaid programs have become victims of inflated health care costs. As these costs have gone up, gaps in benefit coverage have widened. "The increase in costs to the individual has created a situation which deters preventive medicine and stimulates the use of more expensive services," said a spokesman for the American Association of Retired Persons.

The history of Medicare and Medicaid should be viewed within the context of the U.S. health industry in general, which in 1980 employed more than seven million people (as compared to around four million in 1975) and was continuing to grow at a fast pace. National health expenditures, both public and private, were estimated to exceed $218 billion in 1980. This compared to national health expenditures of $25.9 billion in 1960 and $118.4 billion in fiscal 1975. An increase in federal financing of health programs has paralleled this rise in total national health expenditures. Federal expenditures for Medicare and Medicaid were expected to total more than $53 billion in 1981 (up from $37 billion in 1977), accounting for nearly 9 percent of the federal budget.

One of the major reasons for the growth in the cost of the two plans has been that they are entitlement, or what has been characterized as "uncontrollable spending," programs. Of the estimated $219.3 billion in fiscal 1981 outlays by the new Department of Health and Human Services (HHS, formerly the Department of Health, Education and Welfare), fully 95 percent would go to the big entitlement programs — Medicare and Medicaid, as well as Social Security, Supplemental Security Income (for the aged, blind and disabled) and Aid to Families with Dependent Children.

Entitlement programs must provide mandated benefits for everyone who meets eligibility standards. Built-in cost-of-living increases, coupled with rising numbers of aged and disabled persons, have been responsible for the tremendous growth in their costs, said HHS Secretary Patricia Roberts Harris.

The basic reality of the health budget, as in past years, was that inflation in medical costs and an aging population would again push Medicare and Medicaid costs upward, squeezing existing programs and leaving little extra for new initiatives.

It would cost the federal government 12.5 percent more in fiscal 1981 to take care of some 47 million Medicare and Medicaid beneficiaries, including some 700,000 new Medicare enrollees. Of the estimated $62.4 billion fiscal 1981 outlays for health, $53.2 billion would be for the two public health insurance programs. Medicaid outlays were estimated at $15.9 billion, for its 23 million poor beneficiaries. Medicare expenditures would be $37.3 billion, for 25 million aged and three million disabled.

In addition, because of a major flaw in the department's estimating method for fiscal 1980, the administration underestimated Medicaid costs and needed a supplemental appropriation of $2.3 billion to cover program costs for the fiscal 1980 year.

Inflation in health care costs has taken its toll on both the Medicare/Medicaid programs and on the people they were intended to serve. Expenditures for the programs have been projected to outstrip incoming funds by the late 1980s, with inflation consuming most of new Medicare and Medicaid funds. About three-quarters of the increase in expenditures is attributable to rising hospital costs (Medicare and Medicaid accounted for 40 percent of total hospital spending), with the remainder accounted for by the increase in the number of people eligible and the increase in use by those eligible for the programs.

Medicare/Medicaid History

What may have been the first government health insurance program in the United States was established by Congress in 1798 when merchant marine personnel were required to contribute a few cents a month to pay for hospital care provided by a new marine hospital. It was not until the early 20th century, however, that the idea of compulsory health insurance for the general public gained serious attention. At that time, several states debated health insurance proposals and the American Association for Labor Legislation (AALL), a group of lawyers, academics and other professionals, made several attempts to push its bills through state legislatures. Bills introduced in New York and Massachusetts were drafted by the American Medical Association (AMA), which had published several articles in favor of compulsory health insurance. In 1917, the AMA's House of Delegates endorsed a health insurance plan comparable to the model bill of the AALL.

However, opposition to the idea of compulsory health insurance grew. The opponents included Samuel Gompers and a group of other labor leaders who felt that a national health insurance system would increase government control over laborers. In addition, they feared such an insurance plan would cause fewer employees to join unions and give management a reason for not granting raises. Employers also opposed compulsory health insurance, for fear they would have to contribute a disproportionate amount of money to the plan. By 1920, the AMA, reacting to pressure from the state medical societies, had reversed its position and opposed compulsory health insurance.

Interest in a government-sponsored health program was not revived until the 1930s when the Depression stimulated a greater concern for social welfare. In 1934, President Roosevelt established the Committee on Economic Security to devise a bill to provide a minimum income for the elderly. The committee's report led to passage of the Social Security Act of 1935, which provided for a broad range of social insurance and public assistance programs. The act did not include a health insurance program although the committee had endorsed the principle of compulsory national health insurance. Roosevelt dropped the idea for fear its inclusion would endanger passage of the entire act.

From 1935 on, compulsory health insurance bills were introduced in Congress annually. One of the more important bills was proposed in 1943 by Sens. Robert F. Wagner, D-N.Y., and James E. Murray, D-Mont., and Rep. John D. Dingell, D-Mich. The "Wagner-Murray-Dingell" bill called for a sweeping revision of the Social Security Act, including the creation of a compulsory national health insurance system for persons of all ages to be financed through a payroll tax. No action was taken on the measure during the 78th Congress.

President Truman in 1945 made the first proposal for enactment of a federally operated health insurance program. The Truman plan would have covered the entire population, not just the elderly. The proposal immediately brought forth the lobbying might of the AMA. The AMA was joined in opposition by the insurance industry and conservative business groups. Labor unions and liberal organizations worked for enactment of the Truman proposal and the more limited Medicare plan that followed, but there was no one organization that was as important in support of a Medicare program as the AMA was in opposition.

The lobbying campaign for and against the Truman proposal reached a peak when the president pushed for congressional action in 1949-50. Hospital insurance became one of the major issues of the session; when Congress adjourned without taking any action, the AMA was considered to have won a notable victory. Its warnings that national health insurance would mean "socialized medicine" and government interference in medical practice were generally credited with being the major factor in the outcome.

After 1950 the issue subsided for a time; the Eisenhower administration, which came to office in 1953, opposed any such plan. But in 1957 the issue returned to public prominence with introduction by Rep. Aime J. Forand, D-R.I., of a bill which covered hospital and surgical costs of the aged under the Social Security retirement system. This became a major part of the legislative program of the AFL-CIO, and the AMA began another nationwide publicity campaign in opposition. This marked the start of the struggle that ended with enactment of Medicare and Medicaid in 1965.

Revival of Interest

By 1960 the Forand bill (as Medicare was then tagged) had become a very hot political issue. However, the rules of the House were such that the proposal could not be brought to the House floor for debate unless it was reported by the House Ways and Means Committee. The committee in 1960 voted 17-8 against the proposal, and was not to vote in favor of it until 1965.

Medical Peer Review Groups

In 1972, Congress established a network of professional standards review organizations (PSROs), composed primarily of physicians and charged with the responsibility of overseeing the cost and quality of health care provided by three government programs: Medicare, Medicaid and maternal and child health.

The theory underlying the establishment of the organizations was that doctors themselves were best qualified to monitor their colleagues' practices and set standards for the profession. The legislation called for the PSROs to establish treatment standards and review them on a case-by-case basis. In 1978, Congress strengthened the authority of the organizations, giving them the power to make binding decisions on the necessity of medical treatment.

"I think if I were a doctor ... I would work very hard to make that PSRO program work," said former Health, Education and Welfare Secretary Joseph A. Califano Jr. in November 1977. "It's one of the opportunities the doctors have to police their own overutilization of medical facilities, their own prescribing problems, their own hospitalization problems, their own overloading of laboratory tests.... If the doctors can't do it, then somebody else is going to do it.... So we intend to work to try and make that program more effective than it's been."

But eight years after they were established, assessments of the effectiveness of PSROs in controlling costs were mixed. There remained considerable resistance to the concept among physicians and, at best, a lack of enthusiasm among organizations such as the AMA. According to the administration's fiscal 1981 budget, "a 1979 study of PSROs operating throughout the country found wide variations in savings attributable to their review of hospital stays of Medicare beneficiaries, but suggested that substantial savings could result from broader application of the procedures of effective PSROs.... Improved management techniques reduced average operating costs of PSROs from $14 per case in 1977 to less than $9 per case in 1981."

With House action blocked, Medicare supporters worked on getting the bill through the Senate, even though there seemed to be little chance of enactment.

Kennedy administration bills covered only hospital and post-hospital costs, not surgical bills as proposed by Forand. Medicare produced another major Senate fight in 1962. Concessions were made to win five Republican votes, but the administration nevertheless suffered a stunning defeat when the plan was tabled, 48-52. Medicare finally passed the Senate for the first time in 1964, as an amendment to a House-passed bill raising Social Security retirement benefits by 5 percent. But the bill died in conference when a majority of House conferees opposed any Medicare plan and a majority of Senate conferees held firm in favor. As the 1964 bill died, President Johnson spoke of hopes for a mandate in the November election and pledged that he would try again for Medicare.

Enactment of the Programs

As finally passed by Congress July 28, 1965, the bill (PL 89-97) provided for two additional titles to the Social Security Act — numbered 18 and 19. The first section of Title 18 provided persons over 65 with insurance to cover the costs of hospital and related care. The program was to be financed by a Social Security trust fund to which employers and employees were required to contribute. Part B of Title 18 called for a voluntary system of supplemental medical insurance covering doctors' fees and certain other health services. Title 19, the Medicaid section of the bill, provided a program of federal matching grants to states that chose to make medical services available to welfare recipients and the medically indigent.

Two days after Congress cleared the bill, President Johnson flew to Independence, Mo., to sign the legislation in a televised ceremony with Harry S Truman at his side. A few days later, the Association of American Physicians and Surgeons, a group which had been fighting "socialized" medicine since the 1940s, urged its members to boycott the Medicare program. The AMA, however, refused to endorse a boycott by professional organizations. The fight against Medicare and Medicaid was slowly winding down.

Legislative Changes in the Early 1970s

Major amendments to the Medicare and Medicaid program were included in the Social Security Amendments of 1972 (PL 92-603). The bill extended Medicare eligibility to an additional 1.7 million disabled Social Security beneficiaries; enabled Medicare beneficiaries to enroll in health maintenance organizations (HMOs) providing comprehensive prepaid health care with the government paying the premiums if the plans provided federally approved services; covered payments to chiropractors under Medicare; provided coverage under Medicare for most Americans afflicted with chronic kidney disease (end-stage renal disease) with specific protection against the costs of hemodialysis or kidney transplants; and established professional standards review organizations (PSROs) representing local practicing physicians to review Medicaid and Medicare services. *(PSROs, box p. 74)*

During the 93rd Congress, several technical measures were enacted that coordinated Medicaid eligibility requirements with the new federal Supplemental Security Income (SSI) program.

In 1975, legislation was passed (PL 94-182) that allowed local medical groups an extra two years to set

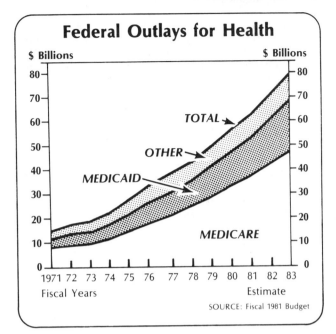

Federal Outlays for Health

$ Billions — $ Billions

TOTAL
OTHER
MEDICAID
MEDICARE

1971 72 73 74 75 76 77 78 79 80 81 82 83
Fiscal Years   Estimate

SOURCE: Fiscal 1981 Budget

up PSROs and provided that prevailing charges for physician services under Medicare could not be lowered. *(See appendix, p. 34-A)*

Two years later, in 1977, Congress moved to clean up fraud and abuse in the two programs when it cleared legislation (PL 95-142) increasing penalties for fraud and abuse, strengthening the oversight responsibilities of PSROs and requiring more ownership information from program providers. The bill was a result of three years of congressional consideration following discovery by federal and state investigators that kickbacks, fraudulent billings, unnecessary medical treatment and other problems were occurring in the federal health programs. (In 1976, Congress had enacted a bill establishing an Office of Inspector General for HEW.) *(1976 act, p. 56-A; 1977 act, p. 57-A)*

Also in 1977, the president signed into law a bill (PL 95-210) that authorized reimbursement under Medicare and Medicaid for services provided by nurse practitioners and physician assistants in rural clinics. In 1978, legislation was cleared (PL 95-292) that would amend the end-stage renal disease program under Medicare to provide incentives for use of self-dialysis. *(1977 legislation, p. 59-A; 1978 legislation, p. 71-A)*

1979 Congressional Action

Rising costs and the need for administrative reforms of Medicare and Medicaid were the primary focus of attention in the 95th and 96th Congresses. The debate centered on hospital cost control, although a number of bills were introduced that would expand the scope of services available under Medicare, lower or eliminate certain Medicare cost-sharing charges, and improve and expand long-term care services available under Medicare and Medicaid.

In July 1979, the Senate Finance Committee voted to reject President Carter's hospital cost control plan and to report instead a "Medicare-Medicaid Administrative and Reimbursement Reform Act" (HR 934) that would limit control efforts to inpatient routine operating costs under Medicare and Medicaid.

The House Ways and Means Committee also reported legislation (HR 3990, HR 4000) making some changes in the programs. The House Interstate and Foreign Commerce Committee, which shared jurisdiction over the legislation, reported its version in early 1980.

Neither the House bills nor the Senate measure had come up for floor votes as of mid-1980.

Senate Finance Committee Bill

The Finance Committee bill was based on a Medicare-Medicaid reform measure (S 505) sponsored by Herman E. Talmadge, D-Ga., chairman of its health subcommittee, and several other bills and committee staff recommendations. Talmadge insisted his plan was not an "either-or" alternative to President Carter's cost control proposal, but the committee basically regarded it as such.

The major feature of the bill was a "prospective" payment system that limited federal payments to hospitals for Medicare and Medicaid patients to the "average" costs for each type and size of hospital.

Under the existing system, the federal government simply paid a portion of a hospital's total expenses after they were incurred on behalf of Medicare and Medicaid patients. Under HR 934, hospitals would be paid at a set rate per day for their routine costs, such as supplies, food and non-supervisory labor. The rate for each type or size of hospital would be determined by comparing costs of similar hospitals and finding an average level of expenditures. Hospitals coming in under the average could keep part of the difference as a bonus; those exceeding the average by more than 15 percent (in the first year) could not recover those "excess" costs. The reimbursement limit would be lowered in future years.

To ease the transition into the program, during the first two years only half the penalties and bonuses would be applied. Other Medicare-Medicaid payments to hospitals for "ancillary" services, such as X-rays, and for reimbursement for health facilities, such as nursing homes, would be brought into this system administratively as cost data became available.

The bill included numerous other provisions designed to induce doctors to accept Medicare reimbursement as full payment for patients' bills, encourage them to practice in medically underserved areas by reducing the existing urban-rural payment differential, and bar most percentage-based reimbursement for hospital-based physicians such as pathologists.

The bill created a new $50 million program to help hospitals convert underused acute-care beds to long-term care beds, and liberalized Medicare payments for home health care. It also barred disclosure by HEW or PSROs of data relating to physician performance or Medicare and Medicaid payments to them.

House Committee Action

The House Ways and Means Committee reported its "thrift package" Medicare-Medicaid legislation (HR 3990, HR 4000) on Nov. 5.

Similar legislation passed the House in 1978 but died without Senate action in the 95th Congress. The legislation originated when the House Budget Committee in effect told Dan Rostenkowski, D-Ill., then chairman of the Ways and Means Health Subcommittee, that the panel could "spend" up to $100 million on Medicare improvements; members then added up options until they reached that ceiling.

The bills made some benefit improvements for Medicare, such as eliminating annual limits on home health care services and liberalizing coverage for psychiatric and certain medical services. HR 4000 authorized a new demonstration project to provide the elderly and disabled with home health and homemaker assistance, and established a voluntary federal certification program for private health insurance policies supplementing Medicare. (Medigap, box p. 78)

HR 4000 authorized federal payments to HMOs enrolling Medicare beneficiaries at a prospectively determined rate of 95 percent of what it cost to provide Medicare benefits through regular fee-for-service doctors and hospitals.

Under existing law the government reimbursed HMOs at a rate of only 80 percent of fee-for-service costs. Partly as a result of the lower payment rate, only one of the nation's 217 prepaid group health plans had taken Medicare members on a risk basis, and only 1.5 million of Medicare's 25 million elderly beneficiaries were enrolled in such organizations. The HMO plans provided health care to members for a fixed annual fee.

The formula change appeared to mean more money for the plans than they could get under existing law, but it also required them to spend any excess funds on improving benefits or reducing co-payments for their Medicare members.

The Carter administration proposed the new reimbursement, as had the Nixon administration. Backers of the provision included the American Association of Retired Persons and prepaid plans such as the Kaiser Foundation Health Plan. They maintained that prepaid plans saved money compared to traditional fee-for-service medicine and that those savings could pay for more health care for the elderly. Some congressional aides questioned the potential for savings and for fraud or reduction in services, however. (See HMO chapter)

Medicare: The Plan and Its Problems

Providing health care for the nation's elderly has become an issue of increasing concern, partly because of the growing proportion of citizens aged 65 and over and because the process of aging is associated with the prevalence of chronic conditions and disabilities. According to the National Center for Health Statistics in an article in the June 1978 Social Security Bulletin, the elderly had about two and one-half times as many restricted activity days as the general population and more than twice as many days in bed and in hospitals.

While the need for medical care increases with age, the cost of that care weighs more heavily on the elderly, because they tend to have fewer economic resources than other age groups. According to a 1976 Census Bureau report, the income for families with elderly heads-of-households was 18 percent below the corresponding figure for all families. In sum, age, low income, chronic disorders and the need for medical care all contributed to the need for a national health care program for the aged.

Medicare was created in an attempt to meet this need. A nationwide program, it provides health insurance to individuals age 65 and over, to persons under 65 who have been entitled for a period of 24 months to Social Security or railroad retirement benefits because they were disabled, and to certain workers and their dependents who need kidney transplants or dialysis. It is a federal program with uniform eligibility and benefit structure throughout the nation. No physical examination is needed for coverage, and protection is available to insured persons without regard to their income or assets.

The vast majority of people age 65 and over are automatically entitled to protection under Part A of the plan. Those over 65 who are not automatically covered may elect to obtain Medicare insurance by paying the full actuarial cost of such coverage ($69 in 1980) — Part B of the plan. Also eligible (after receiving Social Security or railroad disability benefits for 24 months) are disabled workers, disabled widows, disabled dependent widowers between ages 50 and 65, beneficiaries over 18 who receive benefits because of disability prior to reaching age 22, and disabled railroad annuitants. Insured workers under Social Security and their dependents with chronic renal disease may be considered disabled for purposes of coverage.

Although Medicare provides a broader range of benefits than most private health insurance plans, it has a number of serious shortcomings. It has been confined primarily to paying hospital and doctors' bills; it does not pay for prescription drugs, routine eye and dental care, dentures, hearing aids and routine physical examinations and immunizations. It has not served to correct the imbalance in the nation's health care delivery system which often requires elderly persons, particularly those living in rural areas, to travel long distances to seek aid. Nor has it solved the problems of the need for long-term care or the tendency of some physicians to charge higher fees than the program will cover.

As health care costs have soared, Medicare beneficiaries have had to pay greater "out-of-pocket" amounts for deductibles, supplementary insurance policies and the monthly premiums under Part B coverage. In fiscal 1969, Medicare paid 43.9 percent of the elderly person's health bill, which averaged $735; in 1974, it paid 38.1 percent of an average $1,218 yearly bill; in 1977, it covered about 44 percent of a per capita health bill of $1,745 (compared with a $661 annual bill for beneficiaries between the ages of 19 and 64 and $253 for those under 19). When the Medicare program began in July 1966, the monthly premium paid by enrollees in Part B was $3. In 1980, it was $8.70. In addition, the amount a hospital inpatient must pay before Medicare takes over increased from $40 to $180.

Because these "Medigaps" in coverage have continued to widen, more and more persons age 65 and over have turned to private health insurance policies to supplement their Medicare insurance. It has been estimated that more than 50 percent of the elderly have at least one private insurance policy, paying total annual premiums of between $500 million and $1 billion. However, according to a July 1978 report by the Federal Trade Commission, "most supplemental policies will not pay for pre-existing conditions or the major gaps in Medicare, such as nursing home care ... and prescription drugs." Moreover, according to the report, "The lack of consumer information in the Medicare supplement market is so great that it is almost impossible to make rational purchase decisions." Both the Carter administration and the 96th Congress addressed themselves to this problem with legislation that would protect beneficiaries from overpriced, inadequate policies and deceptive sales practices.

In their 1978 study of Medicare/Medicaid and other programs to assist the poor, Davis and Schoen pointed

How Medicare/Medicaid Work

Medicare provides hospitalization and medical insurance for those age 65 and over who are eligible for Social Security or railroad retirement benefits.

Since 1972, this coverage has been extended to disabled Social Security beneficiaries and persons afflicted with chronic kidney disease, regardless of age. The Medicare program is divided into two parts:

Part A. Financed principally through a special hospital insurance tax levied on employees, employers and the self-employed (in 1980, each paid a tax of 1.05 percent of the first $25,900 of covered earnings). Part A pays for 90 days of inpatient hospital care subject to $180 deductible; a $45 a day co-payment is required for the 61st through the 90th day. An additional lifetime reserve of 60 days (subject to a $90 a day co-payment) may be drawn upon when a person exceeds 90 days in a benefit period (defined as beginning when an insured enters a hospital and ending when he has not been in a hospital or skilled nursing facility for 60 days). Part A also pays for 100 days of post-hospital skilled nursing facility care, subject to a $22.50 a day co-payment after the first 20 days; and 100 medically necessary post-hospital home health visits. Part A does not cover doctors' services even though they may be performed in the hospital.

Part B. An optional supplementary insurance plan covering doctors' fees and other outpatient services. Those who enroll pay a monthly premium ($8.70 in 1980). All persons age 65 and older and all persons enrolled under Part A can choose to participate in Part B. The plan pays 80 percent of "reasonable charges" for the following covered services after the insured pays the first $60: services of independent practitioners (primarily physicians), 100 home health visits (exempt from coinsurance), medical and related services, outpatient hospital services, and laboratory services.

In general, reimbursement under the Medicare program is based on "reasonable costs" for hospitals and other institutional providers, and "reasonable charges" for physicians and other non-institutional providers of health care.

Medicaid is a public assistance program that uses state and local tax money as well as federal funds to provide medical care for the poor. Each state is required to provide health care benefits to those persons who qualify for public welfare. If they desire, states may also extend coverage to the "medically indigent" — those persons who do not qualify for public assistance but whose incomes are too low to cover medical expenses. The federal share of state Medicaid funds ranges from 50 to 78 percent depending upon the state's per capita income. Each state administers and operates its own program and, subject to federal guidelines, determines eligibility and the scope of benefits to be provided. The programs vary considerably from state to state, with Arizona having no Medicaid program.

Lobbyists Fight Federal Regulation...

Margaret Dickson got some unsettling advice from health insurance agents when she asked them to look over her collection of supplementary policies for Medicare. Dickson was overinsured, but most of the agents insisted that she buy even more coverage. Some dismissed her policies as "garbage" without even looking at them, and pressed her to replace them with as many as eight new, overlapping plans. One agent grilled her "about my tax bracket, my banks, my general financial situation, and then suggested — oh heavens, I cannot say it — euthanasia as a solution to long-term health problems." He also asked her to give him power of attorney over her affairs.

What these agents didn't know was that Dickson, a retired receptionist for Rep. Clauae Pepper, D-Fla., was working with congressional investigators. Her "son," who took photographs of the meetings, and the insurance sales "trainee" sitting in on them were Pepper staff aides.

In 50 such interviews, conducted during the fall of 1978, only eight agents honestly advised, "Gee, lady, I think you've already got too much insurance."

Dickson's case was not unique. Investigators found widespread misrepresentation of what policies pay for, high-pressure sales tactics, agents posing as federal employees, persuading elderly persons to replace adequate policies with new ones just so the agent could get a higher commission, and companies that paid out very little in benefits compared to the large amounts they collected in premiums.

Compromise Certification Program

More than a year after the investigations by Pepper's Select Committee on Aging, Congress passed legislation that would establish voluntary national standards for "Medigap" health insurance. The Medigap amendment was attached to a bill (HR 3236) aimed at holding down costs of the Social Security disability insurance program. Under the agreement, states would have until July 1982 to enact their own laws on Medigap insurance that met the standards of a model state law designed by the National Association of Insurance Commissioners. The laws would have to provide for minimum loss ratios of 60 percent for individual policies and 75 percent for group policies.

A panel of four insurance commissioners and the secretary of the Department of Health and Human Services (HHS, formerly HEW) would decide whether state laws met the standards. In states that did not comply, the voluntary federal standards would be implemented. Companies would not be required to meet the federal standards, but those that did could say so in their advertising.

Background

Insurance officials insisted they had been treated unfairly by Pepper and the media. They said abuses were not nearly as widespread or serious as charged, and that states should be given time to adopt the model state insurance regulatory code drawn up in 1979 before federal regulation was imposed.

Certification program sponsors said only a handful of states had enacted and enforced adequate Medigap standards as of early 1980. They said the "seal of approval" the new program would give to reputable policies would at least assure buyers that minimal standards had been met.

Of the $4 billion spent each year on supplementary Medicare policies, Pepper said $1 billion was wasted on duplicate or useless coverage. Senior citizens could ill afford this loss, but they were vulnerable to high-pressure sales tactics because they accurately perceived that Medicare was not enough. Medicare, according to estimates, was paying only 44 percent of the medical bills of the elderly, because of its requirements for cost-sharing and because of major exclusions. In addition, the Medicare benefit structure was so confusing that it was difficult for many elderly persons to understand. That confusion and the proliferation of many variations on basic private insurance plans made comparison shopping extremely difficult.

In 1980, Medicare would pay for up to 60 days of hospitalization for each spell of illness, but a beneficiary must pay for the first day each time — a $180-a-day "deductible".

out that "these gaps in coverage are particularly burdensome for the elderly poor. Unlike the other Great Society ... health programs, Medicare is not solely, or even predominantly, a program for the poor. Yet as an integral part of the overall federal health care effort, it has important implications for the poor. Although eligibility is not dependent on income, a large portion of Medicare beneficiaries have modest or low incomes."

A major difficulty in the program, documented by several studies, has been the uneven distribution of Medicare benefits by race and geographical location. According to the National Center for Health Statistics, whites age 65 and over were hospitalized 14 percent more frequently than elderly blacks in 1975. Moreover, older citizens in rural areas and in both urban and rural areas of the South have generally received a smaller proportionate share of Medicare benefits.

Restrictive policies concerning the "reasonable charges" permitted under Medicare have been accompanied by an increased reluctance on the part of doctors to accept the amounts payable as payments in full and to reject assignment rates. In 1978, 73.6 percent of the bills submitted for Part B benefits were reduced because they exceeded the allowable Medicare charge. The percentage of assigned bills (on which the physician agrees to accept the allowable charge as payment in full) was 50.6 percent.

Another problem has been the fee differentials that exist between physicians in different areas of the country — for example, the often relatively high fees paid in urban areas compared with relatively low fees paid in rural and inner-city areas.

"Medicare has without question been an important force in improving the medical care of the elderly and

...Of 'Medigap' Health Insurance Abuses

Medicare began paying doctor bills after an individual spent a deductible of $60 each year; it then paid 80 percent of what it considered "reasonable" fees. but about half of U.S. physicians charged more than Medicare's reasonable fee. So, if a doctor charged $100 for a procedure Medicare valued at $80, Medicare would pay 80 percent of the lesser amount ($64); the patient might have a supplementary plan to pay the remaining 20 percent, but since carriers followed Medicare guidelines for doctors' fees, the payment would be only $16, to make up the $80, leaving the elderly person with a bill for $20 — or much more in cases of expensive surgical procedures.

Insurance carriers also coordinated benefits — meaning that a person could collect only from one company for a given benefit no matter how many policies he had. Yet many advertisements for "indemnity plans" hinted that beneficiaries could actually make "extra cash" during hospitalization by piling up payments from different policies.

For the major items Medicare did not cover, private policies were expensive or non-existent. Medicare did not cover prescription drugs used outside the hospital, routine physical examinations, eyeglasses, hearing aids, dental care or long-term nursing home care.

Typical abuses of Medigap salesmen, according to a 1978 House Aging Committee staff study, included:

● "Twisting" — inducing senior citizens to let adequate policies lapse and buy new coverage instead so the salesman could earn a larger commission. Unfortunately for the insured, new policies might have lengthy waiting periods for eligibility, particularly for treatment of conditions existing at the time the policy was bought.

● Scare tactics. Elderly customers requesting time to consider a policy might be told they could get sick before they make up their minds. One agent for so-called "dread-disease" policies routinely began his sales pitch with the phrase, "when you get cancer," not "if." These policies have been outlawed in a few states because their loss ratios — the amount they pay to beneficiaries compared to the amount paid for premiums — are very low.

● Outright fraud, such as salesmen posing as federal employees or pocketing customers' premium payments.

The Legislation

The Carter administration supported Medigap legislation, and on Jan. 30, 1980, the Senate adopted a proposal by Max Baucus, D-Mont., to create the voluntary federal certification program for Medicare supplemental policies and establish criminal penalties — $25,000 fines and up to five years in jail — for agents who deliberately sold older people more insurance than they needed, posed as federal employees, or misrepresented plans, and for companies selling mail-order plans not meeting state standards or submitting false data to win certification.

Both the House Ways and Means Committee and the Commerce Committee had approved voluntary certification and criminal penalties in their Medicare-Medicaid bill (HR 4000). However, a majority of House conferees on the disability legislation felt that the Medigap provision would be a dangerous precedent for future federal regulation of insurance. They repeatedly referred to "the camel's nose under the tent," arguing that the effort to set voluntary federal standards would grow into full-scale federal regulation.

Moreover, the Medigap legislation was vigorously opposed by lobbyists for major insurance companies, joined by state insurance commissioners. One of the strongest opponents of the provision was Rep. William R. Cotter, D-Conn., who was Connecticut's insurance commissioner before entering the House.

In the end, however, chief sponsor Baucus came up with a new version, acceptable to House conferees. To win their approval, he had to agree to give more authority to state insurance commissioners in the process of implementing the voluntary federal standards. However, he was able to retain the idea of including in the standards minimum rates for "loss ratios" — the percent of health insurance premiums that was returned to policyholders in the form of claims. The final version of the bill containing the compromise Medigap provision cleared Congress May 29 and was signed into law June 9, 1980 (PL 96-265).

reducing its financial burden. But complacency about the program is unwarranted," concluded Davis and Schoen. "Reform of Medicare to correct the program's uneven and socially undesirable effects on the delivery of services is crucial. Five areas particularly in need of re-examination are the cost-sharing structure of Medicare; the range of benefits covered and requirements for eligibility; methods of reimbursing providers of services; methods of financing the program; and supplementary measures that need to be taken to improve the access of minority groups and residents of underserved medical areas to adequate care."

Medicaid — In Need of Overhaul

The Medicaid program, unlike Medicare, is a federal-state matching program, with administrative responsibility and about half of the financing burden vested in state and local governments. It provides health care to low-income persons who are aged, blind or disabled, and to families with dependent children. All states except Arizona participate, but because each state operates its own program, benefits and coverage vary considerably.

Eligibility for Medicaid depends on actual or potential receipt of payments under the government's Aid to Families with Dependent Children (AFDC) program and the Supplemental Security Income (SSI) program for the aged, blind and disabled. States must cover the "categorically needy" under their Medicaid programs — generally, those persons receiving aid under AFDC or SSI. However, states are permitted to limit Medicaid coverage of SSI recipients by requiring them to meet a more restrictive eligibility standard than was in effect on Jan. 1, 1972. Thirty-four states and the District of Columbia cover all persons eligible for SSI.

Medicaid requires states to provide the following services: inpatient and outpatient hospital services; laboratory and X-ray services; skilled nursing facility services for those over age 21; home health services for those entitled to skilled nursing facility care; early and periodic screening, diagnosis and treatment (EPSDT) services for those under age 21; family planning services and supplies; and physicians' services. They may also provide additional medical services such as prescription drugs and intermediate care facility services.

In addition, each state is allowed to place limitations on the amount of care it will provide under a service category (such as the number of hospital days or physicians' visits covered).

Except for hospital care, which is generally governed by the Medicare cost payment system, states have considerable freedom to set reimbursement levels.

Medicaid complements Medicare by providing about four million persons age 65 and over with benefits. While Medicare has benefited one in nine citizens, Medicaid has reached one of every five Americans — primarily children and all poor. Yet it has been estimated that the program covers no more than half of the poor population at any one time.

A 1980 report by the Congressional Research Service delineated some of the major problems confronting the Medicaid program. Like Medicare, it has been plagued by increasing costs and instances of fraud and abuse (the latter consumed an estimated 7 percent of federal outlays for the program). Although fraud on the part of recipients is thought to be less extensive than abuses on the part of providers, it still does occur. Part of the problem has been due to administering the program's complex eligibility requirements.

Rising costs of the Medicaid program have caused states to cut back on primary health care services for the poor, although there have been few curbs on the expensive provision of hospital and nursing home services. During the first half of 1978, six states reduced or temporarily cut back their Medicaid programs. A number of states have also set limits on physician reimbursements that were considerably lower than those authorized under Medicare, resulting in many doctors' refusing to accept Medicaid patients.

Lax and inefficient administration of state Medicaid programs — including delays and errors in making eligibility determinations and inadequate reporting systems and review procedures — have also contributed to the program's problems.

Another difficulty has been the complexity and wide variations in eligibility requirements as well as in the scope of benefits. There has also been concern that the major emphasis of the program has been on institutional care. In fiscal 1977, only 1.1 percent of program payments went for home health services, while about 39.2 percent of program payments went to care in long-term care institutions, which in many cases did not meet required federal standards.

"Frustration with rising costs has eclipsed some substantial achievements of the program," wrote Davis and Schoen. "Most of the recent gains of the poor — greater access to adequate health care services, reduced mortality rates, and other improvements in health — must be credited to Medicaid." Nonetheless, the authors recommended substantial reforms in the program that would integrate it into a national health system.

Outlook

As the costs of Medicare and Medicaid continued to soar, the Carter administration took a number of steps designed to make the programs more cost-efficient.

In March 1977, then-HEW Secretary Joseph A. Califano Jr. announced the establishment of the Health Care Financing Administration within the department that would integrate the two programs, eliminate duplication in operations, and facilitate the development of consistent federal policy in financing health care.

In 1978, the new agency circulated a strategy paper that called for a number of major changes in the Medicaid program: broadening of eligibility standards; establishment of uniform minimum benefit standards and statewide physician fee schedules; and measures designed to encourage more doctors to accept the Medicare and Medicaid programs' patients.

The administration's fiscal 1981 budget included a number of proposals that would improve Medicare and Medicaid benefits, including liberalization of disability insurance, expansion of home health services benefits and liberalization of Medicare mental health benefits. The administration also proposed legislation that would encourage Medicare enrollment in HMOs.

The fiscal 1981 budget contained several measures that, according to the administration, would result in savings of almost $1.7 billion in federal health care costs. Among them was a proposal to open Medicare payments to walk-in surgery centers not affiliated with hospitals. Other legislative proposals for savings in the Medicare and Medicaid programs, estimated at $780 million in fiscal 1981 if enacted, were the following:

● Requiring that hospitals bid competitively for services such as laboratory work.

● Inhibiting fraud and abuse through institution of civil penalties.

● Eliminating the existing Medicare practice of paying hospitals more for nursing care costs for the elderly than other patients paid.

● Making Medicare payments for no more than the actual level of care that institutions provide. (For example, for elderly persons hospitalized in acute care beds but receiving only nursing treatment, the government would pay only the nursing home rate.)

● Requiring employers of elderly workers to include them in the company's insurance plan, thus making Medicare insurance only supplementary.

Although some of these proposals had already been contained in legislation considered by the Senate Finance and House Ways and Means Committees, the fate of many of them was uncertain in mid-1980. Spokesmen for hospitals worried that the new regulations would impose a heavy reporting burden and would increase costs. Others were worried that the proposed legislation could curtail access to hospitals for Medicare and Medicaid beneficiaries. Spokesmen for elderly groups were apprehensive that the proposal to require employers to provide insurance for workers age 65 and over might discourage employers from hiring older workers.

Despite these concerns, there was general agreement that the programs needed reform. "Medicare and Medicaid have not only been unsuccessful in curbing program costs, but they have also failed to protect the poor and elderly from devastating medical care costs and to provide all low-income groups with access to care," concluded Davis and Schoen. "Reform of Medicare and Medicaid could begin to remove many of the programs' internal inequities, but it will be unable to control costs if undertaken alone, without broader reform of all health care financing. . . .

If federal policy is to begin to influence expenditure levels withut hurting the poor and elderly, coordinated public and private efforts and a health care policy that affects all population groups will be required." ∎

Mental Health Care: States v. Communities

The mentally ill, it is said, have no constituency. Everyone seems to want them out of sight and out of mind. But when President Carter sent Congress his message on mental health care one key constituent was on hand to endorse his legislative proposals. Rosalynn Carter, who had had a long and abiding interest in mental health matters, was at her husband's side as he spoke with news reporters on May 15, 1979, in the White House press room. She had served as honorary chairperson of the President's Commission on Mental Health whose report laid the groundwork for the legislation he was asking Congress to enact.

The commission report drew together many of the facts and enigmas surrounding the ill-defined but devastating cluster of disabilities grouped within the term mental illness. If the definitions were elusive, the problems were all too apparent. But the president's legislative prescription for mental health care did not evoke the optimism that infused the war on poverty, the missionary zeal aroused by civil rights, or the compassion inspired by the mentally retarded or physically handicapped.

There were a number of reasons why it was hard to mobilize public interest in the mentally ill. One was the nebulous nature of the population involved. The commission suggested that as many as 15 percent of the American people — some 32 million — might need mental health services at any one time. A figure of 10 percent had previously been used by federal health officials to project the need for services. It was not always clear how many of those persons were too severely ill to meet the everyday requirements of survival in society: to secure an education, hold a job, and relate in some satisfactory manner to others. To make any estimate required arbitrary decisions about whom to include.

Another obstacle to the support for mental health services might stem from public ambivalence toward the people who needed them. There was a continuing stigma attached to mental illness. A "normal" person rarely wished to identify with the problems of the mentally ill, and found it painful to admit that he or she or a family member was afflicted. It has been safer, and more comfortable, to view the mentally ill as people distinctly different. Finally, the needs of the mentally ill had to compete for limited state funds in an atmosphere of taxpayer revolt and for national funds in a sluggish economy.

According to the Carter administration's fiscal 1981 budget, mental disorders accounted for an estimated 8 percent ($20 billion) of the economic costs of ill health in 1975. The 1978 report by the President's Commission on Mental Health stated, "for the long run, the nation will need to devote greater human and fiscal resources to mental health. We now devote only 12 percent of general health expenditures to mental health. This is not commensurate with the magnitude of mental health problems and does not address the interdependent nature of physical and mental health. We must begin now to

seek a realistic allocation of resources which reflects this interdependence."

Based on the commission's recommendations, the administration submitted to Congress the Mental Health Systems Act (HR 4156, S 1177) on May 21, 1979.

'Revolving Door' Mental Patients

Whether there was more mental illness in 1980 than ever before, or whether people were simply more willing to seek help for their mental and emotional problems, one trend was clear: more often help was provided on a temporary, outpatient basis. Often cited to illustrate the trend was a decline in population of the state mental hospitals from 600,000 in 1955 to 160,000 in 1980. Thirty years ago, three out of four mental patients were treated in hospitals; in 1980, three out of four were treated as outpatients.

The discovery in the 1950s of psychoactive drugs that help to control the symptoms of some mental illnesses gave impetus to a movement already under way. With the help of such drugs, one million or more long-term patients were released into their communities. Mental hospitals throughout the United States began to turn away patients, to shorten stays, and to liberalize their discharge policies.

An earlier commission report placed its imprimatur on the goal of providing care in the least restrictive setting, preferably close to home and with relatives — often referred to by the shorthand term "deinstitutionalization." The findings of a Joint Commission on Mental Illness and Health, published in 1961, led to passage in 1963 of legislation establishing community mental health centers (CMHC) and federal funding.

The law envisaged an integration of formal treatment with a complete range of social and human services. A key element of this system of mental health care was the community center. The 1963 program recommended the establishment of 1,200 to 2,000 such centers; but by 1980, only about 700 were in operation, providing services to an estimated 2.4 million persons and serving areas where half the nation's population lived. Deinstitutionalization, termed psychiatry's favorite project of the 1960s, had become dogma among mental health professionals and policy within the government. But how that policy had been executed had become a troublesome political issue at every level of government.

A principal issue was the "dumping scandal" — the release of patients into communities that were unable or unwilling to provide for their continuing care. News reports provided numerous examples, such as the following by Peter Koenig in *The New York Times Magazine*, May 21, 1978:

"Because of a decline in physical conditions and staffing, five California state mental hospitals lost their national accreditation in 1976. It was charged that former inmates had been ejected into flophouses, jails and nursing homes. Gov. Edmund G. Brown Jr. promised to bolster

Evolution of U.S. Psychiatric Profession

For hundreds of years western society has groped for a satisfactory way to deal with disturbed people in its midst. Medical science, particularly public health, has made great strides in treating physical illnesses, but the cause and cure of mental illness are still shrouded in mystery. Even more shadowy is the line between mind and body, and the nature of their interaction.

In America, state institutions built at the turn of the century as safe havens for the mentally ill had grown notorious as warehouses for people who were troublesome or dangerous. The public was shocked by stories of institutional neglect and abuse, and weary at the failure to find cures for mental illness. World War II disclosed a high incidence of mental disorders among men rejected by the draft, and produced casualties among those who served.

As part of a great postwar social stock-taking, the public looked for a better and more humane solution to the problem of mental illness. Several developments gave support to these hopes. Psychiatric medicine had expanded along with other branches of caring for the injured and ill. Research promoted new and apparently more effective forms of therapy. To help meet the growing demand for treatment, new categories of mental health workers were created. Psychologists, psychiatric nurses, and social workers acquired skills and treatment practice in outpatient and child-guidance clinics.

The profession of psychiatry, whose original practitioners were the medical superintendents of mental hospitals, saw its field explode as the boundaries between the well and the ill grew blurred. The number of psychiatrists in U.S. practice shot up from 5,800 in 1950 to 27,000 in 1979. With so many people seeking treatment, they could choose their clientele. The seriously ill in state institutions were largely abandoned in favor of patients more likely to recover. *Time* magazine reported April 2, 1979, that there were 3,200 unfilled jobs for psychiatrists in these hospitals, and over half the staff physicians were foreign-born and foreign-trained.

However, after a remarkable ascent, there were signs that the profession had been oversold and overprescribed and was coming back to earth with a jolt. One symptom was the drop in the percentage of medical school graduates going into psychiatry. Twelve percent entered in 1970, but by the end of the decade only 4 to 5 percent were entering the field. (Some attributed the drop to higher earnings in other specialties.)

Psychiatry has been asked to justify the harsh treatment therapies sometimes used on very sick patients. The most drastic and controversial method of treating psychological or behavioral abnormalities has been brain surgery (lobotomy) — the destruction of brain tissue for the purpose of altering behavior. Another means of treatment that has lost favor was electroshock treatment. Although the development of psychoactive drugs that alter mood and behavior revolutionized the treatment of agitated patients, drug treatment was being reassessed due to mounting evidence of serious physical and mental side effects.

By the end of the 1970s, psychiatry's franchise to treat the problems of everyday living was increasingly being challenged by other mental health professionals. Because of the high cost, typically $50 an hour, psychoanalysis traditionally had been limited to the well-to-do. But with more practitioners in the field, psychiatrists might have to adapt to a different clientele. A University of Michigan study showed that between 1957 and 1976, the biggest increase in patients was among those with low and middle incomes, probably due both to expanded insurance coverage and community services.

As Congress began debate on enacting a national health insurance program, a major turf war was shaping up over who may be reimbursed directly for professional mental health care services. Some psychiatrists maintained that only a physician could recognize organic causes of mental illness, and prescribe drugs. They warned that a lack of medical knowledge could result in overlooking an organic cause of a mental disorder.

---

spending for community care facilities, but most of the increases proposed were dropped after passage of Proposition 13, the tax-cutting measure, in June 1978.

"Thousands of chronically ill discharged mental patients clustered in 'welfare' hotels and halfway houses on New York's upper West Side where they are preyed upon by criminals."

These were not isolated incidents. Thousands of patients who suffered severe and chronic mental disorders had been cast adrift to live alone in squalid rooming houses with no psychiatric, social or medical care other than drugs. Many were more isolated, forgotten, and miserable than they were in the crowded back wards of institutions. Two-thirds were readmitted to hospitals, some more than once, and became known as "revolving door" patients.

Perhaps most painful of all has been rejection by family and community. Social research related mental health to the quality of personal and community support systems such as schools, friends, relatives, clubs, and churches. Yet those persons whose stability was most fragile were often most isolated. Rather than sharing support systems, a cohesive neighborhood might bind together to exclude the discharged mental patient. The number of halfway houses remained virtually the same during the 1970s because of community resistance.

Problems with Community Care

The message that emerged was that deinstitutionalization might be good theory, but in many cases it had been badly — even disastrously — executed. All levels of government have been reluctant or unable to pay the costs involved. Some critics charged that the states used deinstitutionalization as a rationale for reducing the high costs of maintaining mental institutions, and to shift the burden to the federal government.

When the population drops in large institutions, they

said, public funding does not follow patients into the community. As an example, a report prepared for the New York City Council president in June 1979 said, "The state [of New York] continues to pour almost 80 percent of its mental health dollars into large, isolated and often antiquated chronic-care psychiatric institutions" which house 25 percent of the state's mental patients. "The consequences are severe for the tens of thousands of deinstitutionalized state hospital patients as well as for financially strapped localities responsible for funding community-based mental health care."

Another problem has been poor coordination of available resources. In many cases, state-operated hospitals and federally subsidized mental health centers have operated as separate rather than complementary systems. Payment restrictions in the health and welfare assistance available to discharged patients have been built-in incentives to place people inappropriately in nursing homes instead of group homes, or in single rooms instead of with their families. They were also incentives to unscrupulous operators in the "boarding home" industry to keep patients sedated and docile, since a client who got well moved out or commonly had his or her medical and welfare benefits reduced.

Although community mental health centers in 1980 provided 29 percent of the nation's mental health care, they were not effective in coordinating community services for the discharged patient. Their resources were spread thin to provide a wide variety of services. A shortage of staff sometimes resulted in treatment inferior to private care but comparable in cost. In other cases, centers emphasized preventive or "crisis" care rather than the needs of the chronically ill, or conspicuously failed to meet the needs of such underserved groups as the aged, children and ethnic and racial minorities.

The centers were under financial pressure. They were created with the understanding that they would become self-supporting after eight years, but states were not always willing to pick up the tab for non-reimbursable services when federal aid ended. Recognizing these problems, the presidential commission proposed that payments for mental health care be included in any national health insurance plan; that states require better coverage from private insurers; and that Medicare provide for the elderly, and Medicaid for the poor, mental health benefits more nearly on a par with other health benefits.

Despite disappointments with community care, virtually nobody suggested that the solution lay in massive reinstitutionalization. If state hospitals were less crowded, they were still pressed for funds and were short of professional staff. Many remained primarily custodial, as storage centers for the hopelessly ill.

Commission Report, Administration Bill

The commission's final report in April 1978, based on written and oral testimony and the work of its specialized task forces, set as national goals a continued phasing down of state mental hospitals, improvement of care in those that remain, and a comprehensive, integrated system of care in communities. To meet these goals, the commission called for a large increase in the national resources devoted to mental health. Acknowledging a lack of information on causes and treatment, the president's commission focused on problems in the delivery of services.

Cited as major problems were inadequate care of the chronically ill and lack of sensitivity and limited

Other Mental Health Programs

In addition to revising the Mental Health Systems Act, the Carter administration proposed a number of other mental health improvements in its fiscal 1981 budget, among them:

● A joint $65 million demonstration project by the Department of Health and Human Services and the Department of Housing and Urban Development to provide housing and support services for an estimated 3,500 mentally disabled persons.

● A proposal that Medicare copayments for mental health care be the same as for other outpatient services — 20 percent rather than the existing 50 percent — and that the $250 annual reimbursement limit be raised to $750. *(See Medicare chapter, p. 73)*

● A requirement that states provide mental health services for Medicaid-eligible children under the proposed Child Health Assurance Program. *(CHAP story, p. 87)*

● A requirement that mental health professionals who received federal aid in their training pledge to work in underserved areas in return for support. *(See Manpower chapter, p. 41)*

● Establishment of an "Operation Outreach" program for Vietnam-era veterans to offer general mental and psychological assessments and provide treatment or referral services to those who served during the Vietnam War and experienced problems returning to civilian life. *(Veterans' programs, p. 93)*

access that characterized mental health care for certain groups, including rural residents, aged and poor people, women, members of racial and ethnic minorities, and children. The administration's bill, sent to Congress May 15, 1979, drew heavily on the commission's recommendations.

Sen. Edward M. Kennedy, D-Mass., introduced the bill on May 17 and, as chairman of the Senate Human Resources Subcommittee on Health and Scientific Research, conducted a hearing a week later. The bill would authorize more money and reorder policies to achieve the continuing goal of the most appropriate care in the least restrictive setting. The cost for the first year was fixed at $99.1 million, of which about $30 million would be transferred from existing programs. The bill envisioned a rise in the federal mental health budget of $542 million in 1979 to $612 million in 1980.

The main purposes of the bill were to encourage states to develop a comprehensive, integrated system of care for the mentally ill, direct more resources to the chronically mentally ill and underserved, emphasize preventive care, and promote coordination among national, state and local efforts and between primary and mental health care providers.

The Senate Health Subcommittee had been scheduled to mark up the administration bill Oct. 3. But the markup was pushed back to Oct. 18 after mental health interest groups besieged subcommittee aides with proposed changes in the administration plan.

The proposal became caught up in a major dispute over who would control the flow of federal money for community mental health programs in the states. The fight was between different segments of the mental health profession: advocates of community centers who wanted money going directly to them, and supporters of state programs who wanted federal funds channeled through state agencies.

Under the existing Community Mental Health Centers Act (PL 88-164), the federal government has provided direct grants to community mental health centers (CMHCs) that agreed to provide inpatient, outpatient and 10 other mental health services. The money was phased out gradually over eight years, at which point state and local governments frequently picked up part of the tab.

Under the administration proposal, HHS would channel money to facilities that promised to provide at least one service to minorities, children or some other underserved group. It would provide grants to groups that agreed to provide all 12 of the services that CMACs had to offer under existing law. The plan also would make money available to support the continued operation of CMACs already in existence.

Although some members of Congress and representatives of mental health interest groups found fault with an administration plan to allow a clinic serving minorities and other needy groups to offer as little as one service, the principal point of dispute concerned the states' role in mental health programs.

Reservoir of Distrust

The funding dispute reflected longstanding antagonism between community-care advocates and state mental health authorities. The states said they backed attempts to treat the mentally ill as outpatients in facilities close to their homes. But community mental health activists said the states' continued support of large mental hospitals cast doubt on the strength of their commitment to community care.

The issue dividing the state and community mental health representatives went deeper than who controlled the funds, however. It tapped a reservoir of distrust that for years had colored the relationship between community care advocates and state mental health authorities.

"States are not sympathetic" to the notion of community-based care, charged David Sandler, lobbyist for the National Council of Community Mental Health Centers. Sandler said many states still devoted a large portion of their mental health budgets to funding large state mental institutions, rather than outpatient services in community clinics.

Sandler said that states should be allowed to share with the federal government planning and grant approval authority. But he expressed fear that if states controlled the funds, they might bypass CMHCs in favor of state, local or other community-based programs.

"Massachusetts doesn't even mention CMHCs in its state mental health plan," Sandler explained. Moreover, passing the money through another layer of bureaucracy would dilute the funds going toward actual services, he added.

But Harry Schnibbe, spokesman for the National Association of State Mental Health Program Directors, said states ignored CMHCs for good reason. "CMHCs are a nothing program," said Schnibbe. He added that state,

local and private nonprofit clinics provided the bulk of community-based care around the United States.

1980 Action

The administration's fiscal 1981 budget, submitted in January 1980, included a request for $380 million for fiscal 1981 to continue and expand the community mental health programs. Under the request, budget authority for state and local mental health services would increase 55 percent over 1977, and the number of people served annually by the programs would grow to an estimated 3.6 million.

Both the Senate Human Resources and House Interstate and Foreign Commerce Committees reported their versions of the legislation May 15, 1980 (S 1177, S Rept 96-712; HR 7299, H Rept 96-977). Both bills would extend the programs under the act through fiscal 1981 and would establish a revised, broadened and more flexible program in fiscal 1982. Under the bills, state agencies would be allowed to decide which new proposals they should fund to provide outpatient and other mental health services in community settings. The shift to state control would mark a major change in the existing program which sent federal funds directly to community mental health centers.

Other than the heightened state role, the House and Senate versions of the bill maintained the basic thrust of the original Carter proposal. Like the original administration plan, the bills would tailor mental health services to meet the needs of minorities, children, chronically mentally ill individuals and other so-called underserved groups. They would place greater emphasis on prevention of mental illness and promotion of mental health. However, whereas the House bill would authorize appropriations of $152 million for the act in fiscal 1982, the Senate version would authorize $436 million.

"Since 1963, millions of mentally ill Americans, who would once have been sent to remote, restrictive state mental hospitals or simply denied treatment altogether, have been provided with mental health care of high quality in their home communities," said the Human Resources Committee in its report on the bill. "This enormous progress in caring for those with mental illness is due in large part to the Community Mental Health Center program.

"But the very success of the CMHC program has pointed out the weakness of its statutory framework.... Many of those weaknesses could be — and have been — repaired without replacing the act itself; however, it is now clear that certain fundamental mental health needs in our society cannot be addressed until a new legislative framework is created....

"Today, local private nonprofit groups, local governments, state governments, and the federal government are part of a chaotic, inefficient and wasteful mental health system. It is, in fact, a mental health non-system. Now that state governments and the federal government share a commitment to community-based mental health care, this non-system is no longer acceptable. To bring about the coherent mental health system our nation requires, a Mental Health Systems Act is necessary." ∎

Congress Debates Child Health Programs

"Many children are not making it through the front door of our health care system ... because it isn't clear where the door is," commented Hillary Rodham, chairman of the Children's Defense Fund (CDF) lobby in testimony before the House Subcommittee on Health in May 1979. The occasion was hearings on a proposal to step up efforts to locate poor children needing medical care — and to make sure they got it.

After two years on congressional back burners, legislation to replace a much-criticized Medicaid children's health program with a new version known as the Child Health Assurance Program (CHAP) had begun to move. But, despite the political appeal of children, the movement was slow. In 1979 only the House passed a program to expand and upgrade the preventive health care program for children. The Senate Finance Committee had reported a narrower version of the bill, but the Senate did not take it up that year. And, although the Carter administration had pushed for CHAP legislation, by early 1980, budget-cutting consciousness had led to administration and House Budget Committee recommendations that the proposed funds for the program be slashed from $400 million to $40 million.

The idea of revamping the federal child health program arose in 1976, when several members of Congress introduced legislation that would set up a national maternal and child health program as the next step toward comprehensive health insurance coverage for all.

"In 1965, with the passage of Medicare and Medicaid, we provided coverage for our elderly and our poor," House sponsors of the legislation said in a June 1976 letter to their colleagues. "Now we must look to the future of this country, our children."

"The children and mothers of our nation cannot wait for the promise of national health insurance — a promise which has been on the legislative agenda for a long time," added Sen. Jacob K. Javits, R-N.Y., a cosponsor of 1976 child health legislation in the Senate.

The proposed "reform" was of a relatively rare type. Instead of trying to pluck ineligible "cheats" out of tax-funded aid programs, the plan focused on finding needy individuals who were missing out on benefits to which they were entitled.

Supporters of the plan recognized that it could run into opposition because it entailed new spending. But they argued that Congress made the basic decision to go beyond merely paying needy children's medical bills in 1967, and that the new legislation was intended to correct problems in the children's program authorized more than a decade ago.

Advocates of the program also contended that it had several natural advantages. First of all, they noted, it would invest health dollars in the young, who can benefit most fully from preventive care. The program also would give the federal government a chance to experiment with innovative approaches to cost containment before they were locked into a full-scale program. From an operational standpoint, the bill would be more in keeping with the federal government's existing administrative abilities than a universal program. In addition, it had been argued that pediatricians and obstetricians/gynecologists — the doctors most affected by the bill — were more "social-minded" than the medical profession as a whole and were therefore more likely to cooperate with the government. And, too, given little or no growth in the birth rate, the number of persons covered by the program was likely to remain relatively stable. It was also suggested that children were less apt than other groups to misuse or overuse services and drive up costs unnecessarily.

Problems in Existing Programs

In 1979, only one in six eligible children was actually screened for health problems under the existing Medicaid Early and Periodic Screening, Diagnosis and Treatment (EPSDT) program, and 40 percent of the health problems picked up in these checkups did not get treated, according to the CDF.

The program's problems were blamed on administrative neglect in its early years, and a financing structure that had discouraged states from aggressively seeking out eligible children.

Another complaint was that EPSDT, only one of more than 30 public health programs for children, had failed to fulfill its mandate to coordinate these programs. The result had been duplication — or gaps — that cost money and kept confused parents from getting care to which their children were entitled.

To remedy these problems, the Carter administration

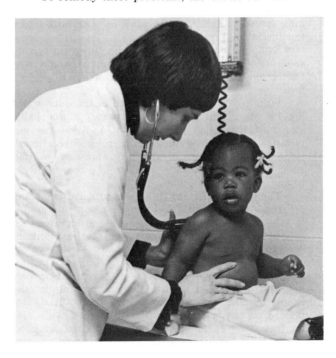

Child Nutrition Programs Face Cuts

While Congress was wrestling over issues of child and maternal health, it was also contending with another controversial topic — child nutrition programs.

Principally at issue in 1980 was the school lunch subsidy program, although in previous years, the supplemental feeding program for women, infants and children (WIC) — a controversial entitlement program — had been the target for cutbacks. *(See appendix, 1978 chronology, p. 73-A; 1979 chronology, p. 80-A)*

Indeed, the hamburgers and pizza that were the mainstays of the school lunches of 27 million children could cost substantially more, if the Carter administration had its way. The Agriculture Department was asking Congress once again to save money — some $400 million in 1981 — by raising the price of federally supported school lunches and breakfasts for children from all but the poorest families.

The vehicle for the battle between the Carter administration — and other budget-cutters — and nutrition advocates was a bill (HR 27) extending the authorization for certain relatively minor child nutrition programs, including nutrition education and summer feeding programs.

The administration's 1980 proposals followed the same lines as those submitted in 1979, but with some changes aimed at making cutbacks in what was easily the biggest and most popular feeding effort in the country more palatable politically. The administration's bill would:

● Reduce by five cents the federal cash subsidy for each meal served to students from middle- and upper-income families, who paid full price for their lunches.

● Lower the income eligibility standards for free and reduced-price meals.

● Reduce to five cents, from 8.6 cents in existing law, the federal subsidy paid for each half-pint of milk served to children who paid for their milk under the special milk program.

● Exclude from the summer feeding program private sponsors, such as churches or community groups, that contracted with profit-making food suppliers to provide food.

Winning congressional approval of the cuts would not be easy, considering the previously untouchable status of the lunch program. But in 1980 the administration was holding a stronger legislative hand. Congressional backers of the program were worried enough that they spurred formation of a new coalition to lobby against the proposed cuts.

The coalition formed to oppose cuts in the feeding programs ranged from anti-hunger groups to groups of school administrators and lobbying groups for food suppliers. Besides the common aim of the coalition, each group had its own individual goals — goals which, on other subjects, were sometimes in conflict. For producers, the school feeding programs were a major market, and one that was particularly important because it was reliable from year to year. School officials depended on the federal payments as essential subsidies for their food operations. Whatever was not supplied by the federal government or the children had to come from their own state and local budgets. Anti-hunger lobbyists, who were supported by a number of church groups, were most concerned with improving the nutrition of children. But because they had often been at odds with producers on other nutritional issues, the coalition was for them something of a Faustian bargain, and they emphasized that it would not lead them to compromise their positions on other issues.

Meanwhile, the frozen food industry wanted to use the bill as a way to get at the 20 percent of the school food market that was made up of government-supplied commodities. It wanted the federal government to substitute money for the 15.75 cents worth of commodities it gave to schools for each lunch served.

Backers of that method for providing food assistance to schools were unsuccessful in their first attempt to win congressional approval, before the House Elementary and Secondary Education Subcommittee. Under existing law, schools bought 80 percent of their food from local suppliers. The remainder was supplied by the federal government in the form of commodities — turkey rolls, apples, canned corn and so on. The government has been required by law to purchase surplus agricultural commodities, and the schools have been a place to dispose of them.

One proposal, offered by William D. Ford, D-Mich., would replace the value of those commodities with "letters of credit," similar to cash. The government would send the letters to schools, which would use them to purchase food from local suppliers. Backers of Ford's amendment, which was rejected by the House education subcommittee, argued that the existing system of commodity distribution was inefficient and expensive.

Arguing against the amendment, subcommittee and committee chairman Carl D. Perkins, D-Ky., warned that it would ultimately destroy the school lunch program. Other opponents of the amendment included some industry groups, such as turkey producers, that had enjoyed substantial business through the commodity system.

"I didn't realize there were so many people making money off of child nutrition," said Ford.

After rejecting Ford's amendment, the House Education and Labor Committee approved the bill, filing its report (H Rept 96-1030) May 19. The panel did not even consider the administration's proposals to cut the cost of the program by increasing the cost of lunches to children from all but the poorest families.

In the Senate, however, nutrition program sponsors swallowed hard and proposed a bill to cut nutrition spending by $413 million in fiscal 1981. The Agriculture and Budget committees voted to accept the full package of administration-proposed cuts. Introducing the bill (S 2675), Nutrition Subcommittee Chairman George McGovern, D-S.D., said, "It pains me deeply to be proposing cuts in the child nutrition program."

On June 11, the Senate Agriculture Committee cut $500 million from child nutrition spending. The House Education and Labor Committee followed suit June 26.

asked Congress to provide financial bonuses for effective state programs, broaden eligibility and improve Medicaid benefits for needy children, and provide Medicaid coverage for low-income women during first pregnancies.

The CHAP plan had few visible opponents. Its most active supporters, the CDF and certain specialized health groups, argued that the bill made sense at a time of heightened cost-consciousness because "its emphasis on preventive and primary care is the essence of cost containment," as CDF director Marian Wright Edelman told the Senate Finance Committee in June 1979. "It's one of the most cost-effective things we can ever do," said Rep. Andrew Maguire, D-N.J., during House debate on the bill. Another factor favoring passage was that "it's hard to vote against kids," as one Finance Committee aide noted.

Background

By the end of the 1970s the federal commitment to children's health had grown from a single Children's Bureau, established in 1912, to some 35 tax-supported programs targeted on low-income mothers and children, or for which they were eligible as part of a larger targeted group.

The two major sources of federal funds for poor children reflected two different philosophies of public aid. The older one — grants to states — began with the 1935 maternal child health program that was authorized as part of the original Social Security Act. These "Title V" programs were the preferred funding vehicle for the American Medical Association (AMA), which argued that they "create capacity" by supporting public health departments and special clinics, and by coordinating existing resources for target populations. Title V funds were focused on two types of programs: preventive services, such as public well-baby and prenatal clinics, and special services for crippled children.

The problem with relying wholly on a grant approach, according to Leonard D. Schaeffer, former chief of the Health Education and Welfare (HEW, now Health and Human Services) Department's Health Care Financing Administration, was that grant projects only "cover children with specific conditions . . . or who live in certain geographical locations, such as the Appalachian or migrant health programs."

Medicaid, the second and larger major source of health assistance for low-income children, was intended to provide uniform basic coverage regardless of where an eligible person lived. State and federal spending for children in Medicaid was estimated at $3.4 billion for 1978. Coverage varied widely because states could set their own eligibility standards and limit even the basic benefits that must be offered — such as days in a hospital. One state, Arizona, even opted not to have a Medicaid program.

Screening Program Authorized

Two years after enactment of Medicaid, Congress in 1967 added EPSDT, requiring states to offer screening and follow-up services for anyone under age 21 who was eligible for the state Medicaid program. Screened children were eligible for some additional benefits under Medicaid, such as eyeglasses and hearing aids. In authorizing EPSDT Congress was moving, for one population group, beyond the basic financing function of Medicaid.

Delays by the Nixon administration kept EPSDT

The Children's Defense Fund

The pint-sized constituents of the Children's Defense Fund (CDF) won a small but critical beachhead in the 1980 battle of the budget.

Thanks to some effective lobbying, the Carter administration and the House Budget Committee reversed earlier decisions to put off the Child Health Assurance Program (CHAP) for a year. Instead, Carter's revised fiscal 1981 budget sent to Congress March 31, 1980, requested $40 million in minimal start-up funding for the program. CHAP had been on early "delay" lists of the Office of Management and Budget as well as congressional budget panels.

Representatives of the CDF started working early, before budget-cutting decisions had been made. CDF Director Marian Wright Edelman shot off a blistering letter to President Carter March 6, accusing him of "hypocrisy" if he dropped CHAP, long one of his pet proposals. Prominent journalists got copies of the letter, and well-placed news stories suddenly appeared in the press. Key members of Congress and top White House officials Hamilton Jordan, Stuart E. Eizenstat and Anne Wexler also received Edelman's letter.

CDF staff concentrated on OMB, the White House and the Budget committees. "We touch bases with whoever returns our calls," said Judith H. Weitz, adding that she talked with opponents as well as supporters, "so that we know what our problems are." CDF doesn't have a large national membership, but it alerted members of other supporting groups, who called key congressmen from their home districts. Within the House Budget Committee Democratic caucus, Reps. Timothy E. Wirth, Colo., and William M. Brodhead, Mich., defended the bill.

The children's lobbyists made policy arguments for CHAP and also laid out for members the intricacies of the Budget Act, which barred congressional action on the authorization in 1980 unless there was some funding for fiscal 1981.

"CDF is very good. They get to the members directly, they're reasonable and they're very, very knowledgeable," said one budget panel aide.

Weitz was careful not to credit her group with the continued survival of the bill. Health, Education and Welfare (HEW) Secretary Patricia Roberts Harris carried the fight for CHAP within the White House, HEW sources said. And Domestic Council aide Dr. James Mongan said CHAP survived because it was, after all, a Carter administration priority.

"Everybody here, at HEW and on the Hill was not especially happy about not doing anything at all" in the health field, and CHAP offered a chance in 1980 to do something, Mongan said.

from being fully operational until 1973. Apparently states were also cool to the program because Congress in 1972 authorized cuts in matching funds for Aid to Families with Dependent Children (AFDC) to penalize states that dragged their feet on the health screening program. But, "while substantial penalties have been assessed against the states (for failure to fully implement EPSDT), they have not actually been collected," according to a 1979

Provisions of 1979 House-passed CHAP Legislation

As passed by the House Dec. 11, 1979, HR 4962 replaced the existing Medicaid program for children under Title XIX of the Social Security Act, the Early and Periodic Screening, Diagnosis and Treatment (EPSDT) program, with a broader Child Health Assurance Program (CHAP). The bill:

Eligibility. Required states to provide Medicaid coverage for children under age 18, regardless of family structure, who met either state income or Medicaid standards or a new national income standard. To qualify under the national standard, an individual would have to come from a family whose income was less than two-thirds of the official poverty level (about $5,000 for a family of four in 1979).

● Authorized optional coverage for adopted children regardless of the adoptive family's income, if the child had been in foster care or had medical or handicapping conditions that would discourage adoption. Coverage would continue until the child reached age 18 or until medical services were no longer needed. For these children, a state could provide either a full range of Medicaid services, or only care required by a specific condition.

● Authorized optional coverage of children in corrective and other non-medical institutions, if they were eligible before they entered the facility.

● Authorized optional coverage for all financially eligible children under age 21.

● Provided federal matching funds for the additional, optional coverage.

● Required states to provide Medicaid for all pregnant women who met either state income or Medicaid standards or a new national income standard. To qualify under the national standard, an individual would have to have an income that was less than 80 percent of the official poverty level for an individual or family (about $3,000 for a single woman). Coverage would be for the course of pregnancy and the first two months following birth of the child.

● Authorized the secretary of HEW to establish federal "intent to reside" standards for Medicaid, to be used to determine which state was responsible for Medicaid for children of migrant workers and other Medicaid beneficiaries.

Continuity of Coverage. Required states to allow enrolled children four months of coverage after they lost Medicaid eligibility for any reason other than age (for example, when family income went up). For children with treatable — but not correctable — conditions, such as diabetes, this "grace period" would be 12 months instead of four. For children with a correctable condition, eligibility would continue until the condition was corrected.

Services. Required states to provide eligible children (under age 18) with all services for which federal Medicaid law authorized payment, and to provide these additional services: child health assessments, immunizations, routine dental care, diagnosis and treatment of vision and hearing problems, hearing aids and eyeglasses, prescribed drugs and insulin, home health, physical therapy and rehabilitative services, prosthetic devices, outpatient and emergency inpatient psychiatric treatment.

● Prohibited states from limiting the amount, duration or scope of these services.

● Required all Medicaid programs to provide prenatal and postnatal services.

Abortion. Permitted Medicaid payments for medical care following termination of pregnancy by miscarriage or by an abortion to save the life of the mother.

● Prohibited Medicaid payments for abortions, except those performed to save the life of the mother.

● Stipulated that nothing in the Medicaid statute should be construed to require any state funds to be used to pay for abortions.

Ban on Co-payments. Barred states from requiring enrolled children to share the cost of any required services.

Reimbursement, Performance Standards. Raised federal matching rates for the costs of health assessments and outpatient health services for children in the CHAP program by an additional 25 percentage points above the existing matching rate of a state. Under the new formula, the federal share of CHAP costs could not exceed 90 percent except for children enrolled with "continuing care providers." For these children, the federal share could rise to 95 percent of costs.

● Raised federal matching rates for outreach and followup to 75 percent (from the overall administrative matching rate of 50 percent), and required states to allocate a reasonable proportion of these program funds to outreach activities.

● Established standards for both "minimum" and "reasonable" CHAP performance by states. Provided an additional "bonus" federal match of up to 25 percent of Medicaid administrative costs for states exceeding the "reasonable" performance standard. Provided for a 20 percent reduction of federal funds for Medicaid administrative expenses, to penalize states that failed to meet the minimum CHAP standard.

● Prohibited the new, higher matching rates for services for states that reduced eligibility standards or cut services for children during the first four years of the program.

Other Provisions. Repealed authority in existing law for a 1 percent cut in Aid to Families with Dependent Children (AFDC) funds as a penalty for states failing to provide health screenings.

● Set a Sept. 30, 1984, expiration date for all provisions in the bill.

● Required HEW to submit CHAP regulations to Congress for review; provided that implementation of part or all of such regulations could be blocked by either a concurrent resolution of disapproval, passed by both houses within 90 days after the regulations were submitted, or a resolution of disapproval passed by one house within 60 days after the regulations were submitted, if the other house did not reject that resolution within an additional 30 days.

House Commerce Health Subcommittee background paper.

In addition to flaws in its financing, EPSDT also suffered because of problems in developing "tracking systems" that would show whether problems detected during screening were actually treated, the House staff noted. The result was a program emphasis on screening, at the expense of follow-up. And even in screening, EPSDT has not realized its potential. Of an estimated 11 million Medicaid-eligible children, only 2 million were actually screened in fiscal 1977, according to CDF. Schaeffer set the number of enrolled children at 3 million, and claimed that EPSDT has "grown dramatically" and that most children received the treatment they needed once they were screened. But the Children's Defense Fund and other critics found the participation rate and slippage between screening and follow-up to be extremely disappointing.

For an individual mother or child, these policy problems could translate into a confusing and difficult medical odyssey. "It is not uncommon for a poor mother to have to go to a local health department for prenatal care and to a public hospital for the delivery of her baby. The pediatrician who examines the new baby in the hospital will never see the child again. The mother will take her child to a well-baby clinic for checkups — but not the same place where she got prenatal care. The well-baby clinic will not take care of a sick child, so when the baby becomes ill, she must go to a private physician or a hospital emergency room. If the child requires specialty care, services will be provided at still another place, probably under another program," CDF's Rodham told the House panel.

The health of America's children suffers, in part because of flaws in EPSDT, according to Fund and HEW officials. Overall immunization levels against major infectious diseases such as polio declined during the early 1970s, although HEW by the late 1970s was trying to reverse that trend. Eleven other nations had better infant mortality rates than the United States and the rate for black American infants was twice that of their white counterparts. "Poor children have twice as many hospital stays, spend more days in bed, and lose more days from school than children who are not poor," according to Rodham.

Carter Administration Proposals

The Carter administration first proposed a CHAP reform in 1977 but the bill was largely ignored until late in 1978, "because it was everyone's second priority," according to a CDF official. The House Commerce and Senate Finance committees both reported amended versions in 1978, but time ran out before either bill could come to the floor. Objections of former Sen. Carl T. Curtis, R-Neb. (1955-78; House, 1939-54), that the legislation would set an undesirable precedent for welfare reform played a role in the Senate delay. The far more generous House version also ran into some budgetary objections from the Carter administration.

In 1979, the administration tried administratively to improve coordination among children's programs and to crack down on states that were skimping on EPSDT. And on May 10 it sent up its 1979 request for new CHAP legislation, incorporating coverage for pregnant women and other changes, largely picked up from the 1978 House bill.

Major features of the 1979 administration CHAP bill would have:

● Mandated improved Medicaid coverage for all children up to age 18 in families with incomes below 55 percent of the federal poverty level or below a state income standard for determining Medicaid eligibility — whichever was higher. The coverage would have been for a specified set of benefits, more generous than the basic Medicaid package, and states would have been barred from limiting use of these services or requiring beneficiaries to pay any of their cost.

● Mandated Medicaid coverage for women pregnant with their first child, meeting the 55 percent national standard or a higher state income standard. Most states in 1979 covered prenatal care only for women with dependent children.

● Authorized higher Medicaid reimbursement levels for physicians and other providers willing to commit themselves, by written agreement, to both screen and provide all subsequent care and checkups for a child. These "continuing care providers" would also have been responsible for making sure their CHAP patients followed up on referrals for treatment.

● Spelled out performance standards for states, such as percentage of all eligible children being seen by continuing care providers. The legislation would have authorized a sliding scale of higher Medicaid reimbursement rates, for outpatient health services for children, for states performing well, and would have authorized a cut in these funds for states performing poorly.

1979 Congressional Action

After a series of delays, the House Interstate and Foreign Commerce Committee reported the CHAP bill (HR 4926 — H Rept 96-568) Oct. 26, and it passed the full chamber by voice vote Dec. 11. The House passed-bill expanded and upgraded the EPSDT program to require states to cover children up to age 18, including those in intact families as well as those living with one parent and to provide prenatal care for poor women during first pregnancies. It set new national income standards, and raised federal Medicaid contributions to the states to help meet the increased costs.

The bill barred states from putting limits on the mandated medical services for children in the program, as they could do for other Medicaid beneficiaries, and from requiring any co-payments for services.

The two major issues that arose during House floor debate on the legislation were abortion and the potential cost of the new program. Despite the popularity of the plan, the future of CHAP became clouded with controversy because the House made the bill a vehicle for two anti-abortion amendments. One of the House-passed amendments asserted that states could refuse to spend their own funds on Medicaid abortions, even if courts had ordered them to do so. The other amendment would, for the first time, change the basic Medicaid statute to prohibit the use of federal funds to end pregnancies, except those which endangered the life of the mother. Both abortion amendments were expected to encounter stiff Senate opposition.

The other controversy surrounded the costs of the program, which could bring as many as five million additional children and 220,000 women into Medicaid, at a cost of nearly $2 billion a year by 1984. House members who warned against the potential expense of CHAP did not ask their colleagues simply to vote against the bill. They offered amendments that, they maintained, would allow Congress to control spending without depriving children of help.

The first cost-control amendment was soundly defeated when the House refused, by a 152-226 vote, to convert CHAP from an open-ended entitlement to a three-year authorization with fixed spending ceilings. (Through the annual appropriations process Congress has a chance to restrict spending for an authorized program; an entitlement requires the government to pay for mandated benefits for any person meeting the statutory eligibility standards, whatever the cost.)

However, the House did agree to a "sunset" amendment that would end the CHAP program at the end of fiscal 1984 unless Congress agreed to continue it.

Meanwhile, the Senate Finance Committee in July had abruptly decided to report a CHAP bill identical to its 1978 version. The Senate version (S 1204 — S Rept 96-274) provided no new coverage for pregnancy, mandated new benefits only for children up to age 6, and did not set a national eligibility standards. It had

no provisions relating to abortion, and its estimated cost — $9.3 million in new federal spending in fiscal 1980 — was much more modest than the House version.

Viewing the bill as a potential addition to a broader health insurance measure, committee chairman Russell B. Long, D-La., delayed floor action on the measure in 1979. Long was also concerned about the program's cost in relation to other health matters.

Indeed, it appeared that cost containment was one major obstacle to enactment of a new child health program. This was apparent in the Carter administration's March 1980 decision to scale down its request for a $400 million CHAP bill to a $40 million pilot project. CHAP had been on early "delay" lists of both the Office of Management and Budget (OMB) and House Budget Committee Chairman Robert N. Giaimo, D-Conn., for a number of reasons. It had not always been treated as an urgent priority even by its advocates in the administration and Congress. It was an entitlement program, a form that had become increasingly unpopular among budget balancers. And the legislation had serious political problems — the controversial abortion amendments added by the House.

Veterans Resist Cutbacks in VA Programs

Congress in mid-1980 appeared ready to give President Carter the unpleasant choice of vetoing a veterans' bill in an election year, or letting a measure already condemned by administration officials become law.

Passage seemed virtually assured for legislation providing hefty pay increases for Veterans Administration (VA) doctors, while early feedback from the Carter administration indicated a veto might be likely because of the bill's cost.

By a whopping 406-1 vote under suspension of the rules, the House May 20 agreed to a 65 percent overall increase in special incentive pay for VA doctors and dentists.

Under existing law, up to $13,500 in various "special pays" could be added to VA physicians' base salaries, which generally ranged from just under $40,000 to just over $50,000. The bill (HR 7102) would boost the maximum special pay to $22,000. It also would create a new $14 million-a-year scholarship program that would require young doctors and nurses to pay back educational support with service in the VA medical system.

The legislation was needed, said House Veterans' Affairs Committee Chairman Ray Roberts, D-Texas, because the VA medical system was having increasing trouble recruiting and retaining young physicians. The expiring special pay system, approved in 1975, was no longer attractive to VA physicians because of inflation, Roberts said.

The reluctance of members of Congress to vote against the powerful veterans' lobby groups, particularly in an election year, was also expected to produce an overwhelming vote in the Senate for a somewhat different bill (S 2534) that also raised the special pay for VA doctors.

Senate Bill

S 2534, reported May 15 by the Senate Veterans' Affairs Committee (S Rept 96-747), followed the House measure in making the special pay system permanent and permitting cost-of-living adjustments. Its maximum for special pay was $23,500, with a different structuring of the various types of bonuses. Both bills would allow an additional bonus, on top of the maximum, to induce physicians to work at VA facilities experiencing severe staff recruiting problems.

The Senate bill differed from the House version in that it did not include a scholarship program or salary hikes for dentists. The Senate veterans' committee had long maintained that VA dentists, in some cases, were treating individuals not strictly eligible for VA care. The Senate measure also included, in a somewhat revised form, the substance of a bill (HR 4015) passed by the House in 1979 that gave statutory basis to existing VA geriatric health centers.

Limits on Free Care

HR 7102 authorized new limits on the free care provided by VA medical facilities, a change that bill advocates said would offset the new costs of the scholarship and special pay programs. Under existing law, veterans with non-service-connected disabilities could be admitted to VA hospitals if space was available and if they said under oath they could not afford to go elsewhere. The bill would, for the first time, permit VA officials to review such a patient's financial status, including health insurance coverage, rather than simply relying on his oath.

The House Veterans' Affairs Committee, which reported the bill May 14 (H Rept 96-958), chose this option instead of a proposal by President Carter that would have authorized the VA to collect from health insurance plans for treatment of insured veterans. The House bill's provision could save the government about $109 million in fiscal 1981 and nearly double that by 1985, according to the Congressional Budget Office (CBO).

The Senate committee also rejected the president's plan, opting instead for studies to determine how much health insurance veterans had and how much money could be saved by the Carter proposal.

The cost of the pay hikes in the House bill would be $40 million a year, CBO analysts said, while the first-year cost of the scholarship program was put at $14 million, with some savings in later years as the scholarship students began serving their obligated time. Because of these costs and because certain other relatively minor provisions were objectionable to the Carter administration, "enactment of this legislation would not be in accord with the program of the president," VA Administrator Max Cleland wrote the House committee.

During debate on the bill May 19, House veterans' committee Chairman Roberts said its overall effect would be to save money — $52.5 million in federal outlays in fiscal 1981 and substantially more than that in later years. He said the new bonuses and scholarship program were needed because the VA "is constantly faced with an ever-increasing number of good, young physicians leaving ... after a short period of time." He also noted that the VA spent over $15 million a year for contract services of radiologists and certain other specialists.

Rep. John Paul Hammerschmidt, R-Ark., warned that the VA system was "in danger of becoming overrun with part-time and foreign-trained physicians." Forty percent of VA physicians were part-time, and 38 percent were graduates of foreign medical schools, he said.

The lone House member to vote against the legislation, Anthony C. Beilenson, D-Calif., said budget considerations and an expected physician surplus suggested to him that the extra VA spending was not needed. Beilenson also said in an interview, "I've not believed in the continuing buildup of this parallel health system, especially since the majority of what the VA treats is not battle injuries."

Provisions of House Bill

As passed by the House, HR 7102:

● Raised to $22,000, from $13,500, the maximum annual special pay for VA physicians, and to $11,000, from $6,700, the maximum special pay for VA dentists; made the special pay system permanent, and provided for cost-of-living adjustments in these amounts. Among the changes in the different components making up the total special pay for an individual was a boost to $6,000, from $2,000, in the incentive pay for full-time physicians. The bill also authorized special bonuses for individuals achieving certification from medical specialty boards and for those working in certain remote areas with health manpower shortages.

● Created a new scholarship program for physicians and nurses, who would be required to pay back each year's support with a year's service with the VA. Medical students could receive $19,320 a year for tuition and living expenses, for four years; nursing students would receive $6,500 a year for four years. Provided for cost-of-living adjustments.

● Required individuals postponing their VA service in order to take graduate training to serve an additional six months with the VA for each year of deferral. The maximum period of obligated service for physicians would be six years; for nurses, four years.

● Permitted special pay only for physicians obligated for more than three years of VA service, and only after they had completed three years of VA service. Until the end of the obligation period, the physician would receive half the normal special pay.

● Authorized financial penalties, ranging from $1,500 for scholarship recipients who failed to complete their medical education to as much as three times the scholarship for individuals failing to fulfill their service obligation. Doctors taking postgraduate training in specialties not needed by the VA, such as pediatrics, could have their service obligation transferred to other federal programs, such as the National Health Service Corps.

● Authorized the VA administrator to review the financial status of veterans seeking admission to VA medical facilities for treatment of non-service-connected disabilities, to determine whether they could use non-VA facilities instead. Veterans eligible for Medicaid and those with service-connected disabilities or VA pensions would not be subject to the financial status review.

● Eliminated VA authority to lease land, property and equipment to other institutions.

1979 Congressional Action

Veterans' lobbies and their friends in Congress won a victory in 1979 when Congress rejected moves by the Carter administration to shrink the medical staffs of Veterans Administration hospitals and clinics and, in December, cleared legislation (HR 3892 — PL 96-151) requiring the VA to maintain staffs at the full levels set by congressional appropriations committees.

The bill also made some changes in health benefits for veterans and their dependents, and continued VA grants for medical schools and aid to state-run nursing homes and other long-term care facilities for veterans.

The administration had proposed cutbacks in veterans' health benefits, and opposed many of the congressional changes as too costly. Veterans' groups strongly objected to any cutbacks. The final version of the bill dropped most of Carter's money-saving proposals; Congress accepted a few in return for administration agreement to restore some of the hospital staff cuts and abide by the levels set by Congress in the future.

HR 3892 also mandated a study of the health effects of "Agent Orange" on Vietnam veterans. "Agent Orange" was a defoliant used in Vietnam from 1962 to 1971 to clear jungle cover concealing enemy troop positions. About 5,000 veterans had sought VA aid for ailments, ranging from dizziness to cancer, which they blamed on certain chemicals (dioxins) in the herbicide. *("Agent Orange" controversy, p. 112)*

In what one senator called a "bitter pill" of a compromise, the Senate swallowed House demands that the study be conducted by the Veterans Administration (VA) rather than the Department of Health, Education and Welfare (HEW, now Health and Human Services). The VA had remained officially skeptical that the chemicals caused anything more than a persistent skin rash, and some senators questioned its ability and desire to do a thorough, objective investigation.

While the VA was to do the study of veterans, under the compromise HEW was to study the health effects of dioxins on civilians. However, President Carter vetoed the bill mandating the HEW studies (S 2096) because it required HEW to have its design for the studies approved by Congress' Office of Technology Assessment. Carter said that was a form of legislative veto over the administrative authority of the executive branch, and therefore unconstitutional. *(Dioxins veto, appendix, p. 76-A)*

HR 3892 contained an identical provision affecting the VA's study, but Carter signed the bill anyway because it extended veterans' health benefits and embodied the compromise on hospital staffing and benefit cuts. He said he would instruct the VA to ignore the objectionable provision.

Staffing Controversy

Administration moves earlier in 1979 to cut VA medical staffs had angered veterans' lobbies and their friends in Congress — particularly since the cuts flew in the face of a 1978 congressional mandate to hire more VA doctors, nurses and other health personnel. The administration had used funds in the fiscal 1979 appropriations bill (PL 95-392) that were earmarked for new staff to "defray the costs" of the October 1978 pay raise for VA employees, according to the Senate Veterans' Affairs Committee.

House Veterans' Affairs Committee Chairman Ray Roberts, D-Texas, said about 6,800 VA medical positions were being cut in fiscal 1979 and it was rumored that more were still to come. He told the House a plan was being implemented "to phase out the VA hospital program."

The result was a House bill that flatly ordered the VA to keep medical personnel at a set level. The Senate compromised somewhat; its bill (S 1039) required the administration to keep health staffing at levels acceptable to Congress (as set in appropriations bills) if it wanted some dollar-saving cuts in health benefits for veterans.

In addition to cutting back on VA medical staffs, the administration wanted to end certain dental benefits for veterans and limit outpatient non-prescription drugs and medical supplies to only extremely needy veterans, those over age 65 or those who were chronically ill. It also wanted to limit transportation reimbursement for veterans to ambulance or other special transportation approved in advance. The changes would not apply to service-disabled veterans or those meeting the VA income test.

Psychological Aid for Vietnam Vets Approved

President Carter June 13, 1979, signed into law a bill (S 7 — PL 96-22) establishing a new psychological counseling program for Vietnam veterans — something sponsors had been seeking for nearly a decade.

The bill also contained a controversial provision empowering the House and Senate Veterans' Affairs committees to approve or disapprove the construction or leasing of Veterans Administration (VA) hospitals. The House committee had insisted on the provision in exchange for supporting the counseling program. It was opposed as a "pork barrel" power grab by the Office of Management and Budget, by some members of Congress and by the congressional appropriations committees, which previously held the power themselves.

Controversial Compromise

Four times since 1971 the Senate had approved a special counseling program for Vietnam-era veterans, together with drug abuse, alcoholism and preventive health programs.

But old-line veterans' groups and their House supporters were cool to the package, particularly since Vietnam veterans' groups pushing the concept wanted much of the program to be conducted outside the VA. They said many younger veterans distrusted the VA, which the older groups staunchly defended.

Sentiment for such a program had grown, however, due in part to a number of popular movies and television shows dramatizing the problems of Vietnam veterans. President Carter, unlike his Republican predecessors, called the program a high legislative priority and included funds for it in his fiscal 1980 budget. And a new congressional caucus of Vietnam-era veterans lobbied for it.

What actually got the program off the ground was a 1978 compromise worked out by Senate Veterans' Affairs Committee Chairman Alan Cranston, D-Calif., and David E. Satterfield III, D-Va., chairman of the House Veterans' Affairs Subcommittee on Medical Facilities and Benefits. In return for House backing of the Senate package, Cranston agreed to support the House plan to give authorizing committees the power to approve or kill major construction projects for VA hospitals and other medical facilities. The House had approved this authority as separate legislation in the 95th Congress.

The House endorsed the compromise intact, although the Senate balked at the medical facilities approval provision and dropped it. Conferees restored it, however, and adjusted other comparatively minor differences.

Background

Studies had shown that, even years after the end of the war, many Vietnam veterans were suffering psychological scars — stress, depression, problems with alcohol, drugs, marriages and jobs. The VA estimated that more than 30 percent of the 8.7 million Vietnam-era veterans faced "serious problems related to readjustment to civilian life." (Only 170,000 probably would actually seek aid under the new program, however, according to estimates.)

According to a 1978 presidential message to Congress, Vietnam-era veterans under age 34 had a 23 percent higher suicide rate than non-veterans of the same age, and the number of problem drinkers among this group had "more than doubled, from 13 percent in 1970 to 31 percent in 1977."

Vietnam veterans had two problems that differed from those of earlier wars: they were much more likely to have survived, but with disabling injuries, and they were "more likely to have doubts about the validity of their sacrifice." The psychological impact of these problems could show up long after discharge, according to VA Administrator Max Cleland.

Cleland said Vietnam veterans needed a special readjustment counseling program because the psychiatric wards of VA hospitals were often understaffed or staffed with foreign doctors, and because many veterans distrusted the VA or feared the stigma of being a psychiatric patient. Under existing law, counseling for most veterans could come only after they checked into a VA psychiatric ward for evaluation.

Major Provisions

As signed into law, S 7 (PL 95-22):

● Authorized the Veterans Administration to provide dental care for veterans of World Wars I and II and the Korean conflict, for Vietnam era veterans who had been prisoners of war for more than six months and for veterans rated as totally disabled.

● Required the VA to provide outpatient counseling and mental health follow-up services for Vietnam-era veterans experiencing difficulty in readjusting to civilian life, if veterans sought the aid within two years of discharge or within two years of enactment of the bill, whichever was later. The services were to be provided directly by the VA unless a veteran lived very far from a VA facility, or a facility could not provide appropriate care. Members of veterans' families also could receive counseling.

● Authorized the VA to conduct a pilot program of contracting with halfway houses and similar community-based facilities to treat veterans with alcohol and drug use problems, and to report to Congress on the program by March 1983.

● Authorized the VA, with the Department of Labor and the Office of Personnel Management, to promote hiring of rehabilitated veterans from the alcohol and drug abuse programs.

● Authorized the VA to start a pilot program of preventive health care services, such as medical checkups, for certain veterans with service-connected disabilities. Authorized $64 million for fiscal 1980-84. Required a study on the cost-effectiveness of the program.

● Barred appropriations for construction or renovation of VA medical facilities costing more than $2 million, or leases of more than $500,000 a year, unless the House and Senate Veterans' Affairs committees had each approved a project by resolution.

The final version of the bill, worked out in informal negotiations and appoved by voice vote in both houses Dec. 6, adopted the Senate version of the hospital staffing requirement but dropped most of the administration's money-saving proposals.

The VA Health System: Background

The veterans' health system was established by Congress in 1924, at a time when hospital shortages were common and health insurance rare. There was no visible federal commitment to provide health care to any segment of the population. The primary mission of the VA system was to make sure World War I veterans received adequate medical treatment, and the system's top priority since then has remained treatment of service-connected disabilities — medical problems stemming directly from an individual's military service. However, the VA has also been authorized to care for non-service-connected medical problems.

By the end of the 1970s, the VA was running the largest medical care delivery system in the nation, employing nearly 181,000 people and spending about $5.6 billion (for fiscal 1980). In fiscal 1980 the system was caring for about 1.3 million inpatients and 18.1 million outpatients, either directly or through contract with private providers. There were 172 VA hospitals, 91 nursing homes and in-hospital chronic care facilities, and 220 outpatient clinics.

Theoretically, nearly all the nation's 30 million veterans were eligible for VA medical care. But VA officials pointed out that a veteran seeking care for non-service-connected problems must certify that he could not find treatment elsewhere, and must find a facility willing to treat him. Despite these barriers, the vast majority of VA patients were not being treated for problems connected with their military service. Fewer than 30 percent of VA medical patients were under care for service-connected conditions.

In 1976, Congress passed a veterans' health bill (PL 94-581) altering outpatient care procedures by VA hospitals to give priority to treatment of service-related medical problems over treatment of problems not connected with the veteran's military service. The bill also authorized total VA health care benefits for any veteran with a service-related disability rated at 50 percent or more — lowered from 80 percent under existing law. The bill broadened eligibility for total health care benefits but restricted benefits for home-bound and other veterans who could not get to VA hospitals.

Conflicting Priorities

Consideration of the 1979 VA health bill revealed conflicting opinions that reflected deep generational divisions between veterans who served during the Vietnam War and those who fought in earlier conflicts. That division was in part responsible for controversy surrounding a bill establishing a counseling program for Vietnam veterans that also cleared in 1979. (*Box, p. 95*)

The various veterans' groups were united on the need for substantial federal benefits for veterans, but often differed on priorities for that spending. The established groups — among them the American Legion, Veterans of Foreign Wars (VFW) and Disabled American Veterans — tended to favor pensions, chronic care and other lifetime benefits for their aging members. They argued that their military service had earned them the right to a separate

health care system, and they bitterly resisted anything that looked like erosion of that system.

However, younger veterans from the Vietnam era "don't exactly warm up to the VA system," said VA Administrator Max Cleland. They have often found it impersonal and incompetent. For some it represented the war they wish they had never fought in. Groups like the Council of Vietnam Veterans were less interested in old-age benefits than in more immediate programs like jobs, education and readjustment counseling. They did not automatically bristle at the concept of meshing the VA system with civilian health care. For instance, many veterans with readjustment problems would rather seek counseling at community mental health centers and other non-VA facilities, said an aide to Rep. David E. Bonior, D-Mich., who helped organize the congressional Vietnam veterans caucus.

Underlying many arguments about veterans' health benefits were two highly emotional issues: the U.S. involvement in the Vietnam War itself, and the future of the VA health system if the nation were to opt for national health insurance.

Groups like the Legion and the VFW were smarting from a 1977 study that suggested preparing the VA for integration into a national health program. The study, by the National Academy of Sciences, also was highly critical of the VA medical system. The heart of the controversy over the report was its conclusion that a separate VA system might not be needed, since most of its treatment was not for service-connected disabilities and since veterans with alternatives avoided it.

Factors Favoring Passage

In addition to securing a legislative compromise, there were other factors that ensured favorable congressional action on the general VA health bill. They were related to the Vietnam veterans counseling program.

● President Carter, unlike his Republican predecessors, asked for funds for the counseling program in his fiscal 1980 budget.

● The presence of Vietnam veteran Cleland in the top VA position meant continuing, visible pressure for the counseling program and the concept that Vietnam veterans had special needs that were not met by existing VA programs.

Cleland lost both legs and an arm in combat. He was convinced that, even years after the conclusion of the Vietnam War, its veterans had unique psychological problems that should not be dealt with on VA psychiatric wards. But, he warned, "If these problems go untreated now, in 10 or 15 years we will have to treat them there and it will be much more expensive."

● Creation of a congressional caucus of Vietnam-era veterans that was pressing for the counseling program and other aid for Vietnam veterans.

Major Provisions of 1979 Veterans' Health Bill

The major provisions of HR 3892 (PL 96-151):

State VA Facilities. Authorized matching grants to states for construction and renovation of state veterans' care facilities such as nursing homes. Authorized $15 million for fiscal 1980 and funds as needed for fiscal 1981 and 1982. Raised the per diem rate of federal payments to state veterans' facilities by 15 percent; limited this raise for fiscal 1980 by stipulating that only the amount appropriated for that purpose could be spent.

Medical Education, Information. Extended the VA medical information-sharing system through fiscal 1982 and authorized $4 million a year for it. Authorized joint information-sharing educational activities between public or non-profit private institutions and VA hospitals that were remote from major medical centers.

● Terminated VA authority to help establish new state medical schools, effective Sept. 30, 1979.

● Extended for three years authorizations for grants to existing medical schools and other health professions training programs affiliated with the VA; authorized $15 million for fiscal 1980, $25 million for fiscal 1981 and $30 million for fiscal 1982. Eliminated a requirement that the schools must increase the number of individuals in training as a direct result of VA grants.

Benefits for Veterans. Eliminated an existing provision for VA payments for travel expenses to VA medical facilities for persons who certified that they could not pay these expenses themselves; instead, required the VA to provide by regulation for partial payments for persons who could not afford travel costs. Provided partial VA payments for travel expenses for veterans with service-connected disabilities and for veterans meeting VA pension income standards.

● Authorized VA reimbursement for non-VA emergency medical care, for non-service-connected problems, under certain conditions. A VA physician must determine that the care was needed, and the care could continue only until the individual could be transferred to a VA facility. Existing law provided for non-VA treatment only if a VA facility could not provide the needed care.

● Required the VA administrator to pay for non-VA dental care costing more than $500 a year, if a VA dentist approved the treatment on the basis of need and of cost.

● Authorized direct (VA) and contract outpatient care in certain circumstances for veterans of the Mexican border period and World War I.

● Broadened health insurance coverage for veterans' survivors and dependents in certain circumstances.

Personnel. Required the Office of Management and Budget (OMB) to keep VA health staff at levels set by the congressional appropriations committees; required OMB and the comptroller general to make periodic reports to Congress on compliance.

Agent Orange Studies. Required the VA administrator to conduct an ongoing epidemiological study of the health effects in veterans of exposure to the chemicals known as dioxins. The study was to be conducted according to a protocol (design of the study) approved by the Office of Technology Assessment. Required a second VA study of the medical literature on long-term health effects of exposure to dioxins.

Funding of Emergency Services Continued

According to President Carter, it was time in 1979 to make state and local governments foot the bill for upgrading and coordinating their own emergency medical services (EMS).

But members of Congress were in no hurry to turn off federal dollars for the program that brings emergency helicopters and other dramatic improvements in emergency care to constituents. Ignoring a presidential request to phase out federal matching funds for regional emergency medical systems, Congress Nov. 29, 1979, cleared legislation continuing the popular program for three years, and authorizing a total of $196 million for it.

Despite this rejection of presidential policy, Carter did not veto the bill (S 497 — PL 96-142), because "the point has been made to the White House that EMS is one of the most favored programs in Congress," as one Health, Education and Welfare (HEW, now Health and Human Services) official said.

"EMS is very popular.... EMS is effective, and people know it. People all over the country know what ambulances are," Richardson Preyer, D-N.C., told the House in Sept. 24 debate on the bill. "Let us tell the communities of America that we are behind them by passing this bill."

Indeed, Preyer's comment reflected widespread congressional reluctance to clamp down too tightly on a program that has bankrolled:

● Emergency helicopters and ambulances, some equipped to monitor a victim's heart rate or other vital signs and transmit the data to a hospital-based doctor, who can prescribe preliminary care for a victim en route to a hospital.

● Sophisticated communications and transportation systems that can route injured or critically ill persons directly to specialized burn, heart attack or accident units.

● Funds for training physician and nurse specialists and emergency vehicle paramedics.

● The 911 "emergency" telephone number and other components of improved communications systems.

● CPR (cardiopulmonary resuscitation) programs that train citizens to give emergency aid to heart attack victims.

● Improved survival and recovery rates for victims of accidents and critical illnesses in EMS regions with the most advanced type of program.

"It's a very sexy program. You can document the results. You can see the helicopters flying overhead. And, it's the kind of federal involvement a lot of people like; we're not delivering the services, just making it possible for them to be there," said HEW official Wayne Mara.

Background

The 1973 legislation (PL 93-154) that set up the EMS program assumed that eventually the nation would be organized into regional emergency medical systems, which would support themselves without federal subsidies. Federal start-up money was needed to overcome a col-

lection of uncoordinated programs in cities, untrained or poorly prepared ambulance and emergency room personnel and outdated equipment, Congress decided.

Under the 1973 law, each EMS region was to progress through a five-year sequence, from preliminary planning to a fully functioning, advanced system. Federal matching funds would shrink and local contributions increase over the five-year period; the completed system was expected to be self-supporting.

A 1976 reauthorization (PL 94-573) required grant applications to show they had the support of volunteer groups and local governments. It also created new authority to support research, training and treatment programs dealing with burn injuries.

The original 1973 act anticipated a national network of 304 advanced regional systems. At the end of 1978, only 17 of those systems, covering 26.2 million people, were complete. Progress had been slow because of relatively low appropriations, but, according to Henry A. Waxman, D-Calif., chairman of the House Commerce Subcommittee on Health, the program itself was "on firm footing and remarkable progress is being made in every section of the country." Carter's plan would have left three-fourths of regional EMS systems "undeveloped or underdeveloped," according to Waxman.

However, according to James M. Collins, R-Texas, the only House member to side with the president during debate, "any community with a will to work" could set up its own system without federal aid. Collins urged members to drop EMS and "get on with more critical concerns in this day of limited budgets."

Funding Phase-out Debate

An "orderly phase-out" of federal EMS spending was appropriate because the national network of these systems was "rapidly nearing completion," according to Carter's fiscal 1980 budget, which would have provided only $76.3 million for the program through fiscal 1982. By the end of fiscal 1979, all but 13 of the 304 EMS regions would have received some federal aid, according to the administration. Appropriations totaling $184 million since 1974 had offset local expenses for planning, equipping and staffing regional emergency systems. An additional $22 million in appropriations supported EMS research.

Earlier in 1979, Carter sought a $6 million rescission in emergency medical services training funds for fiscal 1979. Congress granted only half of the cut.

The congressional committees considering the legislation contended that the EMS network was far from complete and that an early cutoff of federal aid would jeopardize further progress.

If Congress followed Carter's funding recommendations, only one-fourth of the nation's 304 emergency regions would have functioning, advanced systems, according to an April 30, 1979, report (S Rept 96-102) of the Senate Labor and Human Resources Committee.

Postponing the cutoff date until 1985 would permit 85 percent of the regions to complete the sophisticated communications, transportation and treatment systems envisioned by the 1973 law, the committee said.

The House Interstate and Foreign Commerce Committee, in its May 15, 1979, report (H Rept 96-185), agreed that Carter's phase-out proposal was premature.

Both committees cited progress in emergency care that could be credited to federal investment in improvements. Since 1972, for example, 15 percent fewer people had died from accidents, while the nation's population grew 3 percent. "Although no single factor can be credited with causing this decrease ... some credit can be attributed to improvements in the quality of emergency care," the Senate committee said. Deaths from heart attacks and accidental poisoning were down, as was infant mortality. These victims were "particularly dependent on good emergency care," the committee observed.

"When the EMS Act was first introduced in 1972, many ambulances did not have attendants who had been trained in even first aid . . .; in many communities the undertaker's hearse doubled as an ambulance." Now most accident victims can be assured "they will not be further injured through improper handling by the ambulance attendant. Most heart attack victims now receive experienced and knowledgeable help within minutes of their attacks," according to the Senate report.

Bills Compared

The House-passed bill generally followed the Senate version in continuing grants and contracts for planning, operation and improvements of regional EMS systems. But funding levels were higher throughout and distributed somewhat differently. For example, matching funds for basic EMS grants were authorized at $40 million annually for fiscal 1980-82, as in the Senate bill, but HR 3642 added $5 million a year more for a new, separate "extension and improvement grants" program.

The House measure also authorized two additional grants to EMS applicants, thereby lengthening an individual system's eligibility for federal matching funds to seven years, from five years under existing law.

Both bills continued a burn control program and authorized new spending to integrate existing poison control centers with the emergency system and create new centers.

The House bill omitted some administrative program changes of the Senate bill, and did not include a separate two-year, $12 million reauthorization for federal information and counseling programs on "crib death" (sudden infant death syndrome, SIDS) added by the Senate to its bill. The Senate SIDS provision overlapped existing authorizations, but also included administrative changes.

Major Provisions

Following are the provisions of S 497 relating to the EMS program worked out by key House and Senate committee members in informal negotiations. The compromise, authorizing a total of $196 million over three years, was approved Nov. 15 by the Senate and Nov. 29, 1979, by the House. It continued, at about existing appropriations levels, federal support for organizing and upgrading regional emergency transportation and communication systems, and for training specialists in emergency care. The bill:

● Authorized $40 million annually for grants and contracts for planning, initial development and expansion of emergency medical services systems in fiscal years 1980-82. That was a $30 million reduction in the fiscal 1979 authorization level.

● Provided that up to 5 percent of appropriated funds would be earmarked for planning grants and contracts; set a minimum earmark for this purpose of 1 percent for fiscal 1980, three-fourths of 1 percent for fiscal 1981 and one-half of 1 percent for fiscal 1982.

● Required priority treatment for applicants for planning grants or contracts who had not previously received federal aid. Deleted a requirement that no more than half of appropriated funds could be used for second-time planning grants or contracts.

● Permitted a third expansion or improvement grant for systems meeting certain conditions. (Existing law permitted only two grants of this type to any entity.) Authorized $6 million for fiscal 1981 for these grants.

● Continued a requirement that one-fifth of appropriated funds for emergency systems development must be earmarked for initial operations projects, and one-fifth for expanding existing systems.

● Extended authorizations for grants and contracts for research in emergency medical services as follows: $3 million for fiscal 1980 and $3.5 million a year for fiscal 1981 and 1982.

● Expanded a demonstration program for research and training in burn treatment and rehabilitation to include trauma and poison programs as well. Authorized $6 million for fiscal 1980, $12 million for fiscal 1981 and $10 million for fiscal 1982. Earmarked half of the fiscal 1980 funds for poison control programs, and 25 percent for these programs for fiscal 1981 and 1982. Also specified that at least 25 percent of these funds must be spent each year for trauma programs.

● Authorized $5 million for fiscal 1980, $7 million for fiscal 1981 and $8 million for fiscal 1982 for emergency medical services training programs.

● Authorized $5 million for fiscal 1980 and $7 million for fiscal 1981 for SIDS programs. ∎

Disease Prevention Programs Under Review

"Many of our nation's health problems can be prevented, and studies indicate that future improvements in our health are more likely to come from greater attention to disease and injury prevention than to their treatment," according to the Carter administration's fiscal 1981 budget. "Health research on the causes, prevention, and treatment of disease, and the promotion of preventive measures are critical components of the administration's health strategy for the 1980s."

Disease prevention: the phrase can cover a variety of measures, depending on how one defines it. And the Carter administration's definition has been a broad one, including:

● A new program to provide health care for young children and pregnant women. *(Child Health Assurance Program, p. 80-A)*

● Family planning, and counseling for pregnant teenagers. *(Appendix, p. 65-A)*

● Programs to reduce environmental hazards, including air and water pollution control and regulation of the treatment, storage and disposal of hazardous wastes and toxic substances.

● Consumer product safety, covering regulation of products intended for use or affecting children; reform of federal drug laws; regulations to ensure the safety and effectiveness of medical devices; and guidelines for use of X-rays and other exposures to radiation. *(Drug law reform, p. 131)*

● Traffic safety measures, such as the 55-mile-an-hour speed limit, mandatory safety belts and recalls of defective automobile equipment.

● Community water fluoridation efforts.

● Health promotion efforts — anti-smoking and physical fitness campaigns, and a program to educate and screen Americans for hypertension (high blood pressure).

● Research into the causes, effects and possible cures of diseases such as heart attack, cancer, birth defects, infant and childhood disease, mental retardation and illness and diabetes. *(Mental health, p. 83; cancer research, p. 69-A)*

● Regulation of food quality. *(Food laws, p. 119)*

● Programs to prevent and treat drug and alcohol abuse. *(Appendix, p. 79-A)*

● National immunization against childhood diseases. *(Appendix, p. 59-A)*

● Nutrition programs, including general federal education efforts, school lunch and breakfast programs, and a special supplemental food program for women, infants and children (WIC).

● Workplace health and safety standards administered primarily by the Occupational Safety and Health Administration (OSHA).

These were among the programs cited by the administration as measures that would reduce the more than $400 billion in annual direct and indirect costs of injury, illness and premature death. According to the August 1979 Surgeon General's report *Healthy People,*

preventive actions by individuals, corporations and government at all levels represented the most likely means by which dramatic health status gains could be made in the future.

Despite this prognosis for the nation's health system, disease prevention efforts in 1980 accounted for only a small portion of the administration's health budget, and at least two of the programs, workplace safety and child nutrition, were under critical review, the latter by the Carter administration itself. *(See chapter on child health, p. 87)*

The Disease-Prevention Coalition

Beginning in 1978, a handful of members of Congress and an ambitious Carter administration task force began the massive job of reorienting the nation's health care system to prevention — as well as cure — of disease. But, by 1980, their efforts had amounted to no more than a modest addition to the existing federal commitment to preventive health programs.

Although Congress in 1978 passed a handful of new disease-prevention programs, by the standard Washington measure — money — these programs were minor. They probably would add only $300 million, over two or three years, to the federal health budget. That compared with a fiscal 1979 health care budget of $49 billion.

But the process of passing the programs established a potentially important link between environmental interests and health institutions. That linkage also showed up in the Prevention Initiative task force in the Department of Health, Education and Welfare (HEW, now Health and Human Services), which made workplace and en-

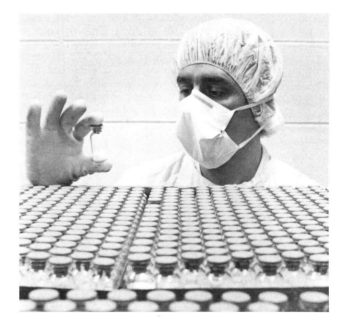

vironmental health issues a top priority.

A third, related development was the emergence of a new "disease prevention and environmental health" coalition of more than 100 health, environment, labor, insurance, consumer and public interest lobbies. Boosters of the loosely structured coalition hoped that it would be able to marshal the resources of such powerful organizations as the American Medical Association (AMA), the AFL-CIO and effective environmental and consumer groups behind disease-prevention policies.

Obstacles

But preventive health efforts faced some formidable obstacles.

● Budget austerities were a certainty, and new programs had to contend with an increasingly cost-conscious Congress and administration.

● Contributions to public-interest lobbies, a large component of the coalition, reportedly were drying up.

● The medical establishment had long doubted the effectiveness of large-scale disease-prevention efforts.

● Agency resistance could sandbag some of the newly passed measures.

● The environment and workplace initiatives that were central concerns of both the administration task force and coalition fell into one of the most embattled areas of federal policy.

Chemical manufacturers and other industrial interests bitterly protested the expense of complying with environmental and occupational health laws and regulations. The president's inflation fighters also were hostile to apparently costly regulatory efforts.

And industry had created a multimillion-dollar coalition to combat Occupational Safety and Health Administration (OSHA) moves to adopt carcinogenicity standards for ranking suspect substances by potential hazard.

The principals in the disease-prevention efforts conceded the magnitude of these problems. But they insisted that disease prevention and health promotion should be a top health priority, with or without a national health insurance system.

Congressional aides who developed the 1978 preventive health programs also suggested that cost concerns could be useful political vehicles for future disease-prevention efforts. Advocates of so-called "personal" preventive measures, such as screening and other services for the well population, could benefit from support of environmental lobbies. And stressing the preventive health role of environmental regulations could recruit important support for their implementation, they hoped. "How could the AMA, for example, come out against something labeled 'disease prevention'?" asked one coalition organizer.

A cautionary note was sounded by former Rep. Paul G. Rogers, D-Fla., one of the most committed disease-prevention advocates. He warned a Nov. 15, 1978, meeting of the coalition against uncritical adherence to the "bogus economics" of strict cost-benefit analysis in health policy. This premise could lead to the conclusion that "if getting sick is cheaper, then maybe we should not try to prevent illness," Rogers said.

But the developing effort extended beyond cost issues — although a major strategy of the cost-conscious HEW task force was use of existing resources, from the neighborhood school on up, to promote preventive health measures.

Michael McGinnis, a deputy assistant secretary for health responsible for the task force, discounted the skepticism that was associated with the concept of preventive health services. Major efforts to change Americans' personal health behavior had never really been tried, and a couple of experimental efforts to reduce heart disease by persuading people to take better care of themselves had had promising results, McGinnis said.

Background

Many doctors have been skeptical about the effectiveness of major disease-prevention efforts.

"We don't really know what preventive medicine is, except immunization and things we already know about keeping healthy," AMA board chairman Robert B. Hunter told a group of journalists in Washington in January 1978. "I can't think of a single person in the United States that doesn't know that cigarette smoking is bad for your health," but his patients rarely quit or cut down, Hunter added.

Hunter also said that studies by Kaiser-Permanente and other prepaid group health plans cast doubt on the cost-benefit of annual physical examinations, a key element of traditional preventive medicine philosophy.

This brand of medical skepticism had been compounded over the years by several factors: traditional medical education, health financing systems and fear that scarce resources would be diverted from care of the ill to vaguely defined preventive programs.

Critics of the cure-oriented American medical system said that U.S. doctors were trained to medicate, operate and soothe the pain of illness, but not to think about systematic strategies for preventing it. They added that federal and private health insurance programs reinforced this philosophy by paying doctors on a per-service — per-sickness — basis, and not paying them for preventing illness.

The nation's health laws had been largely shaped by this conservative attitude and by political realities. They tended to fund proven prevention strategies such as innoculation of children against infectious diseases such as polio.

Disease prevention had not been omitted from federal law. But it had not been a very high priority except for the constituencies of the venerable, targeted public health programs, sometimes collectively referred to as "disease-a-month" programs. These programs included family planning, rat control, lead-based paint poisoning and genetic disease screening, screening and information programs for hypertension, and immunization. The authorization for the stepped-up "war on cancer" included prevention as a statutory goal, but environmentalists complained that the resulting research and service programs focused too narrowly on treatment and cure, to the exclusion of prevention.

McGinnis and other advocates of the new initiatives cast a very broad net, however, when they talked about disease prevention. In this view, nutrition programs scattered through HEW and the Department of Agriculture were disease prevention, and the Food and Drug Administration (FDA) and Center for Disease Control (CDC) were wholly preventive agencies. Alcohol and drug abuse efforts also were categorized as preventive programs, as was control of carcinogens and other toxic substances.

This broad view sometimes moved critics to ridicule. One health planning agency that urged strict enforcement of speed laws was criticized for straying beyond its jurisdiction. But national health statistics ranked accidents in the top five leading causes of death. (The others were heart disease, cancer, stroke and pneumonia and influenza, according to the National Center for Health Statistics.)

1978 Congressional Action

Historically, medical and environmental interests have traveled different paths that only occasionally paralleled each other.

The separation extended even to the staff of the Rogers subcommittee on health and the environment. "Environment people worked on their bills, health people worked on their bills. We said 'good morning' in the hall, but we really didn't start putting things together until this year," recalled one aide.

For several related reasons, 1978 was different. First, there were the pressures — industry pressures to weaken environmental health laws and regulations, and pressures from national health insurance advocate Sen. Edward M. Kennedy, D-Mass., to begin to create a meaningful commitment to disease prevention and health promotion.

A third source of pressure was New Jersey Rep. Andrew Maguire, D, whose heavily industrialized state showed a high incidence of cancer on the ominous "cancer maps" of federal health statisticians.

Late in 1977 Maguire introduced a cancer prevention bill that was the product of several years' drafting by health aides with substantial academic credentials. Maguire pressed hard for enactment, and most of the original bill's provisions were adopted as part of reauthorizing legislation (S 2450) for the National Cancer Institute. There were some changes, however, since the institute and its powerful friends let it be known that it did not want direct responsibility for preparing the required annual list of known or suspected carcinogens and certain other responsibilities that the Maguire bill gave it.

Kennedy also introduced a disease-prevention bill that stressed fitness programs and other personal or behavioral measures. Many of its provisions were adopted, but not those providing for stiff anti-smoking measures and nutritional labeling of food. These "ran into flack early on" and never emerged from Kennedy's Human Resources Health Subcommittee, aides reported.

These developments, and renewed labor interest in occupational health issues, came at a time when about 85 percent of federal health programs were up for reauthorization — and during a relatively quiet year for environmental staff on the House Commerce Committee.

The result was that, at the behest of Rogers, committee staff began combing through health law, looking for appropriate places to inject a new environmental-disease prevention thrust. Congress finally passed three major health reauthorizations (categorical health programs and health centers; biomedical research and service programs for cancer and heart, lung and blood diseases; health statistics and health care delivery research) that included new environment-related and disease-prevention authorizations.

The new thrust was also in a House bill (HR 11488) to reauthorize the federal health planning system that failed — for other reasons — to pass the House under suspension of the rules and died for lack of a second House vote. The bill directed state and local health planning agencies to involve themselves in "disease prevention needs and resources," including occupational, environmental and nutritional health.

Late in the session, Rogers also introduced a health manpower bill (HR 14264) designed to survey the needs created by environmental health laws for toxicologists, epidemiologists and other health professionals, and to fund training programs where needed.

The 96th Congress did little in its first session (1979) to strengthen disease prevention programs, and with administration and congressional moves to cut down on discretionary domestic programs in the fiscal 1981 budget, it appeared likely that efforts to prevent disease would be overridden by other perceived priorities.

Administration Task Force

Two intensive campaigns, in a California town and a county in Finland, to reduce the incidence of cardiovascular (heart and blood vessel) disease had lessened both the measurable risk of the disease and the actual onset of symptoms in the targeted populations, according to health researchers.

The projects used existing social structures and institutions — schools, local health services, clubs and other voluntary groups — and media advertising to heavily promote four strategies known to be effective in cutting down on heart disease: exercise, nutrition, smoking reduction and control of high blood pressure.

The administration's Prevention Initiative task force hoped to duplicate these results in 15 demonstration

---

Disease Prevention Efforts

Three health bills passed by the 95th Congress (S 2450, S 2466, S 2474) mandated the following preventive health efforts:

• The first comprehensive listing of all known or suspected carcinogens, including estimates of how many people have been exposed to the substances, where the exposures occurred, and the effectiveness of regulatory efforts.

• An ongoing national survey of the total costs of death and illness linked to pollution and other environmental conditions. In addition to toting up the costs of patient care, statisticians were instructed to estimate such indirect economic losses as absenteeism, lowered productivity, and human grief and suffering. The intangible factors were difficult to quantify but an important "cost" to the nation, according to the legislation.

• A statistical picture, updated periodically, of death rates and behavioral and environmental causes of "preventable" diseases in the United States.

• New stress on environmental and occupational causes of cancer in federal cancer research programs.

• New state-level preventive health programs, targeted on leading causes of death in each state, with funds earmarked for media campaigns.

• New national programs to deal with unwanted teenage pregnancies, which often adversely affect the health of both immature mothers and their infants.

• New national campaigns to discourage teenage smoking and alcohol consumption.

Reducing Health Hazards in the Workplace . . .

The first major attempt to legislate changes in the 10-year old Occupational Safety and Health Administration (OSHA) in 1980 created expectations that the agency would face continuing legislative challenges in the future.

According to Sen. Richard S. Schweiker, Pa., ranking Republican on the Labor and Human Resources Committee, the much-criticized agency should concentrate on businesses with bad safety records. To that end, he introduced legislation (S 2153) that would exempt an estimated 90 percent of businesses from OSHA safety inspections.

OSHA was established under 1970 legislation (PL 91-596) that authorized the federal government to set and enforce safety and health standards covering all businesses engaged in interstate commerce. Over the years, limitations on appropriations whittled that jurisdiction down — but the Schweiker bill was the first to provide a statutory exemption from coverage for whole groups of businesses. The bill had the support of Labor Committee Chairman Harrison A. Williams Jr., D-N.J., and 19 other cosponsors.

Even if the Schweiker bill were not enacted, it raised a basic question about the future direction of federal job safety efforts: Should regulation concentrate on the workplaces where injuries were most likely to occur, or should it protect all workers, through the threat of inspection of every business, no matter how safe? One basic idea behind the Schweiker bill was that OSHA was spread too thin — only 1,600 agents to inspect about five million workplaces. That was too few, supporters of the bill argued, to waste on inspecting businesses with good safety records, when they could focus instead on the most dangerous jobs.

An indication of the weakness of existing inspection policies, according to Schweiker, was that serious accident rates had risen since OSHA was established. One statistic that measures accidents, the number of job-related injuries that lead to lost time from work, increased 38 percent between 1972 and 1978.

Even more important politically was the frustration felt by business owners who must submit to repeated safety inspections no matter how injury-free their workers had been in the past. Inspections cost businesses time and money even when no fines were handed out for safety violations.

The solution to both these problems, backers of the Schweiker bill said, was to replace the "stick" of inspections and fines against employers with the "carrot" of exemptions for businesses that were successful in protecting workers through their own efforts. Under the bill, businesses that reported a low rate of injuries for a year would be free, in most cases, from the threat of a routine safety inspection during the next year. On the one hand, supporters of the bill asserted, the new approach would allow inspectors to spend all their time on the 10 percent of businesses that were most dangerous to their workers. On the other hand, it would also relieve most business owners from the trouble and expense of inspection. The bill would not make changes in health inspections. Those mainly involved possible exposure to dangerous chemicals, the effects of which frequently do not show up for a number of years.

Objections to the Bill

Labor unions and OSHA officials attacked the bill as both wrong in theory and unworkable in practice. Actually, OSHA had already begun to adopt one of the ideas underlying Schweiker's bill — that inspections should concentrate on the most dangerous types of businesses. Since taking office in 1977, OSHA administrator Eula Bingham had sought to steer agency efforts away from its former "nitpicking" regulation of minor safety violations, and toward major problems likely to cause serious injuries.

Many OSHA standards had been simplified and clarified. More than 11,000 safety and health rules had been critically assessed, and nearly 10 percent had been revoked as obsolete, overly detailed or irrelevant. In addition, 95 percent of all discretionary safety inspections were being targeted on larger workplaces and more hazardous industries.

But, Bingham told the Labor Committee, the existing orientation still retained the "all-important" principle that all businesses remain under OSHA's legal authority. The threat of inspection, no matter how unlikely, made every business conscious of safety, she said — just as the faint possibility of an audit made most taxpayers file an honest return.

A statutory exemption, however, would leave many workers without any protection, Bingham argued. "The bills before you would create two classes of workers — one entitled to full protection under the law, the other relegated to second-class status," she said.

Moreover, opponents of the bill pointed out, there was no way to assume on the basis of one year that a business would be safe the next. Many businesses experienced considerable fluctuations in their injury rates from year to year, for example, because of the installation of new equipment or the hiring of relatively unskilled new workers. "No statistical analysis yet devised of past experience can assure workers that their work places

projects, sponsored by regional health planning units (health systems agencies, or HSAs) with federal technical assistance funds granted for such programs.

"The challenge is to mobilize community resources. The resources for [much disease-prevention] are in those settings, not in the federal government," McGinnis said.

This plan was one example of the task force's style, which emphasized locating and using existing capabilities

— in new expanded roles. "It is not the year to talk about new money," a McGinnis aide noted in 1978.

Task force legislative priorities in 1978 were to enlarge a health screening program for poor children and to add an adolescent pregnancy prevention component to federal family planning programs. The first plan succumbed to objections from congressional conservatives that it set undesirable precedents for federal welfare policies, but the

... Controversy Over OSHA Prevention

are safe while they are working in them," Bingham said.

From a practical standpoint, critics contended, the bill would base its exemptions on inadequate information. Businesses could prove their safety either with their reports to state workers' compensation systems, or by filing affidavits with OSHA. However, state workers' compensation systems varied widely, and often collected inadequate information. Bingham said that, even with federal financial help, few if any of the state systems could supply OSHA with all the information it needed to separate safe from unsafe businesses. And employer affidavits would be subject to falsification, unions worried, even though the affidavits would have to be posted in the workplace.

Previous Legislation

Business owners had been getting a sympathetic response from members of Congress about their complaints against OSHA almost since the agency was founded. But until 1980, they never had any realistic hope of winning a major legislative revision of their foe.

At its birth, OSHA enjoyed solid congressional support — the 1970 legislation that established it passed by overwhelming votes in both House and Senate. Enthusiasm for the agency quickly waned, however, as members began to hear from businesses affected by the first actions implementing the act. By 1972 three congressional panels were holding hearings on business complaints against OSHA. But none of the panels took any action on legislation that year. In fact, the House and Senate labor committees never seriously considered an OSHA reform bill until 1980.

The lack of action on legislation forced congressional hostility to OSHA into another arena — the annual appropriations bill for the Departments of Labor and Health, Education and Welfare. Each year since 1974, the Labor-HEW bill had been the vehicle for new restrictions on the use of funds for OSHA activities.

In the beginning, OSHA amendments to the Labor-HEW appropriations bills concentrated on things like making OSHA consult with businesses on how to eliminate hazards before they were the subject of fines, and freeing small businesses from having to keep elaborate safety records. But attempts to exempt small businesses from OSHA authority were deleted in conference in 1974 and 1975.

The first big wave of successful OSHA limitations came in 1976. That was the year Congress decided that some businesses should be exempt from regulation be-

cause of their small size. Over the next few years this was to be a recurring issue, with business arguing that small businesses should not have to put up with the burden and expense of inspections, and labor responding that a small business was not inherently safer than a large one.

The first size-based exemption, added to the fiscal 1977 Labor-HEW appropriation, applied only to farms with 10 or fewer employees. The other amendment approved that year prohibited inspectors from fining a business for health and safety violations the first time they were detected, unless the violations numbered 10 or more, or involved serious hazards to the workers.

The next qualitative change in congressional OSHA limitations came in 1978, when the idea of basing exemptions on past safety records first appeared. That new idea came not on the appropriations bill, however, but on Small Business Administration (SBA) authorization. Sen. Dewey F. Bartlett, R-Okla. (1973-79), proposed an amendment to the SBA bill that relied on both business size and safety. His amendment, which was approved by the Senate but subsequently gutted in conference, allowed an exemption for businesses with 10 or fewer employees, provided they were in a category of business that, on average, had fewer than seven job injuries a year for every 100 employees.

The same idea reappeared in 1979, this time on the Labor-HEW bill. Sen. Frank Church, D-Idaho, offered an amendment to prohibit inspections of a business with 10 or fewer employees, as long as it was in a category of business experiencing no more than six injuries a year for each 100 employees. That blanket exemption probably would have passed, had not Schweiker proposed an additional amendment allowing continued inspections in cases of imminent danger or fatality.

Another limitation on the Labor-HEW bill that year prohibited OSHA from inspecting businesses that had been inspected by a state safety and health agency in the preceding six months.

The Schweiker bill followed from the ideas presented in Bartlett's and Church's earlier amendments, but with two important differences. Instead of providing exemptions only to small businesses, it would give them to all businesses, regardless of size, provided they met safety requirements. And, instead of basing the exemptions on industry-wide injury statistics, it would make each business qualify on the basis of its own individual safety record.

Given the intensity of labor's opposition, the chances for passage of the Schweiker bill in 1980 appeared slim, although some of the ideas behind it might become law through the vehicle of other legislation.

---

second survived the hostility of anti-abortion members and was enacted. (Appendix, p. 58-A)

Task force subgroups were also working with the Office of Education on a school-based health promotion program, trying to coordinate nutrition programs in HEW and the Department of Agriculture, and planning national conferences on health promotion and nutrition education.

The task force also tackled one of the most difficult

problems in environmental health — testing of industrial substances for carcinogenicity and other health hazards. What testing was done was scattered through federal research and regulatory agencies, and some of the research entities, notably the National Cancer Institute, were criticized by environmentalists for being unresponsive to regulatory needs. (Researchers intent on preserving a basic research capability responded that priorities should come from the scientific data, not the political arena.)

The disease prevention group established a new HEW toxic substances program, combining the testing resources of the National Cancer Institute, the Food and Drug Administration, the National Institute for Occupational Safety and Health and the National Institute of Environmental Health Sciences. Priorities would be set by an advisory committee bringing together the participating research agencies and the regulatory agencies with toxic substances responsibilities — OSHA, the Environmental Protection Agency and the Consumer Product Safety Commission.

Dr. David Rall, director of the environmental health institute and head of the new toxic substances program, said that its work would not duplicate that of an existing interagency liaison group. Participating HEW agencies would each lead in their areas of expertise, but their work would be coordinated to prevent duplications or omissions.

Writing in the May 26, 1978, issue of *Science* magazine, professors Ernest Saward and Andrew Sorenson of the Rochester School of Medicine and Dentistry, concluded, "The most effective means of disease prevention and improved health status lie outside the medical care process and are related to reducing hazards and adopting appropriate personal habits. The medical care process itself has significant measures to offer through both immunizations and secondary prevention by early detection of disease. But partly because of the anticipated restrictions on resource allocation to the health sector in its entirety, the latter approach will be less effective in relation to the funds expended. The conventional view that physicians must do more or that we must have more physicians certainly misses much of the problem that faces us. . . .

"The responsibility for the prevention of disease and disability through health education, improved life-style, and environmental control permeates all aspects of society: the individual, the family, the school, the workplace, and every voluntary agency and level of government. We believe that we can elevate our collective sensibility to that responsibility without further medicalization of our society." ∎

Victims of Environment Hazards Seek Aid

Vietnam veterans exposed to a herbicide so powerful it could strip the leaves from every tree in a forest in 24 hours.... Farmers who pastured their sheep downwind from the U.S. nuclear test site in Nevada.... Soldiers who were marched into the radioactive fallout for "stress tests".... Families living above the buried chemicals at New York's Love Canal.... Farm workers sprayed with agricultural chemicals ... uranium miners, chemical workers....

The number of groups was growing — people who claimed they were victims of harmful health effects from radiation, toxic chemicals or other environmental factors, and wanted help. They wanted the federal government, or someone, to pay their medical bills and compensate them for disabilities they said they had suffered, or might suffer, through no fault of their own — cancer, miscarriages, sterility, birth defects in their children.

In 1980, they were putting new pressures on Congress and the courts for that help. The Vietnam veterans claimed that the potent herbicide Agent Orange sickened them and caused defects in the children they later fathered. Western ranchers and soldiers exposed to radioactive fallout from the Nevada nuclear tests claimed a heightened incidence of cancer. These two groups, apparently the most organized, filed sizable lawsuits and persuaded members of Congress to introduce bills on their behalf. *(Details on agent Orange exposure, box, p. 112; radiation exposure, p. 108)*

Their demands came at a time when the issue of compensation was also surfacing in "superfund" legislation. Bills introduced in the 96th Congress dealing with cleanup costs for chemical spills and waste dumps also contained provisions authorizing either a special compensation fund for "victims" or procedural changes to ease the burden of proof for individuals suing for damages.

In trying to push environmental law beyond disease prevention efforts into the area of compensation, the veterans and other self-identified victim groups were venturing into a legal-scientific quagmire that environmental groups and their congressional allies had generally avoided, for several reasons.

One problem was that illnesses blamed on environmental agents might actually be developed from multiple causes, acting over a long period of time. Victims might never be able to prove the strict cause-and-effect relationship required by most existing legal systems — tort law, state workers' compensation programs, the Veterans Administration (VA) disability program. Another major problem was cost. Compensating an unknown number of victims for illness, long-term disability, and possibly even the lifetime earning losses of their children born with defects, could run into billions of dollars. The federal government has been no more anxious to assume such a burden than was private industry.

But the increasingly militant "victim" groups argued that they should have special help because:
- They were involuntarily exposed.
- They were not informed about possible hazards.

- They could not get aid through existing legal systems because of stiff evidence standards and time limits.

What they wanted was either direct compensation payments or changes in certain legal "presumptions" so that they could more easily collect damages in lawsuits or from existing programs such as those of the Veterans Administration. That would mean major changes in the systems themselves, to accommodate the new concept of environment-related disease.

Legislative Proposals

The victim groups' demands were reflected in a number of bills introduced in 1980:

Agent Orange. Vietnam veterans' education and readjustment bills introduced by Sen. John Heinz, R-Pa., and Rep. Thomas A. Daschle, D-S.D. (S 1872, HR 6050), also established a "presumption" that Agent Orange was a potential cause of compensable disabilities for veterans.

Radiation Exposure. HR 4766, introduced by Gunn McKay, D-Utah, declared the federal government "liable" — financially responsible — for leukemia, thyroid, bone cancer and any other illnesses that might be linked to radiation exposure, for residents of a specified area in Utah, western Nevada and Arizona who lived in the path of radioactive fallout from atmospheric nuclear weapons testing.

In the Senate, Orrin G. Hatch, R-Utah, and Edward M. Kennedy, D-Mass., introduced a broader version (S 1865) that also covered uranium miners.

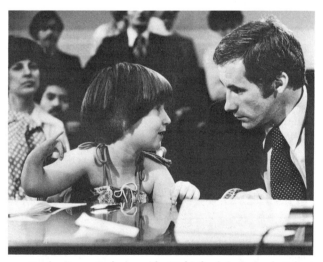

Kerrie Ryan, 8, born with 18 birth defects, and Robert Muller, chairman of the Council of Vietnam Veterans, at House Commerce Oversight and Investigations Subcommittee hearing in June 1979. Kerrie's father was exposed to Agent Orange in Vietnam. Muller's group is seeking compensation for veterans exposed to the toxic chemical.

Compensation for Radiation Damage . . .

"During the time the radiation was out, we worked and we played in it, but we thought it would be okay because we believed it was safe like we were told. . . ."

—Agatha Barnum to Sen. Jake Garn, R-Utah, at St. George, Utah, April 20, 1979

* * *

Between 1945 and 1963, the year of the nuclear test ban treaty, the United States exploded some 235 nuclear devices in atmospheric tests in the Pacific and in Nevada.

The trials at the Nevada test site began in 1951, and radioactive fallout is thought to have drifted into that state, neighboring portions of Utah and Arizona, and perhaps farther. The major population groups exposed to fallout — and who were seeking compensation from the government — were civilians who lived in the path of the drift and civilian and military personnel — as many as 250,000 soldiers, according to one estimate — who took part in the tests.

"Many units were marched or helicoptered to ground zero soon after the explosion. . . . At one test, six volunteers stood at ground zero under an airburst some 20,000 feet above them," Sen. Alan Cranston, D-Calif., told a 1979 Senate hearing.

These people were exposed to ionizing radiation — radiation that is capable of causing illness. It may have one of several effects on human cells, according to the 1979 *Report of the Interagency Task Force on the Health Effects of Ionizing Radiation* — also known as "the Libassi report" after the chairman of the task force, F. Peter Libassi, former general counsel of the Department of Health, Education and Welfare (HEW). The radiation may pass through a cell; it may cause damage which the cell repairs; it may kill a cell. It may also cause irreparable damage that is reproduced in new cells as the injured one divides, resulting in "cancer, developmental abnormalities or genetic damage," the report said.

Evidence on the health effects of relatively small doses of radiation is confusing and not well developed; most of the data linking radiation with human illness comes from studies of the massive "doses" at Nagasaki and Hiroshima. Scientists have not developed a definitive method for relating the size of a low-level dose to its impact, if any, on human health.

At the time of the atmospheric weapons tests, most researchers thought low doses were safe. However, later studies suggested that the risk at low levels is in fact 10 or 20 times greater than was accepted, according to the Libassi report, which also noted that "scientists

now assume that there is no threshold dose level below which radiation exposure is safe." And because of the extraordinarily long "half-life" of radioactive materials, the exposure may continue long after the actual contact if, for example, a person ingests or inhales radioactive particles.

The major sources of low-level exposure are "background" radiation, from cosmic rays and naturally radioactive substances in the environment, and medical exposures such as X-rays. The next largest source is radioactive fallout. Other sources are nuclear energy and consumer products, according to the task force.

Tests Safe, AEC Said

The Atomic Energy Commission (AEC), which was abolished and had its functions split up in 1974, was responsible both for conducting the nuclear tests and monitoring their health effects.

AEC's public position during the 1950s was that the tests were safe. Utah Gov. Scott M. Matheson, D, remembers that "on occasion, residents were advised to remain indoors for an hour or two" during tests, but "the AEC [radio] announcements were quick to remind listeners that 'there is no danger'."

Those public announcements masked internal warnings, which the AEC disregarded and sought to discredit as "Communist inspired" scare stories, according to evidence produced at joint Senate-House committee hearings in April 1979. The warnings were that actual doses were significantly higher than "safe" levels, and that they could cause human illness.

One dramatic early warning came in 1953, when about 17,000 sheep that had been grazing in the path of test fallout died. Exposed sheep herds also showed large numbers of stillbirths and birth defects. Radiation dose levels for those herds were "almost 1,000 times the permissible count for human beings," and public health officials questioned the implications for human health in internal AEC memos, Libassi testified in 1979.

But the AEC ruled out paying damages for the dead sheep, because, as an AEC official told sheepherders at the time, "If we paid for them, every woman that got pregnant and every woman that didn't would sue us."

Another witness at the hearing, Dr. Harold A. Knapp, testified that his 1962-63 study concluded that the AEC had grossly "miscalculated" — by a factor of 1,000 — radiation doses to infants' and children's thyroids from drinking contaminated cow's milk. Reconstructing the sequence from old memoranda, Knapp found that the AEC refused to lower acceptable exposure

---

Superfunds. S 1480, "superfund" legislation introduced by Edmund S. Muskie, D-Maine, and John C. Culver, D-Iowa, was being marked up in early 1980 by the Senate Environment and Public Works Subcommittee on Environmental Pollution and Resource Protection. *(Details, p. 111)*

In the House, John J. LaFalce, D-N.Y., who represented the congressional district where the much-pub-

licized Love Canal toxic chemical dump was located, had also drafted a series of bills to deal with both cleanup costs and compensation for ill health resulting from those chemicals. One version, HR 5291, would pay benefits from a "superfund" financed largely by industry.

Workers' Compensation. Edward P. Beard, D-R.I., whose House Education and Labor Subcommittee on Labor Standards was confronted with a variety of bills to com-

... From U.S. Nuclear Tests Sought

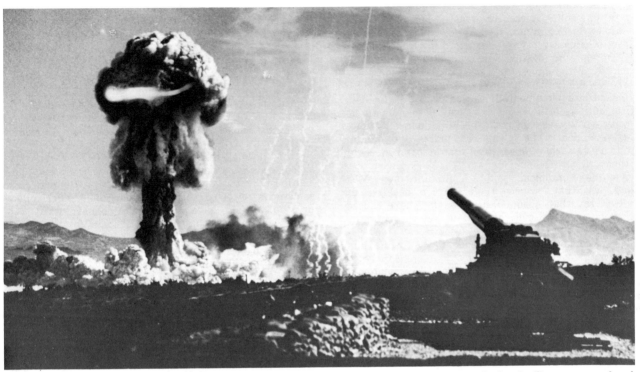

History's first atomic artillery shell was fired at Frenchman's Flat, Nev., in May 1953. Hundreds of military personnel and several members of Congress were present.

levels because a change could create public doubts about the earlier standard, and because of the "world situation." In 1965, Public Health Service officer Edward S. Weiss suggested a link between increased leukemia in southern Utah and the tests, but the report remained an "internal," unpublished document until 1979, said Sen. Orrin G. Hatch, R-Utah.

Over the years, at least 15 congressional panels have concerned themselves with radiation, with hearings on health questions as early as 1963. HEW studies of exposed children for leukemia, bone cancer, thyroid abnormalities and congenital defects were begun, but dropped in 1971. The visibility of the issue in 1979 and 1980 stemmed from 1978 radiation hearings by former Rep. Paul G. Rogers', D-Fla., House Commerce Health Subcommittee. Rogers' hearings, pressures from Utah Gov. Matheson for disclosure of accurate exposure data, and two new studies prompted another round of congressional hearings in 1979.

A 1977 study by HEW's Center for Disease Control found double the expected rate of leukemia among par-

ticipants in a 1957 nuclear test, "Smoky." In 1977-78, Dr. Joseph Lyon of the University of Utah again looked at childhood leukemia rates, and discovered that children born during the test years in areas downwind from the test sites had twice as much leukemia as children born both before and after the tests. The significance of this finding has been questioned by Dr. Marvin Schneiderman of the National Cancer Institute, however. He said other types of cancer in that group dropped during the years leukemia went up — "so did they just get leukemia" instead of another type of cancer they would have gotten anyway?

A Feb. 21, 1980, report in *The Washington Post* raised the possibility that the 1979 Three Mile Island nuclear accident may have produced a new group of "victims." After the accident an unusually large number of children were born with serious thyroid defects in the three Pennsylvania counties near the nuclear plant, according to the story, which also included official denials that the amount of radiation released could have caused the problems.

pensate textile and asbestos workers and uranium miners and revise the "black lung" program for coal miners, opted for a comprehensive approach. His bill (HR 5482) set mandatory federal standards for state workers' compensation programs, including payment for occupational diseases designated by the secretary of labor.

In the Senate, Harrison A. Williams Jr., D-N.J., and Jacob K. Javits, R-N.Y., reintroduced their long-running

proposal (S 420) for advisory federal standards on occupational disease for workers' compensation.

Background

Science has always lagged behind public perceptions that *"something* causes cancer" and other environmental diseases, according to Dr. Irving J. Selikoff, chief of the environmental sciences laboratory at Mt. Sinai School of Medicine in New York and an expert in industrial diseases. He cited a classic, if extreme, example: In 1507 it was reported that women in a German-Czech mining region were remarrying with startling frequency — as many as nine times apiece. The reason: Their husbands, who worked in the mines, died very young. More than four centuries passed before scientists discovered that the miners' premature deaths were caused by radioactive pitchblende in the mines.

The law has been even slower than science to recognize the concept of environmentally caused disease — for both political and scientific reasons. Chemical manufacturers and other businesses that could be hurt financially have resisted the idea, while lawmakers, judges and administrators have sought stronger proof than researchers could give them.

One major problem, said VA Administrator Max Cleland, was that "science can't prove a negative. It can't ever say that Agent Orange *couldn't* have caused these problems. It also hasn't told us yet that it did." Cleland added ruefully that, "Because we can't say yes or no, we get beat over the head in the media and raked over the coals in Congress."

During the 1970s, Congress passed numerous landmark environmental laws — clean air, clean water, toxic substances, pesticide and occupational health statutes, all mandating the elimination or control of pollutants believed to cause illness. But while a basic assumption of the

> *"It may be more costly to litigate on causation and negligence than just to pay, within certain reasonable bounds."*
> —Rep. Bob Eckhardt, D-Texas

legislation was that pollutants harm human health, in only a few cases did Congress go further, to decide that environmental agents had already caused abnormal, compensable conditions.

In 1969 Congress did establish a program to compensate coal miners afflicted with "black lung," a disease caused by prolonged exposure to coal dust. It also compensated a miner's dependents, if he was totally disabled, and his survivors when he died. Originally the federal government paid the claims, at a cost of over $1 billion a year, but in 1978 the law was revised and the responsibility for compensating black lung victims was shifted to the industry. A tax was imposed on all coal mined, to finance trust funds to pay disability and survivors' claims.

Another program, enacted in 1977, compensated Marshall Islanders who were exposed in 1954 to radioactive fallout from a nuclear weapons test and who later developed thyroid cancer and related diseases. In a third instance, the Senate in 1976 approved a bill to compensate Michigan residents who were exposed to polybrominated biphenyls (PBBs) in their food after a 1973 mixup in which livestock feed was contaminated with the toxic chemical. But the House never approved the bill.

In 1978, amid rising concern about the costs of environmental pollution controls, Congress directed the National Center for Health Statistics to begin putting together a national data base on environmental illness, in order to estimate its cost.

Problems in Compensation

Compensation programs for environment-related health problems have been rare because of the unique evidence problems of environmental illness, because of the huge potential expense of such programs, and because concerted support has been lacking in the past.

Evidence

While Agent Orange veterans and other victim groups had emotion on their side, many members of Congress tended to agree with Rep. David E. Satterfield III, D-Va., that "we as legislators ought to leave the decision up to the scientists" on whether specific environmental factors in fact are to blame for various ailments.

But lawmakers have often felt sandbagged when they asked scientists for decisions. Researchers interpreted data cautiously, often disparaged each others' findings, and sometimes retracted their own conclusions after follow-up studies. Said Selikoff, lawyers often have asked "scientists to do something they just hate to do — give quantitative information" about exposure and illness. Members have felt particularly exasperated by scientific ambiguities when their constituents were pressing them to take action. "More study . . . that's all professors want. They never get anything out," observed McKay. "At some point, we [in Congress] have to make decisions."

The chief scientific-legal problem of compensation has been that so little has been known about many serious illnesses such as cancer and birth defects. And the fact that many of these disorders were common made it difficult to prove that a specific case was not an "act of God, and not Dow Chemical," as a congressional aide put it.

For example, some 30 percent of pregnancies ended in miscarriages and up to 8 percent of babies were born with defects in 1980. Pinpointing the cause in every case was beyond science, particularly since Agent Orange and radiation exposures were probably at fairly low levels. Scientists had the most trouble with low-level exposures because it was harder to rule out other "competing" potential causes of cancer. In addition, many of the complaints of Agent Orange veterans and individuals living near toxic waste sites and spills — fatigue, neurological sensations, psychological problems — could also be explained by other factors. Cleland said VA doctors found most of these symptoms in veterans of World Wars I and II.

Against this background, the "victims" have had trouble developing clear proof that their cases were uniquely deserving of special treatment. Many workers' compensation plans have not covered what have been called "ordinary diseases of life." In general, workers' compensation, public assistance, private insurance plans, the VA compensation program and tort law have been far more responsive to acute illnesses and accidents than to chronic, environment-related disease. So that liability can be determined, most required very specific evidence, both of the exposure itself and of the connection between the substance and medical symptoms. (A major problem for both the Agent Orange veterans and radiation victims has been lack of complete records documenting their actual exposures.)

There were also time limits that did not take into account the long latency periods during which chronic diseases develop. For example, the VA had only a one-year "presumption" period under which a veteran could claim benefits for cancer — which usually has a latency period of 20 to 30 years. Senate Labor and Human Resources Committee aide Michael L. Goldberg summed up the problem: "One minute a guy is operating a punch press and he has five fingers, and the next minute he has four. You know when, where, how and why it happened. But cancer...? Did he get it from benzene, or the time he worked in a pesticide plant, or from smoking, or because his father had it?"

Cost

With the rapid escalation of medical costs firmly fixed in members' minds by the three-year struggle over hospital cost control, the expense of medical compensation assumed particular importance to Congress. And the thought of compensating for long-term disability for an unknown number of victims was even more sobering.

Even sympathetic members like Rep. Bob Eckhardt, D-Texas, favored only very narrow relief for specific groups. "In a perfect society, we would take care of victims of disease. But if we can't even provide hospitalization and medical care, we can hardly agree to compensate" on a general basis, Eckhardt said.

To cite just one example, rough estimates for cleaning up the Love Canal chemical dump have been put at $30 million to $40 million, while residents were reportedly seeking as much as $2 billion or $3 billion in damages (health and disability as well as property). Costs for larger groups or more severe health problems could be astronomical.

The 1979 *Report of the Interagency Task Force on the Health Effects of Ionizing Radiation*, put together by a Carter administration group, backed off the compensation issue because of cost problems. Since clinicians were unable to look at most cancer and say what caused it, there were only two policy options, according to the report: to pay for all illnesses that could have been caused by an environmental agent — whether or not they were — or to pay for none. For cost reasons, the administration did not include victim compensation in its superfund bill (S 1341, HR 4566, HR 4571), and the president "certainly would oppose" direct compensation in any legislation passed by Congress, according to an Office of Management and Budget source.

Eckhardt, whose House Commerce Oversight Subcommittee held hearings on dioxin, radiation and toxic substances, suggested that "it may be more costly to litigate on causation and negligence than just to pay, within certain reasonable bounds." But he also suggested a tradeoff to resolve the cost problem. His solution would be to ease evidence requirements, making it easier for a victim to recover damages, but to place limits on the amount of damage awards, and the groups that could qualify for them.

Lack of Support

In the past, environmental groups have not pushed for victim compensation, because their resources were limited and because they regarded prevention and cleanup as more urgent priorities — much as medical researchers have argued that funds spent on discovering a polio vaccine did more good for more people than dollars invested in iron lungs for those who already had the disease. The Environmental Protection Agency (EPA) shared that basic assumption. So did key members of Congress such as

James J. Florio, D-N.J., chairman of the House Commerce Transportation Subcommittee, one of several panels with "superfund" jurisdiction.

Potentially powerful lobby coalitions — for instance, environmentalists, labor organizations and farm workers exposed to pesticides — had not materialized by early 1980, although that could change. Another factor in past inaction was that, until the superfund legislation came along, compensation showed up in Congress as a parochial issue. Members limited their bills to a specific problem in their state or district, or to a special group such as the veterans. "Narrowing the group" to limit the potential cost of a bill has been a respected legislative tactic for softening opposition. But a narrow bill might not attract broad enough support to pass. Such bills have had a high failure rate in the past.

Not only was support for environmental disease compensation weak, but there was strong industry opposition to the idea. The chemical industry continued to raise serious questions about the concept of environmental illness, per se, as well as about the validity of charges against specific substances. Chemical and other companies resisted incorporating the concepts of "environmental" or "occupational" disease into law.

When the Occupational Safety and Health Administration (OSHA) began formulating a "cancer policy" to streamline agency action on suspected carcinogens, a million-dollar lobby, the American Industrial Health Council, was created to fight that proposal.

The Dow Chemical Co. successfully blocked past federal actions to remove the suspect component of Agent Orange from the domestic market, and was in 1980 actively contesting veterans' claims in a major federal court suit in New York. It was not that the product contributed significantly to Dow's profits. "This stuff is .000 percent of a nine-and-a-quarter billion-dollar-a-year business," said Dow spokesman Phillip Schneider. The real issue was the quality of scientific findings on which legal decisions were made, said Dow attorney Don Freyer. After 30 years of manufacturing the herbicide, Dow had "a large data base that just eloquently demonstrates that this isn't harmful. If we can't demonstrate it in this case, then no one can make any chemicals," Freyer warned.

Outlook

The solution most favored by victim groups — direct compensation funds — seemed least likely to succeed in 1980 because of congressional and Carter administration concerns about new spending. Two Senate environment subcommittees narrowed the broad compensation provision in S 1480, the superfund bill — a provision so broad that "every cancer victim in the U.S. could collect," a chemical industry lobbyist charged.

In a key decision Feb. 19, 1980, the subcommittees ruled out direct compensation for cancer or other long-latency diseases from the fund. The fund would provide supplementary payments for individuals who had brought court actions but were dissatisfied with settlements. The panels also approved controversial changes in federal court rules, to ease the burden of proof for individuals suing chemical manufacturers or others for out-of-pocket medical damages. They would allow as evidence materials that had not usually been admitted, such as animal data and small-group epidemiological studies of humans, and would permit a plaintiff to show a "reasonable likelihood"

Agent Orange: 10-Year Controversy . . .

"Each day we would finish our duties absolutely drenched with [Agent] Orange — our fatigues totally saturated and the defoliant actually dripping from our hair. . . . I can attest to excellent health for myself as well as other soldiers with whom I've subsequently maintained contact."

—Maj. Donald R. Taylor, U.S. Army Chemical Corps, in a 1978 letter to Rep. David E. Satterfield III, D-Va.

* * *

"Very few toxic substances have been shown to affect such a wide range of [human] body systems, and nothing in the industrial environment approaches TCDD [the contaminant in Agent Orange] in how very little of it" can affect biological systems.

—Dr. Marion Moses, Environmental Sciences Laboratory, Mt. Sinai School of Medicine

* * *

Agent Orange was a chemical used by the U.S. Army in Vietnam to defoliate the dense jungles that provided cover for the enemy, and to destroy food crops. It was a combination of two herbicides — 2,4-D and 2,4,5-T, which also has been used domestically for about 30 years to control broad-leaf weeds.

Thousands of U.S. soldiers may have been exposed to Agent Orange in Vietnam, according to a General Accounting Office (GAO) study done at the request of Sen. Charles H. Percy, R-Ill. Unlike Major Taylor, many of those veterans blamed that exposure for a long list of health disorders, and they were suing the manufacturers of Agent Orange for damages.

The veterans claimed the chemical caused cancer, liver damage, psychological and neurological symptoms such as depression, sleeplessness, tingling or loss of sensation in limbs, malfunctioning of the body's disease-fighting ("immune") system, miscarriages, stillbirths, and a broad range of birth defects in their children.

The component of Agent Orange that is suspected of causing diseases, TCDD, is a contaminant of 2,4,5-T — that is, a substance inadvertently created, in varying amounts, in the manufacturing process. TCDD is the "most toxic" of approximately 75 chemical compounds known as dioxins, according to Dr. Marion Moses of the Environmental Sciences Laboratory at Mt. Sinai School of Medicine in New York.

"Very few toxic substances have been shown to affect such a wide range of [human] body systems, and nothing in the industrial environment approaches TCDD in how very little of it" can affect biological systems, he told a House Commerce Oversight and Investigations Subcommittee hearing in June 1979.

But the manufacturers insisted the herbicide was safe. Dow Chemical Co. said that in its 30-year history of producing it, there had been only one incident of illness among exposed workers — a 1964 outbreak of chloracne, a persistent and sometimes painful skin rash. That exposure resulted from an accident, not from normal manufacturing processes, and produced no "excess" illnesses or deaths, according to Dow attorney Don Freyer.

Dow and four other manufacturers were fighting the veterans' class action lawsuit, and said the Veterans Administration (VA) should be responsible for any claims.

The only condition the VA recognized as Agent Orange-related was chloracne.

Research Studies, Theories

Dr. Irving J. Selikoff, chief of the Mt. Sinai laboratory, said that dioxins might interfere in the body's basic metabolic processes by stimulating abnormal enzyme production by the liver. Enzymes are essential to such body processes as producing hormones, converting food into energy, and thinking.

Metabolic disorder is a relatively new concept, and many of its effects might still be so novel or subtle as to elude existing analytic techniques. Animal research suggested that almost unimaginably small specks of the substance could have an effect on living organisms.

But animal studies had not yet supported claims of human illness, VA Administrator Max Cleland contended. He wanted scientists to show him "how chronic animal exposure over two years relates to random and incidental exposure of troops on the ground."

Accidental industrial exposures to dioxin have provided the only evidence to date on human health effects. A study by Dr. Raymond R. Suskind, director of the Institute of Environmental Health at the University of Cincinnati, and Monsanto epidemiologist Judith A. Zack, reported in the January 1980 *Journal of Occupational Medicine*, found no "excess" deaths from either cancer or cardiovascular disease in an exposed group from an industrial explosion in 1949 at Nitro, W.Va.

Selikoff dismissed Suskind's study as "terrible," and said his researchers found "excess" cardiovascular deaths reported among workers who cleaned up after a 1963 dioxin accident in Holland. In both instances, however, conclusions were tentative because of the small size of the groups studied.

Decade of Controversy

Dioxins were a subject of controversy throughout the 1970s. There have been efforts to ban them, and objections that there was not enough human evidence to justify a ban.

In May 1970 the Agriculture Department (USDA) moved to end the use of 2,4,5-T products on food crops and near homes, recreation sites and other areas. According to Steven D. Jellinek, who traced dioxin regulatory efforts for the House commerce subcommittee in 1979, the USDA action was based on a National Institutes of Health study linking TCDD to stillbirths and malformations in laboratory animals. Jellinek subsequently directed the toxic substances program at the Environmental Protection Agency (EPA).

The Defense Department also ended its Agent Orange spraying in Vietnam in 1970 — for political reasons, according to Maj. Gen. Garth Dettinger, deputy surgeon general of the Air Force. Between 1965 and 1970 the department sprayed 10.7 million gallons of Agent Orange,

... Over Health Effects on Humans

at a rate of about 3 gallons, undiluted, per acre, in concentrations much stronger than those used domestically.

"I would say purely as a sop to the political, this [spraying] was one of the programs we felt should be removed to decrease the opposition to our involvement" in Southeast Asia, Dettinger told the House Veterans' Affairs Subcommittee on Medical Facilities and Benefits in October 1978.

Also in 1970, the Monsanto Co. ceased 2,4,5-T production — but "not at all" for health reasons, according to spokesman Dan R. Bishop. The subcontractor that fabricated the basic chemical was no longer able to supply it to Monsanto because of Defense Department priorities, and Monsanto's own plant at Nitro, W. Va., was "too old" to be put back into production, Bishop said.

In 1972, the ban on 2,4,5-T products was successfully challenged by Dow in a court suit against the EPA, which had taken over most of the Agriculture Department's regulatory responsibilities for agricultural chemicals.

EPA started up ban proceedings again the following year, but abandoned the process and turned to studies instead. While laboratory data showed that "even ... minute quantities of dioxin" could cause cancer, birth defects and other problems in animals, EPA needed a firm link — then lacking — between that animal evidence and human health risk, Jellinek said. Congress had, by law, required EPA to have such a link as

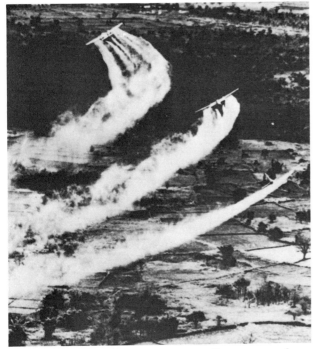

U.S. Air Force planes spray Agent Orange over dense vegetation in South Vietnam in 1966 to destroy enemy cover. A 1979 General Accounting Office study said thousands of U.S. troops were exposed to the toxic chemical.

"reasonable basis" for beginning proceedings to remove substances from the market, Jellinek noted.

A massive 1974 National Academy of Sciences study of Agent Orange found no "definitive indication of direct damage by herbicides to human health," but suggested that was because there wasn't enough research on human exposure to show what the hazards might be. It urged further studies because stories of dioxin-related illness among Vietnamese were "so consistent that they could not be dismissed."

By 1977, Vietnam veterans were beginning to contact the VA about health problems they believed were caused by their exposure to the defoliant. The issue made headlines early in 1978 when a Chicago CBS affiliate aired a program on the veterans' claims.

1979 Developments

In 1979, as the issue heated up further, there were these developments:

● EPA suspended the use of 2,4,5-T on forests, rights of way and pastures on the basis of a study prompted by complaints from women in Alsea, Ore., that they suffered miscarriages shortly after the herbicide was sprayed near their homes.

● Agent Orange victims formed an organization and launched a massive class action suit in New York against the five corporations that had supplied the federal government with the herbicide: Dow Chemical, Monsanto, Thompson-Hayward Chemical Co., Hercules Inc. and Diamond Shamrock Corp. On behalf of themselves and their children who had been born with birth defects, the veterans asked the court to order the companies to set up a fund to pay medical and disability expenses. More than 300 persons had become parties to the suit.

● Two GAO reports, in April and November 1979, urged a long-term study of persons exposed to Agent Orange during military service. The second report also backed up veterans' claims that they had been sprayed directly or moved into areas immediately after spraying, contrary to Defense Department assertions that ground troops did not enter defoliated areas until many weeks after spraying.

● Studies proliferated. The Air Force began developing a six-year study of 1,200 persons who participated in one of the major spraying missions ("Operation Ranch Hand"). Congress ordered the VA to undertake a study of Agent Orange victims. President Carter vetoed a companion bill calling for a study of civilian exposure to the substance, but established an Agent Orange task force to coordinate federal agency studies and directed the Health, Education and Welfare (HEW) Department to study the problem anyway.

The VA ran a quick, small-scale study and found traces of dioxins in the body fat of both Vietnam veterans and a control group of individuals who had not been in Southeast Asia. It then made plans for the long-range study ordered by Congress. The VA and HEW established registries of persons exposed to the herbicides.

● About 4,800 Vietnam veterans had sought VA treatment and 750 had filed compensation claims for illness they attributed to Agent Orange as of early 1980.

that exposure to a substance caused his illness, a much looser standard than the existing requirement for a "preponderance of evidence." It would then be up to the defendant to prove that the exposure did not cause the injury.

Of the various victim groups, the veterans appeared most likely to get some help, because they were organized, they were not asking for something totally new, and because Congress was very sensitized to veterans' demands. The veterans mainly wanted better access to the existing VA compensation system, whose standards of proof were more lenient than those of case law. A veteran did not have to prove that military service actually caused a disabling condition, only that the condition originated during the time he was on active duty. Prodding from Senate Veterans' Affairs Committee Chairman Alan Cranston, D-Calif., moved the VA to liberalize and systematize its consideration of radiation disability claims. The Defense Department also began to reconstruct exposure records, to aid veterans in filing their claims.

The civilian radiation victims, aided by former Interior Secretary Stewart Udall, brought three major lawsuits against the government.

Compared with the radiation victims, who had decades of hearings and studies behind them, the Agent Orange veterans appeared to be starting a very long process. They also were focusing on a major lawsuit, against the chemical manufacturers.

Congress Seeks Greater Role in NIH Research

Efforts to give Congress a greater voice in deciding federal health research spending priorities touched off a heated tug-of-war between a House health committee and much of the nation's biomedical research community in 1980.

At issue was a bill (HR 7036) that would authorize specific dollar amounts over a three-year period for each of the 11 National Institutes of Health (NIH). The bill had been ordered reported by the House Commerce Committee May 6, 1980.

Unlike most federal programs, most of the institutes had not required authorizations in order to obtain appropriations — and the health research establishment wanted to keep it that way. Sponsors said the bill simply was meant to provide guidelines for appropriations — and thus avoid drastic funding cuts, and to ensure that Congress would rationally determine NIH spending priorities. But opponents of the measure were alarmed at the prospect of NIH losing its special funding status, and with it, some of the research community's influence over the distribution of health research dollars.

Some scientists feared that if Congress set research priorities, NIH would tilt more toward diseases with high public interest, such as cancer and heart disease, and away from less visible "pure" scientific research. Opponents also argued that adding another layer of congressional involvement in the funding process — the authorizing committees — could lead to delays and thus endanger ongoing research efforts.

Backers of the legislation accused the opposition of conducting an "hysterical" lobbying campaign against the bill. They said opponents were "reactionary," "overly fearful," and had purposely spread misinformation about what the legislation would do.

Lobbyists opposed to authorizations for the institutes shifted their attack from the Senate to the House after provisions objectionable to them were removed from the Senate NIH bill (S 988). Those provisions had authorized specific spending levels for the institutes and set expiration dates for most of the authorizations. The original Senate bill had provided that the institutes would "cease to exist" at the end of the authorization period unless Congress specifically extended their authority.

Only two of the 11 NIH research institutes had specific authorizations: the National Cancer Institute and the Heart, Lung and Blood Institute. They were reauthorized in 1978, with the authorizations due to expire Sept. 30, 1980. The other nine institutes were funded on the basis of general research authority given to the Department of Health and Human Services (HHS, formerly HEW) by the Public Health Service Act. HHS spent most of the federal government's medical research dollars, with NIH receiving the largest single allocation.

Massive Research Program

There was good reason why the battle to gain or keep control over research funds was fierce. NIH probably was the largest and best funded biomedical research entity in the world. It has provided a consistent infusion of dollars for research across the nation, particularly in academic institutions, which have depended heavily on federal funds.

With an annual budget in fiscal 1980 of almost $3.5 billion, NIH provided over two-thirds of federal funds spent for health research, according to HHS. Almost 90 percent of the budget was used to support research at universities, medical centers, hospitals and other research institutions. More than 1,200 institutions, located in every state and some foreign countries, received NIH funds; about one-fourth of them were education institutions.

NIH's intramural research — work done inside the institution, by NIH staff — employed about 6,400 persons and took up about 10 percent of the NIH budget in 1980. And for almost every major health problem, there existed a constituency — a group of organizations plugging its own health research agenda. Most organizations keyed their efforts to supporting one of NIH's 11 institutes. Other groups, such as those representing medical colleges or social scientists, worked for across-the-board changes or funding increases.

NIH has grown rapidly since the first institute, the National Cancer Institute, was established in 1938, but the authorizations have varied. The cancer and heart institutes have specific authorizations by name and amount, primarily as a result of legislation that was the product of an era of "great cancer scares" and fears about an increasing degree of heart trouble, noted an HHS official. Some institutes have been authorized by name without specific figures, and still others have been funded only on the basis of the HHS department's general research authority.

The Senate June 19 unanimously approved its version of NIH Registration, making some changes in the institutes' structure and makeup.

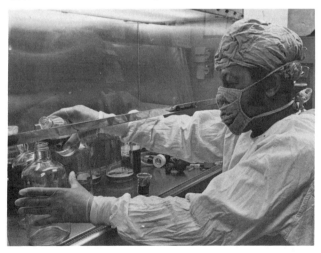

National Cancer Institute Scientist in Hot Virus Laboratory

Opposition to the Bill

The Association of American Medical Colleges (AAMC) led the opposition to the House subcommittee bill. AAMC spokesmen claimed the legislation was both unnecessary and potentially harmful to health research efforts. In a March 1980 letter to the House Commerce Subcommittee on Health, the AAMC attached the names of 37 other organizations that also opposed the bill, most of them associations for health professionals. Some of those groups later reversed their positions to support the legislation. The AAMC, however, remained adamant in its opposition.

AAMC officials contended that by authorizing specific amounts over a certain time period, the bill would threaten the existence of the institutes and place ceilings on the funds that could be appropriated. They feared that if funding proposals underwent more review — particularly if authorizing committees conducted very thorough reviews — requests could be pared down and interest groups would wield considerably less influence. They said they also worried that authorizations might not be passed in

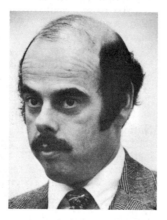

"I've been amazed at the reaction to the bill — somewhat bordering on hysteria. . . . I think [the medical colleges] are afraid of any change in the status quo."
—Rep. Henry A. Waxman, D-Calif.

timely fashion, leading to interruptions in funding. The long-range outcome, opponents contended, would be fewer dollars for health research and a new set of priorities that put popularity above scientific considerations.

Backers of the bill responded that the legislation would protect research funding. Guidelines such as those provided in the bill, they said, would provide a stable base for future appropriations requests. Said Rep. Tim Lee Carter, R-Ky., ranking minority member on the House health subcommittee, "If we cut down on research we'd really be in trouble. At the present time there's just too much flexibility. I think it's customary to have an authorization set by the Congress. This just adds another safeguard to the process."

AAMC spokesmen also argued that by actively exercising their authorizing powers, the congressional committees would take research decisions out of the hands of those most familiar with them — the scientists themselves. Specific authorizations also would limit NIH's ability to follow scientific breakthroughs, opponents said. (To deal with that criticism, the House subcommittee added an amendment authorizing $100 million over the three years covered by the bill to be used for pursuing unexpected leads or discoveries.)

House committee members admitted the bill could

set the stage for a reordering of funding priorities that relied more heavily on public interest. A spokesman for one member, Barbara A. Mikulski, D-Md., said efforts were likely in future years to increase funding for practical applications with more public appeal than basic scientific research. Supporters of the bill contended that it was totally appropriate for Congress to perform that function, since NIH was spending taxpayers' money.

Intense Lobbying

Rep. Henry A. Waxman, D-Calif., chairman of the House health subcommittee, characterized the lobbying against the bill as "intense." "I've been amazed at the reaction to the bill — somewhat bordering on hysteria, by some of the medical colleges particularly," he said. "I think they're afraid of any change in the status quo." Waxman and spokesmen for several key committee members charged that misinformation had been prominent in the campaign against the bill. Committee members received numerous letters from organizations that promote health research, from professional associations and from deans of medical colleges. They expressed fears that the bill would endanger future health research funding and the existence of the institutes themselves. A primary argument was that the committee should take more time to consider the legislation.

The time factor was perhaps the most prominent among AAMC's stated reasons for opposing the bill. Association spokesman Thomas Morgan contended, "There really has been so little time for discussion, for people to take a look at what is being proposed, that almost every day [has] brought a new revelation" about its possible impact. "The more we look at it, the more snakes we discover," said another AAMC representative.

But Waxman said he believed the AAMC, in its zeal to counter the proposal, had purposely spread "misleading" information about the bill. As a result, Waxman said, he resorted to writing medical colleges to explain the bill and to counter charges that it would put permanent ceilings on biomedical research funds and "sunset" the research institutes.

House Committee Action

Despite strong lobbying against the bill, the House Commerce Committee voted May 6, 1980, to order it reported and subject all the institutes to the authorizing process. The measure had been approved by the health subcommittee March 19 by voice vote.

Action on the bill had been held up while the Carter administration revised its position, reversing itself on major points such as the proposal to authorize specific amounts for each institute.

As approved by the committee, HR 7036 authorized a total of $3.8 billion for the 11 institutes for fiscal 1981, $4.4 billion for 1982 and $4.9 billion for 1983. Also authorized were funds for National Research Service Awards (grants to pre- and post-doctoral students of biomedical science) — $719 million over the three fiscal years. The bill also authorized support for cancer research centers for five years; the centers would be funded by the National Cancer Institute without the ceiling on expenditures in existing law.

A total of $100 million was authorized over the three-year period for research on scientific "breakthroughs." The bill prohibited the use of the Department of Health

Fiscal 1980 NIH Appropriations

(millions of dollars, figures rounded)

Institute	Appropriations
Cancer	$1,000
Heart, Lung, Blood	528
Arthritis, Metabolism, Digestive Diseases	341
Aging	70
Allergy, Infectious Diseases	215
Child Health, Human Development	209
Dental Research	68
Eye	113
Neurological, Communicative Disorders, Stroke	242
General Medical Sciences	312
Environmental Health Sciences	84

and Human Services' general research authority as a fallback in the event that funds were not authorized in the future for a particular institute. Instead, HR 7036 provided that if Congress did not act to approve a different authorization for fiscal 1984, the institutes would receive 15 percent more than the fiscal 1983 amount for the next year.

The committee bill required that institute advisory councils would have to review major NIH contracts. In the past, councils have reviewed grant applications, but not other types of research funding. The councils, some of which would be created in law for the first time under the bill, would be composed of biomedical scientists, social and behavioral scientists, lay persons and non-voting administration officials.

During markup, the Commerce Committee adopted a Waxman amendment limiting advisory council review of NIH contracts to agreements costing $500,000 or above. The original bill required advisory council review for contracts of $50,000 or more. The amendment was suggested by representatives of biomedical research interest groups.

In another change in review provisions, the committee accepted a Waxman amendment to clarify that NIH's in-house research would be reviewed as a program, rather than project by project, another change sought by research interests.

In other provisions, HR 7036 established the position of director of NIH and clarified his authority; created a new assistant directorship for promoting prevention, education and health information programs; required an annual report by the director to Congress and the administration, including a five-year plan for NIH activities and policies; and directed the establishment of information centers on certain diseases.

The committee adopted amendments that:

● Added $90 million in fiscal 1981, $108 million in 1981 and $130 million in 1983 for new and existing cancer research demonstration centers.

● Provided that students accepting National Research Service Awards for less than a year's work would not be subject to "pay-back" provisions requiring them to teach or perform a similar service.

● Established a system for collecting, analyzing and distributing information based on studies of diabetes patients and data on the risk to the general population of developing diabetes.

The committee rejected by a 2-11 vote an attempt by William E. Dannemeyer, R-Calif., to cut authorizations for the institutes across-the-board by an average of 6 percent, an estimated $403 million reduction.

Senate Bill

As approved by the Senate Labor and Human Resources Subcommittee on Health and Scientific Research April 24 and by the full committee May 8, S 988 was a skeleton of the measure introduced by Kennedy in April 1979. The revised version was designed to accommodate the concerns of various health interest groups and subcommittee members who sought changes. Amendments knocking out provisions opposed by the research community were made informally through successive redrafts, according to subcommittee aide Robert Graham.

When the subcommittee took up the measure April 24, it simply accepted a motion to consider the revised draft as the bill. No amendments were offered, and the bill was approved by voice vote. Full committee approval also was routine.

David Blumenthal, a former health subcommittee staff member who helped draft the original bill, said the provision setting specific authorization levels and expiration dates was removed "largely because it seemed to aggravate the interest groups, and it really wasn't that important." He added, "It just may not be realistic to provide forced reviews" of the institutes.

As approved by the committee, S 988 authorized the existence of each of the 11 NIH institutes by name and function — but without specific dollar amounts. It also authorized an advisory council for each institute.

The "centerpiece" provision of the bill would establish a 16-member, presidentially appointed council to review health research spending priorities and make recommendations concerning NIH's annual budget to the administration and Congress. This provision, which Graham called the most important innovation in the bill, was opposed by the administration and most of the interest groups that had taken positions on the measure.

The council's recommendations would be in the form of suggested "ranges" — maximums and minimums — for funding levels. The council would play "a major role in advising [Congress] of relative priorities," said Graham.

In addition to developing annual proposals for NIH research goals and spending priorities, the council would conduct a comprehensive study to project health research needs in the years 1985 to 2000. The study, which probably would be done by the National Academy of Sciences, would have to be completed by 1985.

Proponents of the bill said that as a result of these provisions, Congress would be less susceptible to appeals for funding based on the traditional "disease-of-the month" syndrome, under which priorities for NIH funding have been determined in large part by the visibility and emotional appeal of particular diseases.

Administration Position

Initially, the administration had strongly objected to major parts of both the Senate and House committees' bills. HHS Secretary Patricia Roberts Harris, in a March 1980 letter to House Commerce Committee Chairman Harley O. Staggers, D-W.Va., said the department only wanted a simple extension of authority for the two institutes with expiring authorizations. She listed several provisions that "we believe would increase the administrative burdens of the National Institutes of Health and adversely affect the ongoing research programs at the component institutes."

Among them were authorized dollar amounts for each institute, elimination of a provision in existing law allowing shifts of funds under general departmental research authority, and extension of requirements for advisory council review to include contracts rather than just grants.

At one point top NIH officials came up with their own "marked-up" version of the bill as introduced, which they circulated to interested organizations. According to an NIH spokesman, the proposal was simply an attempt to solicit views on what changes should be sought in the legislation. However, the effort was halted after word of it reached committee members and top department officials, an HHS spokesman said.

In addition, some NIH officials individually contacted committee members and major research interests to discuss their opinions of the bill. For example, while visiting Duke University in North Carolina for a lecture, NIH Director Donald S. Fredrickson discussed the bill with university officials. Duke had been receiving some $40 million annually in federal grants and contracts for medical research, the bulk of it from NIH, according to William Anlyan, the university's vice president for health affairs. Duke officials consulted with subcommittee member Richardson Preyer, D-N.C., Anlyan said, but decided not to oppose the bill actively.

Senate Bill

On June 19, the Senate unanimously passed its version of the NIH bill (S 988), providing statutory authority for NIH and creating a 16-member council to make recommendations to the president and Congress on health research priorities and funding levels.

It specifically authorized the 11 health institutes, their directors and advisory councils, and made some changes in their structure and makeup. It did not, as in the original version of S 988, set termination dates for the institutes. Nor did it provide specific dollar authorizations, as did the bill reported by the House Commerce Committee.

Sponsors said the legislation was designed to protect NIH funding and bring more orderly planning to federal health research efforts.

The President's Council for Health Sciences established by the bill was charged with making annual recommendations on health research priorities and funding levels, as well as studying long-range health research needs. This provision, which met at best a lukewarm reception from the administration and interest groups, was labeled the "major element" of S 988 by chief sponsor Edward M. Kennedy, D-Mass., chairman of the Human Resources Subcommittee on Health and Scientific Research.

The only specific dollar authorization included in S 988 was $123.6 million over three years for diabetes and arthritis research and training centers, arthritis demonstration projects and national advisory boards on diabetes, arthritis and digestive diseases.

The bill required experimental programs to provide alternative methods for reviewing research grant proposals to provide an appeals process for applicants rejected for grants, and to try methods for reducing paperwork required of grant applicants. It also authorized the director of NIH to use a certain percentage of funds taken from the individual institutes each year to promote certain priority research.

Floor Amendments. Before passing S 988, the Senate adopted amendments:

● By David Pryor, D-Ark., to extend through fiscal 1981 federal funding for state efforts to identify fraud in Medicaid, the state-federal health program for the poor and disabled. The federal aid was due to expire at the end of fiscal 1980. That would mean a number of the 29 existing fraud control units would have to be shut down, while other states might not open units, Pryor said.

● By Howard M. Metzenbaum, D-Ohio, making the National Institute of Allergy and Infectious Disease responsible for research into Reye's Syndrome, a potentially fatal disease found in people recovering from viral illnesses.

Congress Considers Major Food Law Review

Under pressure from angry consumer activists, farmers and food industry representatives, Congress had been expected in 1979 to undertake a major review of federal food law. In the end, although no action was taken that year, the issue remained a thorny one that was likely to be debated in future Congresses.

The principal target of demands for change in the law was the 20-year old Delaney amendment, which flatly prohibits any food additive that "induces" cancer in man or animals. The growing movement for change coincided with the fact that an 18-month ban on the artificial sweetener saccharin had been due to expire in May 1979. The House voted overwhelmingly to extend the moratorium on the ban, and Food and Drug Administration (FDA) officials said they would wait for a final congressional decision before resuming proceedings to ban saccharin. On May 15, 1980, the Senate Labor and Human Resources Committee approved the House-passed ban (HR 4453); it cleared the full chamber June 9 by voice vote. Added to the saccharin controversy were FDA efforts to ban the meat preservative sodium nitrite and certain animal drugs.

Saccharin helps diabetics and people with weight problems, according to its many advocates. Similarly, meat processors and farmers contended that nitrites and animal drugs had major benefits. Opponents of the Delaney clause said the law was too rigid because it recognized neither the benefits of the suspect substances nor the fact that scientists had developed the ability to measure quantities of those substances far smaller than anyone had imagined in 1958, when the amendment was enacted.

In the following two decades, scientists had so refined chemical detection techniques that they were able to measure unimaginably tiny particles — parts per billion or per trillion of a substance. Such tiny quantities surely could not harm human health, opponents of the Delaney clause argued.

And with the new testing capacity, traces of previously undetected chemicals might start showing up in a broad range of foods previously considered risk-free, opponents added. "It will turn out that everything we eat is carcinogenic at some level," suggested Frank Slover, spokesman for the industry-backed Calorie Control Council.

Former FDA Commissioner Donald Kennedy conceded that common sense suggested that exceedingly small quantities of suspect chemicals were safe. But, he added, "common sense also tells us the world is flat," and certain chemicals are toxic at the most minute level.

At the close of the 1970s, science still had not answered the major question on which the 1958 Delaney clause was based: whether there was a "safe" level of human consumption for substances that caused cancer in laboratory animals. *(Testing problems, box, p. 120)*

Even if a safe level, or "threshold," were established for an individual, "we could not be sure that your threshold was the same as mine, due to differences in genetic background and our inventory of habits, good and bad," Kennedy said.

While industry critics and farmers faulted the rigidity of the Delaney clause, consumer activists found another problem with it: the loopholes. Depending on how a potential carcinogen entered the food supply, regulatory restrictions have been more, or less, tight. Additives approved by the FDA before 1958 were permanently exempt from Delaney. From a health perspective, "there is no particular reason to treat these things selectively," Kennedy contended.

Both sides agreed in principle that Congress should tidy up the inconsistencies in the Food, Drug and Cosmetic Act. But where the Calorie Control Council sought relaxation, consumer activists like Michael Jacobson of the Center for Science in the Public Interest wanted more, not less, protection.

Consumers themselves appeared to have mixed feelings about how far Congress and federal regulators should go to protect them from the potential hazards of food additives. On the one hand, FDA moves against popular substances like saccharin provoked strong protests. But consumers were also convinced that "the American public needs protection from the food industry," according to a preliminary report on food additive hearings conducted in 1978 by the FDA.

Other Pressures

Meanwhile, other developments were also creating pressure for a general review of food law:

● In November 1978 and March 1979, the National Academy of Sciences issued a report that found that saccharin was a weak carcinogen in rats and posed a risk for human health; but at the same time the panel recommended that the existing flat ban on the use of carcinogenic food additives be dropped and that federal food laws should be revamped to take risk factors into account.

● A House subcommittee and at least one group of scientists warned that some Americans might be eating pesticide-tainted meat and produce because of lax monitoring and enforcement by the trio of agencies with responsibility for food safety: the FDA, the Agriculture Department and the Environmental Protection Agency (EPA).

● There were strong economic pressures to revise the Delaney amendment as well.

Saccharin, with about 300 times the sweetening power of sugar, was cheaper for soft-drink manufacturers to use than its high-calorie counterpart, according to a Calorie Control Council spokesman. The no-calorie soft drink market, which accounted for the greatest percentage of saccharin consumption, was growing rapidly.

Beef producers also argued that a drug ban would push soaring beef prices higher. And a nitrite ban, at a time when beef prices were moving up rapidly, would hurt hog producers who might otherwise expect a rise in consumer demand for nitrite-processed pork products like sausages, luncheon meats and hot dogs.

Regulation of Food Additives Brings Congress . . .

The limits of science and statistics have been a major issue in congressional debate on food safety.

Pressures for decisions on saccharin, sodium nitrite and animal feed drug additives pushed Congress and federal regulators into the shifting world of scientific hypothesis, where certainties are rare — and almost always challenged.

Key technical questions remained unanswered in arguments over how far federal regulators can go to remove from the food supply suspected carcinogens or other "-gens" — substances that may damage the developing fetus, or make the body's immune system function less well, or cause permanent genetic changes affecting future generations.

For instance, no one appeared to know with any exactness:

● How environmental exposure, genetic makeup, the disease process and personal habits mix to cause the approximately 110 types of cancer.

● How to predict the magnitude of risk to humans from a substance that causes cancer in laboratory animals.

● How to set a safe level for consumption or other human exposure to substances that cause cancer in laboratory animals.

Affected industries have bitterly resisted regulatory efforts growing out of such an uncertain science base because, as Tobacco Institute official Dr. Charles L. Waite phrased it, "We don't want to be guessed out of business."

One of the few scientists in Congress, Rep. James G. Martin, R-N.C., a former chemistry professor, found statistical translations of laboratory data on cancer in rats to be "exercises in imaginary numbers."

Pressures for Decisions

But the pressures for decisions despite scientific uncertainty remained strong.

Industry officials "are not the people that are going to be held accountable 30 years from now when some crying health effect comes screaming along," said Environmental Protection Agency (EPA) spokesman L. G. Blanchard. Many of the health problems predicted for suspect chemicals have a lead time of decades or longer. Cancer "latency" periods run 10 to 40 years, for example.

Steven D. Jellinek, directing EPA's pesticide and toxic substances programs, agreed that decision-making in the absence of absolutely clear scientific conclusions was "crazy." But, Jellinek added, "the alternative is to not decide anything — in essence, to turn the human population into guinea pigs. There aren't any of us in a public policy role that are ready to do that."

Much of the debate over carcinogenic substances turned on the accuracy of testing, with spokesmen for affected industries arguing that producing cancer in animals simply was not the same as producing it in humans.

The Calorie Control Council's criticism of animal data on saccharin emphasized the enormous quantity of the sweetener that was fed to small laboratory animals to produce a heightened incidence of cancer. In 1977 the council estimated that humans would have to drink about 800 cans of saccharin-sweetened beverages daily to run the same risks as rats in a key study. By 1979, the estimate had been revised upward — to 1,000 cans.

Cancer researchers responded that the sizable doses compensate for built-in shortcomings of animal tests, and that the test results are valid. Rats are smaller, their lives far shorter, and their cells multiply more rapidly than those of humans. Dosage levels must compensate for these differences, researchers argued.

Moreover, low-level risk such as that attributed to saccharin meant that relatively few cases of cancer would show up in an exposed population.

Even if test animals could perfectly duplicate human life-span and size, no one could test a substance on 220 million animals, thus duplicating the size of the U.S. population. Concentrated dosage is need to reveal the probability of risk in smaller test "populations," the researchers said.

There are problems in using animal data to predict human susceptibility to a carcinogen, but ethics bar duplicating animal results by de-

● Many food industry officials insisted that the Delaney amendment should be tempered by permitting — or requiring — a risk-benefit assessment of questionable substances, such as the FDA was doing for some new drugs. But while cost-benefit or risk-benefit analysis appealed to administration inflation-fighters, there was evidence that key health officials might resist that modification of Delaney because it would increase regulatory overload.

The food-safety debate came at a time when there was also increasing interest in requiring more nutritional and other information on food labels and in improving federal capacity to monitor and recall contaminated food. *(See Food Labeling chapter)*

Background

For purposes of regulation, federal law has divided food additives into groups and subgroups, depending on how the additives entered the food supply, or on how powerful their defenders had been in past congresses. For example, a red dye that was part of a group of colors earmarked for special precautions received an exemption in 1956 when Florida citrus growers persuaded Congress they needed it to mask the natural greenish color of ripe oranges.

Regulatory treatment has differed for substances, depending on whether they:

● Were added deliberately during food processing;

● Occurred naturally in food; or

● Were inadvertently added, such as environmental contaminants.

The latter two categories have generally been ignored for regulatory purposes, on the assumption that it was impossible to remove them from the food supply. (If environmental contaminants were found at an unaccept-

...Up Against Uncertainties of Scientific Testing

liberately exposing human subjects to a carcinogen. However, all but two substances known to cause cancer in man also produce cancer in laboratory animals, according to Dr. David Rall, head of the National Institute for Environmental Health Sciences.

It was still considered difficult-to-impossible to conclude from animal data just how many human beings would develop cancer from exposure to a carcinogen.

Improved Detection Methods

A second related testing issue involved the dramatic improvement in the last two decades of methods for detecting the presence of chemicals.

Scientists can now measure quantities as minute as a nanogram — a billionth of a gram. A gram is about a thirtieth of an ounce. They may refine detection techniques even further.

The capacity to measure ever-diminishing quantities means that scientists may never be able to rule out the possibility that a troublesome substance is present, at very tiny, trace levels.

What this means for regulators is a problem sometimes referred to as "the search for a vanishing zero." The Delaney amendment flatly forbids the presence of a carcinogen, no matter how small an amount, and science may not be able to guarantee that absence.

Human susceptibility to carcinogens can only be measured in-

directly, through epidemiological studies of populations who have not been able to avoid exposure to substances in question. For regulatory purposes these studies are broad and imprecise: They often cannot single out the effect of one carcinogen in a population that has been exposed to several hazardous substances. Nor are they reliable for predicting very low-risk carcinogens — substances that might cause very few deaths in a very large population.

These problems worried scientists who were involved in regulatory decisions.

Dr. Sanford Miller of the Food and Drug Administration's (FDA) Bureau of Drugs said he was subject to "the uneasy feeling that the number I'm measuing is real. That there are 120 people out there that are going to develop bladder cancer."

But Rep. Martin claimed the risk from saccharin was "not great, as life goes. It shortens life by 23 minutes."

The science of predicting cancer may never be precise because ethics rule out direct tests on human populations.

The Poison Squad

There was a time when human testing of food additives was federal policy.

Sometime in 1903, a dozen young men in the Department of Agriculture sat down to the first course of what was to become a five-year chemical "feast" that included saccharin, borax, formaldehyde and

other proposed additions to processed food.

The volunteers comprised an early food additive testing project, known officially as "the hygienic table," but quickly dubbed "the poison squad."

Their successors at the FDA have pointed out that, ominous as some of those early chemical entrees sound, they suggested the food industry was trying to respond to a real need for food preservatives.

"Just eating was hazardous to your health in 1900. People got sick and died from eating. They had diarrhea all the time from spoiled food," said Miller.

Part of the hazard, Miller added, was due to uncritical addition of chemicals and other supposed preservatives and colorings to food.

The poison squad ate its way to the conclusion that manufacturers should have to prove both the "need" and "wholesomeness" of additions to food before they were marketed, according to FDA records.

Fifty years later Congress agreed, deciding in 1958 to require pre-market testing of additives.

Although the poison squad's tests of saccharin convinced them that the sweetener should be banned, President Theodore Roosevelt, who took daily doses for unknown medical reasons, responded that anyone "who thinks saccharin is injurious to health is an idiot." In 1912 a saccharin ban did go into effect, but it was later lifted when sugar supplies shrank during World War I.

able level in a given food, however, batches of the product could be recalled.)

Regulatory standards ranged from the unqualified ban in the Delaney amendment, which applied to substances added by manufacturers, to a two-step process for pesticides and animal drugs. Preliminary approval of a substance (by the FDA for drugs or the EPA for pesticides) was followed by monitoring for unacceptable levels in food, and confiscation if food was contaminated.

Tolerance levels were set for pesticides; for animal drugs, the manufacturer had to show that the technology existed to detect traces of it in animal carcasses. (The Commerce Department handled contaminated fish; FDA and the Agriculture Department shared responsibility for monitoring meat and produce.)

Substances that had been sanctioned by the FDA for use before 1958 were exempt from both Delaney and

tolerance-setting, having been "grandfathered" in the food law revision of that year. They were still subject to a general-safety requirement, however.

Past Congressional Action

The history of food legislation has mirrored public distrust that has cut two ways, against both manufacturers and federal regulators. Constituents sometimes have pressured Congress to protect them from apparent hazards. But industry lobbyists and constituents have also persuaded members to block the FDA when it has tried to remove popular substances from the market.

For example, a battle along the same lines as the saccharin fight erupted in 1976, three years after the FDA proposed to set potency limits for vitamins and minerals and to regulate as drugs any diet supplements that exceeded those limits. Members received about as much protest mail on that issue as on the impeachment proceedings that year, according to a Library of Congress legislative history. Opponents, including health food and pharmaceutical groups, argued against "diet dictation" and "Big Brotherism," and Congress responded by severely curbing FDA authority over vitamins and minerals.

First Food Law. Congress first authorized regulation of the food industry in 1906, following muckraking press reports of watered milk (with chalk added to restore white color), canned green beans whose color was maintained with copper, unsanitary meat processing and other disturbing food industry practices. The 1906 law, the basis of the existing Food, Drug and Cosmetic Act, prohibited manufacture of or interstate commerce in foods that were adulterated or misbranded.

For the next 52 years, however, it was up to federal regulators to find violators and make the case that a given additive was a health hazard. A 1938 overhaul of the law tightened labeling requirements and broadened the definition of prohibited additives to anything that was injurious to health. (The 1906 law focused on poisonous additives.)

1958 Act. Not until 1958 did Congress require manufacturers to prove the safety of an additive before putting it into food. (For pesticides, mandatory pre-market testing was enacted in 1954. Color additives, treated separately, were brought under mandatory pre-market testing and the Delaney clause in 1960.)

The 1958 act came six years after a special House committee, chaired by James J. Delaney (D-N.Y., 1945-47, 1949-79), had conducted a two-year review of pesticides and food additives and recommended pre-market testing for additives. Public concern with cancer was high, and the act included Delaney's amendment barring additives that induced cancer in man or animals.

But there were major exemptions to the pre-market testing requirements for two large groups of additives: those that had already been sanctioned for use by the FDA, and those that were "generally recognized as safe" — that is, they had been used for years with neither FDA sanction nor apparent ill health effects. Saccharin was in the second category.

The amendment caused controversy at the time among some scientists and industry spokesmen, who said it was not scientifically valid to bar use of a food additive at safe levels simply because the same substances at much higher levels of use could cause cancer in laboratory animals.

Arguments over whether the requirement was too strict continued to surface from time to time, particularly during the "cranberry scare" of 1959 and in connection with the FDA's bans on cyclamates (another artificial sweetener) in 1970 and red dye No. 2 in 1976.

Opponents argued that the clause was too rigid and that even toxic or cancer-inducing substances should be usable if evidence indicated they were harmless for certain purposes or in certain quantities. Backers of the clause responded that it was unsafe to permit the use of any known carcinogen since there was no way to establish a threshold of danger below which a carcinogen would not cause cancer.

The Saccharin Controversy

In April 1977, after Canadian studies showed that high dosages of saccharin produced bladder cancer in rats, the FDA proposed to ban it as a food additive. The proposed ban was based on both the Delaney clause and on the general food-safety law. The FDA also proposed to permit the sale of saccharin as an over-the-counter drug — temporarily, and with a warning label. Manufacturers would be given six months to prove that it was an effective drug for diabetics and the obese.

"All hell broke loose" after the FDA proposal, one member of Congress recalled. The 1969 FDA ban on cyclamates had been less controversial because there was an alternative artificial sweetener — saccharin. But the proposal to eliminate the last non-caloric sweetener provoked very strong protests. Consumers, the soft drink industry, diet food manufacturers and diabetics ridiculed the Canadian findings, arguing that a human being would have to drink 800 12-ounce cans of diet soft drinks each day to duplicate the saccharin consumption of the affected rats.

The Calorie Control Council, representing soft-drink manufacturers and other industrial users of saccharin, argued that banning the sweetener threatened the health of diabetics and people who needed to control their weight. People would brush their teeth less with unsweetened toothpaste and children would spit out unsweetened medicine, opponents of the ban warned.

In defense of the ban, a few prominent researchers argued that saccharin was of no particular benefit to diabetics and might even harm them, by maintaining their taste for sweets. And Dr. Sidney Wolfe, of Ralph Nader's Health Research Group, told a congressional hearing that saccharin caused laboratory animals to gain, not lose, weight because it increased their hunger by lowering their blood sugar to abnormal levels.

1977 Congressional Action

Congress finally decided to postpone the proposed ban for 18 months, require warning signs and labels on products containing saccharin, and order studies on saccharin and food safety policy (PL 95-203).

The issue of health warnings accompanying advertisements surfaced as the main controversy during Senate floor debate on the bill. Before voting Sept. 15, 1977, to delay the proposed ban, the Senate approved an amendment eliminating provisions that would have required all radio, TV, newspaper and magazine advertisements for products containing saccharin to include warnings that the substance might cause cancer.

The House version did not include the strong advertising requirements for broadcast and print media. In addition, the bill did not require that the secretary of the Department of Health, Education and Welfare (HEW, now Health and Human Services) place a warning label on saccharin products, as the Senate bill did.

The final version of the ban adopted the stronger Senate language, including the Senate provision requiring warning labels on saccharin products. Both chambers routinely adopted the conference report (H Rept 95-810) in November. *(Major provisions of 1977 bill, box p. 123)*

1978 Saccharin Study

In November 1978 the first of the two reports on the safety of saccharin was completed by the National Academy of Sciences (NAS). The academy found that:

● Saccharin by itself or in combination with other substances was a relatively weak carcinogen in rats. Saccharin itself, not impurities in the substance, was the carcinogen.

• It was scientifically valid to conclude that if a substance caused cancer in animals, it would cause cancer in humans. However, animal tests could not predict just how great the risk of human cancer was for a given substance.

• There were no acceptable epidemiological (population) studies linking cancer directly to human consumption of saccharin, but that might be because study methods were too insensitive to pick up the incidence of cancer from a relatively weak carcinogen or separate out the effect of saccharin from exposure to stronger carcinogens like cigarette smoke or asbestos.

• There were no adequate clinical studies of the claimed medical benefits of saccharin for diabetics and the obese; that is, no one had either proved or disproved these benefits with patients.

• Although the cancer risk of saccharin was probably low, "even low risks to a large number of exposed persons may lead to public health concerns."

• Children and women of child-bearing age consumed more saccharin than other population groups.

"The ultimate judgment must be made through the socio-political process," the first report concluded.

Industry Reaction

The Calorie Control Council, to the surprise of some observers, interpreted the first NAS study as a confirmation of its position that saccharin should be left on the market without further restriction.

Slover said the risks for human users of saccharin "have never been demonstrated," and that 90 percent of health professionals thought saccharin should continue to be available for diet control, according to opinion sampling conducted for the council. "I'm confident that anyone who reads the science will not be convinced that saccharin is a carcinogen," Slover said.

The council criticized the NAS report on these grounds:

• It only reviewed existing saccharin studies, and did not present any new evidence.

• It based its finding of the carcinogenic effect of saccharin on a limited number of high-dosage experiments "whose applicability has been questioned by many scientists."

• It "accepted the impossibility of finding that saccharin is a carcinogen in humans."

• It failed to offer evidence to back up its suggestion that saccharin consumption "jeopardizes the health of children."

• It underestimated "the fact that saccharin offers substantial benefits, both physiological and psychological."

1979 NAS Report

In the second part of its two-part study ordered by Congress in 1977, the National Academy of Sciences in effect told Congress to leave the saccharin ban decision up to the FDA regulators. In its March 2, 1979, report, the scientists recommended that Congress drop the existing flat ban on the use of carcinogenic food additives. Instead, they said, Congress should permit regulators to factor health or economic benefits into their decisions on some carcinogenic additives, including saccharin. (Cost-benefit debate, box, p. 124)

The NAS report said Congress should rewrite federal food laws to permit a variety of regulatory options for carcinogenic and other food additives, depending on how

1977 Bill Delaying Saccharin Ban

As signed into law, the 1977 bill (PL 95-203) delaying the proposed Food and Drug Administration (FDA) ban on the artificial sweetener saccharin contained the following major provisions:

• Prohibited the secretary of Health, Education and Welfare (HEW, now Health and Human Services) from banning or restricting for 18 months the sale or distribution of saccharin or any product containing it on the basis of any studies or tests available before the date of enactment of the bill. The provision would not prohibit the secretary from banning saccharin due to new information discovered during the 18-month moratorium.

• Stipulated that the secretary's new authority to require labels and warning signs about the risks associated with saccharin would not be considered as restricting or prohibiting the sale or distribution of saccharin.

• Required that any food product containing saccharin introduced into interstate commerce beginning 90 days after enactment of the bill would be considered misbranded under the Food, Drug and Cosmetic Act if it did not contain the following label in conspicuous and legible type: "USE OF THIS PRODUCT MAY BE HAZARDOUS TO YOUR HEALTH. THIS PRODUCT CONTAINS SACCHARIN WHICH HAS BEEN DETERMINED TO CAUSE CANCER IN LABORATORY ANIMALS."

• Authorized the secretary to revise or remove labeling and information requirements if new information about saccharin warranted it.

• Required manufacturers of products containing saccharin to provide retail establishments selling those products with warning signs informing consumers of the health risks associated with saccharin. Food sold in a store that did not display such signs would be considered misbranded.

• Required the secretary to prepare information on the saccharin controversy to be displayed and distributed by retail establishments selling saccharin products.

• Authorized the secretary to require vending machines containing saccharin products to display in a conspicuous place on the machine a warning of the health risks associated with saccharin usage.

• Required the secretary to conduct studies and report to Congress within 15 months on a number of subjects, including existing technical capability to determine the carcinogenicity of substances added to or normally occurring in food, the health benefits and risks to humans from carcinogenic substances in food, and federal food regulatory policy as it related to carcinogenic substances.

• Required the secretary to report to Congress within one year on the chemical identity of any impurities found in saccharin, their toxicity and carcinogenicity, and the health benefits resulting from the use of artificial sweeteners in general and saccharin in particular.

• Directed the secretary to ask the National Academy of Sciences to conduct the studies; if it declined, authorized him to contract with another public or nonprofit entity.

Cost-Risk-Benefit Analysis: 'Political Arithmetic'

When the National Academy of Sciences, in its March 1979 report on food safety laws, suggested that economic factors might be taken into account in figuring the risks and benefits of hazardous substances, they were riding a rising tide of interest in the traditional economists' exercise.

The Delaney clause flatly forbids any carcinogenic food additive, no matter how small its risk or how substantial its benefits. Some scientists and members of Congress found the risks of the artificial sweetener saccharin negligible, and its benefits to diabetics and dieters compellingly real. They wanted the Delaney clause changed so that the health risks or economic costs of a food additive could be measured against its benefits, case-by-case, substance-by-substance.

The rising anti-regulatory mood in Congress and the administration and competition for scarce federal dollars pushed to new prominence economic techniques for weighing benefits of a proposed action against its expected costs or risks. The traditional tool of public works, military, transportation and environment planners was being promoted as an antidote to "inflationary" regulation in other fields.

President Carter urged "cost-effective" solutions to health problems; his fiscal 1980 budget justified preventive health expenditures on the grounds they would pay for themselves in lowered health costs.

Mandatory cost-effectiveness analyses were part of broad regulatory reform packages introduced by the administration and members of Congress in 1979-80. The bills would require agencies to publish, for comment, a statement of the need, cost, alternatives and other factors of any proposed regulation. By the spring of 1980, committees in the House and Senate had reported regulatory reform bills containing those requirements.

Appropriate in Health Policy?

The notion of calculating cash benefits of health decisions is not new. In 1690, Sir William Petty, a physician and pioneer in what he called "political arithmetic," suggested that the British economy would benefit if plague-ridden Londoners were sent to the country for three months. For every pound spent on the project, 84 pounds would be gained, Petty claimed, since peoples' lives would be lengthened and they could work longer. Office of Technology Assessment researcher Clyde Behney, who cited that story, said the city of Boston used similar arguments to justify public spending on improved sanitation in 1850.

There have been warnings, however, about the use of cost-risk-benefit analysis in health policy.

Former Rep. Paul G. Rogers (D-Fla., 1955-1979), a major figure in health and environment legislation, warned in 1978 against uncritical adoption of such political arithmetic. Strict application of cost-benefit analysis to health policy could lead to the conclusion that "if getting sick is cheaper, then maybe we should not try to prevent illness," Rogers said.

Warnings also came from government and labor officials concerned with health, that economic techniques did not mesh neatly with traditional medical values of saving lives and alleviating pain.

A Difficult Task

The terms cost-benefit, risk-benefit and cost-effectiveness have often been used interchangeably to describe what essentially has been a comparison process. The theory was that with such a comparison in hand, a rational decision could be made on, for instance, whether improved health was worth expensive environmental improvements.

Economists and administrators who had to make the comparisons noted that assessing cost was far different from calculating risk. They added that it was extremely difficult to define any of the three major elements so that they could be compared.

The Environmental Protection Agency (EPA), charged with balancing costs, risks and benefits in administering pesticide and toxic substances laws, found the task "incredibly difficult," according to Steven D. Jellinek, head of the pesticide and toxic substances unit. He said EPA often had to make decisions on "lousy data."

The science of estimating human risk from animal data on cancer was very new and had not "been tested out in a human population," said Stuart Pape, a Food and Drug Administration (FDA) attorney who was drafting the administration's food law proposals. And potential health problems from exposure to hazardous substances often were difficult to measure, or even identify.

"Safety conventionally was defined in terms of death, but now [there were] more complex questions about safety, such as behavior, physical performance, immune response," which could not be estimated accurately, noted Sanford Miller, director of FDA's Bureau of Foods.

Even with the problems of assessing risks and costs, cost-risk-benefit analysts found benefits hardest to pin down. "A man dies early from cancer caused by exposure to asbestos. His wife can't get work, his kids grow up without a father, one maybe goes on drugs, there's a lot of upheaval in the family. It's a real 'cost.' How do you put a dollar sign on it?" asked Frank Greer of the Occupational Safety and Health Administration.

There were a few traditional measures for ill health and death: productivity losses, medical bills, the value of life insurance policies or compensation demands in lawsuits. But none of these included "quality of life" costs.

Organized labor shared the fears expressed by Rogers about attempts to impose cost-risk-benefit analysis on health policy. Anthony Mazzocchi, vice president of the Oil, Chemical and Atomic Workers Union, queried, "Whose cost? Whose benefit? ...They're going to say that it's too expensive" to protect workers' lives.

Mazzocchi pointed up a major problem in cost- or risk-benefit analysis: that the people who gained the benefit might not be the same people who were running the risk or paying the cost.

risky they were for human health. That recommendation seemed to conflict with the conclusion of the November 1978 report, that science could not yet predict human risk for substances that caused cancer in laboratory animals, particularly at low-risk levels (meaning that relatively few individuals would get cancer).

The second NAS report recommended that Congress empower the FDA to classify a substance as high-, moderate- or low-risk, and choose an appropriate response — outright ban, restricting sales, continuing sales with warning labels, or no regulatory intervention at all. In effect, food regulators should have broad, discretionary power to decide how to deal with carcinogens and other health hazards, the panel said.

Decisions on how to classify and regulate suspect substances should be based primarily on health considerations, the panel said, but "perceived" benefits such as those attributed to saccharin should also help determine how strictly a substance would be regulated. The earlier NAS report found no clinical evidence that saccharin improved the health of the obese or diabetics, but that there was still strong demand for it.

The majority report stopped short of a clear recommendation on saccharin, and the overall thrust of its recommendations was to pass the buck back to Congress and, ultimately, to the FDA.

In an unusual development, there was a minority report on the second NAS study. In a strongly worded statement, dissenting members said there was still no "scientifically defensible way to divide carcinogens" or other substances with irreversible health hazards into different risk categories. The dissenters also said that food regulation should be particularly strict, because of the "enormous" number of persons exposed to potential hazards and because the method of exposure — chronic ingestion — was the "optimal" way to cause cancer.

To further confuse the situation, a group calling itself an independent "voice of science on key public health issues" announced Feb. 27, 1979, that saccharin was safe and without risk for humans when consumed in "normal dietary amounts." In a position identical to that of the Calorie Control Council, the American Council on Science and Health recommended that the FDA approve saccharin as a safe food additive, to be sold without warning labels.

Reaction, House Action

These developments brought sharp reactions from many health and consumer advocates who believed that science still had not established a safe level for consumption of carcinogenic substances. "Until that time comes, it is unconscionable for Congress to allow any amount of a known carcinogen to be added to any food product," said Ellen Haas of the Community Nutrition Institute.

Nonetheless, the House voted overwhelmingly in July 1979 to permit products containing saccharin to stay on the market for two more years. The Senate did not act on an extension of the moratorium until 1980, thus leaving the FDA free in the interim to resume proceedings to ban saccharin. However, FDA officials said they would wait for a congressional decision before doing so.

During House floor debate on the measure (HR 4453), Henry A. Waxman, D-Calif., chairman of the Commerce Subcommittee on Health and sponsor of the moratorium extension legislation, said the new legislation did not mean "we are unconcerned about the dangers from saccharin."

But, he added, "we are also not unaware of the concerns of diabetics and others on a sugar restricted diet, who feel that without this substitute they will face a known health hazard from sugar."

Nitrite, Animal Drugs, Pesticides

The controversy over the saccharin ban moratorium coincided with a rising level of debate on several other additives that had been linked to cancer.

The FDA ran into congressional hostility in 1977, when it suggested banning antibiotics and certain other drugs that were routinely added to animal feed to prevent disease and enhance growth in the animals. The fiscal 1979 agriculture appropriations bill (PL 95-448) directed the FDA to hold off on that ban until research and public hearings on the issue were completed.

Cattlemen and other meat producers argued that drugs were essential in volume production of meat, which involved fattening confined animals in crowded conditions. However, in January 1979 a group of scientists renewed warnings that antibiotic feed additives were producing drug-resistant bacteria in animals that could cause human illness. The scientists published their findings along with charges that the advisory group for which they had studied the problem had tried to water down their conclusions. The advisory group, the Council for Agriculture Science and Technology, was supported by chemical, fertilizer and drug manufacturers.

The situation with sodium nitrite was somewhat different than that of saccharin because the Carter administration in 1979 introduced its own legislation to bar any agency action against the preservative for about a year and then permit phasing it out as safe substitutes were developed. FDA spokesman Wayne Pines said the nitrite bill did not really go against the administration's advocacy of a general overhaul of food laws, because nitrite was a "unique" substance requiring special treatment. The bill would not set a precedent for breaching the Delaney clause, Pines insisted. But one congressional aide on food matters called that remark "just whistling in the wind."

Another difference was that the scientific evidence on the carcinogenicity of nitrites was thought to be less well developed than that on saccharin. Scientists in 1979 were still reviewing a Massachusetts Institute of Technology study that had prompted the Agriculture Department to consider banning nitrite, whereas saccharin findings had undergone at least two rounds of reviews.

The Agriculture Department did not formally propose a nitrite ban, but simply asked the Justice Department whether it could choose a phase-out rather than a flat ban if the cancer studies turned out to be correct. The Justice Department replied in March 1979 that under existing law, the phasing approach was illegal, and the administration introduced its bill shortly thereafter.

Lax Enforcement Charged

There have been charges that meat, poultry and produce containing unsafe levels of pesticide residues were showing up on the nation's dinner tables because of inadequate enforcement by FDA, EPA and the Agriculture Department.

The House Commerce Subcommittee on Oversight and Investigations said in December 1978 (H Rept 95-67) that:

● The EPA, in setting tolerances for pesticides, was increasing public health risks by "veering away from the health-oriented language [of federal food law] toward the 'risk-benefit' balancing language of federal pesticide statutes."

● The Agriculture Department, responsible for sampling meat and poultry for pesticide and drug residues, was "doing a poor job of finding residue violations and of preventing . . . the marketing of contaminated meat."

● The FDA was failing to monitor "many chemicals occurring in food" that were suspected causes of cancer, birth defects or genetic mutations.

Taken together, these failings meant that Americans could not be sure that what they ate was not contaminated, the subcommittee chairman, John E. Moss, (D-Calif., 1953-1979), warned in urging stronger regulations.

On the other hand, after his committee in 1978 requested economic impact statements on both the nitrite and animal drug bans, Senate Agriculture Committee Chairman Herman E. Talmadge, D-Ga., warned against causing economic problems "in the pursuit of a minor benefit, or to eliminate a theoretical risk." Increasingly sensitive tests raised "basic policy questions about risk and how far do we go with regulations," Talmadge said. ∎

Food Labeling: A Thorny Issue for Congress

The quirks of federal food regulation have kept Americans confused about what has been in the food they eat.

On that much, consumers, food industry officials and federal regulators themselves have agreed. They even have agreed in a broad way on a solution: a unified national food policy to simplify the regulatory thicket created by three separate agencies overseeing food processing and marketing.

But any consensus that something ought to be done had begun to evaporate when the different groups got down to the details of how to straighten out the system.

Industry groups like the National Food Processors Association and fast-food chains such as McDonald's have urged Congress to prune back cumbersome and costly food regulations. These regulations added millions of dollars a year to the nation's food bills and kept the industry from telling consumers how nutritious their products were, industry officials claimed.

Regulators such as former Food and Drug Administration (FDA) chief Donald Kennedy wanted just the opposite: more power to require uniform, full disclosure of nutritional and other characteristics of food. Uncoordinated, partial industry programs only confused consumers and made it difficult to compare foods, he said. At a minimum, he argued, consumers should have the same information, in an easy-to-understand format, about fresh and processed food from the supermarket and about meals from fast-food outlets.

Meanwhile, consumers themselves were sending Washington a mixed message. Some pollsters said Americans felt they already knew enough about what they were eating. But organized consumer groups and individuals who testified at a series of joint hearings by the FDA, the Agriculture Department (USDA) and the Federal Trade Commission (FTC) demanded full disclosure of ingredients, nutritional data and other food information.

Mixed Regulatory Bag

The FDA, USDA and FTC have shared responsibility for the safety and honest marketing of food. The FDA has monitored processed foods, USDA has been responsible for meat and poultry products, and the FTC has had jurisdiction over food advertising.

Food information rules have been a mix of voluntary and mandatory standards. This has meant different rules for fresh and processed foods and, in some instances, no standards at all. It has also meant oddities like stiff nutritional disclosure standards for cheese pizza, under FDA jurisdiction, and much looser labeling requirements for pizza topped with just enough pork sausage to bring it under the jurisdiction of the Agriculture Department. USDA's Food Safety and Quality Service has no nutritional labeling program. Moreover, the stricter FDA standard applied only if the maker of the cheese pizza fortified his product or made nutritional "claims" for it — such as listing caloric value.

The FTC also got into the act by suggesting that restaurant menus function as "food labels" and should therefore be regulated as nutritional "claims."

"You get confusing regulation where you have unclear mandates," Kennedy observed.

Congressional Action

Congress began rewriting the basic federal food laws in 1970, but was not expected to finish the job until 1980 or later.

Congressional action was expected to move on several tracks, with one cluster of bills on information issues, and a second set on safety matters, including the 1958 ban on cancer-causing additives. The safety issue took precedence over information bills in 1979 because a moratorium on an FDA saccharin ban expired in May. (In July 1979, the House voted to permit saccharin to stay on the market for two more years and the Senate followed suit in June 1980.) *(See story, p. 119)*

The agencies also planned to move as far as they could administratively on food information, but observers thought that decision was based on equal parts of skepticism about what Congress could do and old-fashioned turf protection.

In any case, Congress would probably be asked to make some hard judgment calls on any food information legislation. Among the questions both consumers and industry officials were asking were these:

● When does providing nutritional information, like "low-fat," become a "claim" that your food is more healthful than that of competitors?

● Who should decide what nutritional information consumers should get — the federal government or the food industry?

● How much more information do consumers need, and how much are they willing to pay for it?

Background

Federal involvement in the food industry began in 1906 when Congress banned interstate commerce in adulterated or misbranded foods. The next major expansion of that law, in 1938, broadened FDA authority to locate adulterated foods.

Standards of Identity. The 1938 law also established a type of food regulation known as a "standard of identity" — which by 1980 had become a target of consumer activists. These recipe-like regulations were intended to assure shoppers that they were buying a familiar, recognizable food like one they might prepare themselves. A mayonnaise manufacturer whose product conformed to the standard of identity, for instance, was required to list only ingredients other than those of the standard.

Critics of this type of regulation have said it obscured the nature of many foods. Also, processing has become so sophisticated and products so differentiated that the standards of identity are outmoded, according to the argument.

Makers of non-standardized foods were required by the 1938 law to list ingredients by their common or usual name. But spices, flavorings and colorings can go under those broad designations, without any more specific identification.

That provision gave considerable trouble to individuals with allergies, FDA's Kennedy said. For instance, an estimated 100,000 people had a severe reaction to one yellow dye — "and it's not just hives, it's not a joke," Kennedy said.

Some manufacturers argued, however, that full disclosure of all ingredients would give away trade secrets and that, in any event, a full list of flavoring agents could run to as many as 100 separate and confusing chemical names for one product.

USDA Regulations. Statutory authority to oversee meat, poultry and dairy products moved on a separate legislative track.

These laws, administered by USDA, weigh producers' commercial needs as much as human health issues. For instance, the USDA grading system has not established the nutritional value of foods; its standards for size, aesthetic and other qualities have been used simply to compare products for pricing. The department's food service has used "standards of composition," which set maximum or minimum requirements for certain ingredients.

The 'Vichyssoise Bills.' Beginning in 1971 the Senate passed a series of food bills to beef up federal authority to monitor the food industry for contaminated or hazardous foods and require various types of information on food labels.

Senate action was prompted by public concern over several much-publicized recalls of hazardous foods, including mercury-tainted fish and botulin-bearing vichyssoise soup.

The bills got no further in the House than two bottleneck committees: the producer-oriented House Agriculture Committee and the perennially overloaded House Commerce Subcommittee on Health. The bills also lacked an influential House advocate. Not until the summer of 1978 did the chairman of the House health panel, former Rep. Paul G. Rogers, D-Fla. (1955-1979), turn his attention to food labeling and surveillance issues.

'Affirmative Information' Regulations. Meanwhile, in 1974 the FDA and the FTC moved into "affirmative information" regulations for food processing and advertising. These controversial regulations earned the agencies a reputation among many Washington lawyers for what was known as "creative lawyering" — not a complimentary term.

Even former FDA officials said privately that the regulations were weak because they were not based on an explicit congressional decision that consumers must be fully informed about food. Instead, the FDA and FTC based their regulations on the punitive, decades-old statutes that were meant to prevent fraud and deception in food marketing.

The basic assumption of the government regulations — which regulators have pressed Congress to write into law — has been that manufacturers cannot advertise only favorable nutritional aspects of their products and omit other information. In this view, any nutritional claim for food must include all ingredient information, the po-

tentially negative as well as the positive. For instance, listing the contents of a hot dog as meat, water, salt and sweetener "tells everything one needs to know except the percentage of fat in the product," according to Carol Tucker Foreman, assistant secretary of agriculture for food and consumer services — information important to consumers instructed to watch their weight or cholesterol intake.

Food industry critics have disagreed with this assumption. Officials of McDonald's and Kentucky Fried Chicken told George McGovern's, D-S.D., Senate Agriculture Subcommittee on Nutrition in February 1979 that they had paid independent researchers to work up nutritional profiles for their food, but that they were afraid to advertise or distribute them for fear federal agencies would judge that information to be a health claim and would then require excessive amounts of additional information.

Former FDA Commissioner Kennedy contended that putting some nutrition information on food suggested that that food is good for you, particularly if competitors' products were not labeled. "You are in effect making some health claims. We have some responsibility to make sure they're correct," Kennedy said.

Kennedy said McDonald's could have gone ahead with its nutritional information program if it had agreed to print the information on napkins as well as wallboards, so that carry-out customers could have the same information as those dining in the chain's restaurants. But he also made clear that the FDA would like Congress to give it statutory power to require that any such nutritional information campaigns would have to include all nutritional factors, not just the ones the company wanted to emphasize.

That larger issue, whether manufacturers should choose what information to provide or whether the federal government would set minimum information standards, was the one that would be at the heart of Congress' deliberations on food labeling.

Consumer Attitudes

In recent years consumers have been queried repeatedly about how much and what kind of food information they want. The results have been somewhat contradictory, reflecting complex attitudes about food and lifestyles.

In a 1978 study prepared for the Food Marketing Institute by Yankelovich, Skelly and White, 77 percent of consumers interviewed said they were more interested in nutrition than they were several years ago, but only 24 percent thought themselves "well informed" on the subject; 63 percent said they were "fairly well informed."

Interest in nutrition did not necessarily mean that consumers' buying habits were dominated by health concerns, however. Cost and convenience were also important in food choices. Only 24 percent of interviewees said they felt "very strong[ly] about only eating what's good for you."

Roper surveys cited by Jack Webb of the National Restaurant Association indicated that Americans thought they ate reasonably well and knew about as much as they needed to know about nutrition. But, added Webb, "a 1978 question shows that consumers are making changes in food selection for health reasons."

Preliminary analysis of the FDA-USDA-FTC hearings in 1978 revealed considerable suspicion of the food industry, among other things. A December FDA summary cited these "prevailing" attitudes among individuals who testified at the hearings:

- Consumers have a right to know what is in the food they eat.
- The American public needs protection from the food industry.
- All additives are bad. Or, "if you can't pronounce it, it can't be good for you."
- Much of existing food advertising undermines consumers' efforts to select the most nutritious food possible.
- More nutritious foods can be regulated into existence.

Witnesses thought ingredient disclosure the most important of seven labeling options, Kennedy told McGovern's hearing. There was also substantial demand for information on total sodium (salt) and sugar content, for date-labeling and for understandable nutrition information.

The agencies had not succeeded in getting a very "crisp" answer on how much consumers would be willing to pay for the additional information, Kennedy said. But he said later that uniform labeling "need not be excessively costly."

Outlook

Although FDA and USDA officials and senators who have been active on food legislation in the past — Edward M. Kennedy, D-Mass., Donald W. Riegle Jr., D-Mich., and George McGovern — all planned new bills, Congress had not completed work on the food-information issue by mid-1980.

The principal actors were moving slowly. There were many reasons for the delay. Many members cited the anti-regulatory atmosphere prevalent on Capitol Hill in 1979-80. And, although the FDA had been almost continually taking minor actions against contaminated lots of food, there was no urgent tuna or soup "crisis" to push the legislation along.

Another problem was that the course of any food legislation was difficult because of multiple committee jurisdictions. Producer-oriented Agriculture committees had different priorities than health panels. In the Senate, the Agriculture, Labor and Human Resources and Commerce committees shared responsibility for food statutes; in the House, as many as three Agriculture subcommittees could share with the health subcommittee of the House Commerce Committee jurisdiction over any comprehensive food bill that covered all types of foods.

Meanwhile in December 1979, the FDA, USDA and FTC issued proposed regulations intended to provide further information to consumers in food labeling. The proposed rules would affect most foods except fresh fruits and vegetables and fresh or frozen, otherwise unprocessed, meat, poultry and fish. Foreman said the proposal represented "a major government-wide effort to improve food labeling" and "the most important action in the area in over 40 years." Although the process of implementing the regulations — including a 90-day wait for public comment, preparation of the resulting regulations, and another comment period — was expected to take up most of 1980, FDA and USDA spokesmen said they would in the meantime seek legislation to mandate even fuller disclosure of ingredients in the foods Americans eat. ∎

Senate Approves Major Drug Law Revision

Responding to chronic dissatisfaction with federal drug law in the industry, among consumer groups and in the Food and Drug Administration (FDA), the Senate in 1979 approved a major overhaul of regulations governing the approval and marketing of drugs in the United States. But the fate of the measure remained uncertain in 1980 because the anti-regulation majority dominating the House Commerce Health Subcommittee that would handle the bill could delay action in that chamber.

Although the bill (S 1075) made the most extensive changes in federal drug law since 1962, it slipped quietly through the Senate by voice vote on Sept. 26, 1979, with only a handful of members on the floor and virtually no debate. Edward M. Kennedy, D-Mass., steered it through so adroitly that the bill was already passed before most of its critics could open fire on it.

The measure was denounced, for different reasons, by Ralph Nader's Health Research Group and the Pharmaceutical Manufacturers Association (PMA). The American Medical Association (AMA), the American Pharmaceutical Association (APhA), representing pharmacists, and the public-interest Center for Law and Social Policy also were critical of various provisions. The outcry was notable because, as one Food and Drug Administration attorney remarked, "Anytime you've got drug makers *and* Nader against you, you've got a pretty interesting bill."

The bill won praise from one consumer group, the American Association of Retired Persons (AARP). "Kennedy deserves a lot of credit for making this bill as good as it is," said AARP spokesman Fred Wegner. "He had a very powerful interest group working against him. There was PMA, and each drug company with its own lobbyists — including presidents. They were all over the place, like locusts."

S 1075 was Kennedy's rewrite of a broader 1978 Carter administration proposal, which was stuck in committee until Kennedy and Sen. Richard S. Schweiker, R-Pa., negotiated an agreement on a block of industry-backed amendments.

FDA officials were generally pleased with the Senate bill, which would give them new powers to take drugs off the market, to require monitoring of approved drugs for adverse reactions or abuses and to limit distribution of high-risk medications. "While it does not contain every provision of the administration's proposal, nonetheless [it] is one we can support," said Sherwin Gardner, then acting FDA commissioner.

Major provisions of the bill:

● Shortcut certain approval procedures to hasten the marketing of new drugs.

● Permitted so-called "breakthrough" drugs to be prescribed before broad tests for their effectiveness were completed.

● Permitted export of drugs that did not meet U.S. safety and efficacy standards, in certain circumstances.

● Weakened the criminal liability standard for drug company executives.

● Mandated more drug information, including patient package information (PPI) inserts in most prescription drugs.

● Permitted drug companies to submit summaries — instead of raw test data — on safety and effectiveness testing of drugs for which they were seeking approval.

● Barred promotion abuses such as costly gifts by drug companies to encourage physicians to prescribe their drugs.

● Created a new office to study potential new drugs and evaluate the impact of drug regulation on the market.

Background

Unlike major congressional rewrites of federal drug law of the past, S 1075 was not a direct response to an acute public health problem, although drug manufacturers had been complaining that lengthy FDA procedures impaired the health of Americans by creating a "drug lag," delaying the marketing of needed new drugs.

The first drug regulation laws, of 1902 and 1906, followed muckraking accounts of adulterated drugs and foods. They imposed standards of purity and accurate branding, and empowered the government to seize and condemn drugs that violated these standards.

The next major revision, in 1938, was spurred by the deaths of more than 100 persons from a liquid version of sulfanilamide which had not been tested for safety. Congress that year required that drugs be safe, shifted the burden of proof to manufacturers, who were required for the first time to show that new drugs met federal safety standards, and strengthened FDA enforcement powers.

Until 1962, drugs automatically entered the marketplace after a fixed period of time unless the FDA found them to be unsafe. The only loophole — administrative delay — was dramatically highlighted when FDA official Dr. Frances Kelsey used it to block thalidomide, a sedative found to produce birth defects in children of mothers who took it during pregnancy.

The thalidomide scare, following extensive and well-publicized hearings by Sen. Estes Kefauver, D-Tenn. (1949-1963) on drug company profits and price-fixing, prompted Congress to act — although not on Kefauver's controversial drug patent proposals. The 1962 amendments required pre-market approval of new drugs and required manufacturers to demonstrate a drug's efficacy as well as safety. Congress also authorized the FDA to order immediate withdrawal of very dangerous drugs from the market.

1978 Carter Proposal

On March 16, 1978, the Carter administration proposed a massive revision of federal drug law. The bill included a number of ideas that had been circulating in Congress for years.

The industry had long wanted swifter approval procedures, requiring less exhaustive data, like those used in European countries. Useful and important drugs moved to patients much more quickly abroad, without any harmful effects, the drug companies argued. Excessive data requirements and bureaucratic foot-dragging were driving U.S. drug firms overseas, they claimed.

The FDA maintained that it must be very conservative about letting drugs onto the market because it lacked adverse reporting systems and summary powers to take hazardous drugs off the market that were common in Europe. FDA officials also suggested that the movement of drug-development capital abroad might be due to other factors than FDA performance, such as favorable tax climates in other countries, requirements that a drug be manufactured within a country in order to be sold there, and lower costs of clinical research in nations with publicly funded health insurance.

Then-FDA Commissioner Donald Kennedy argued that while the United States lagged behind Europe in the total number of new drug introductions, the numbers relating to significantly new or improved drugs were not very different. While personally disputing the reality of the drug lag, Kennedy produced a bill in March 1978 that was designed to speed up pre-marketing approval procedures and to give the FDA new powers to move against drugs already on the market.

The administration proposed to replace the existing procedure, under which each drug producer must go through FDA approval processes, with a new "monograph" system. A monograph on a drug would establish a single, federal generic standard for that drug, based on the application of the first manufacturer. Subsequent manufacturers would simply be licensed to produce the drug according to the federal standard.

The major drug companies reacted sharply against the monograph's requirement for publication of a company's data on a drug's safety and effectiveness. They said that would destroy incentives for the very costly process of developing and promoting new drugs, because competitors could raid the data and market cheaper versions.

The data disclosure and other provisions intended to open up the drug approval process to public participation reflected a second major source of pressure on the FDA, Nader's Health Research Group. FDA's own discovery of false and misleading data submissions by drug companies made public scrutiny of the data essential, the group argued.

The administration bill also reflected changes sought by the FDA itself, to provide statutory authority for procedures it had already adopted administratively. For instance, FDA, without any statutory definition of what "safe" or "effective" drugs were, had been using risk-benefit criteria for about eight years in its drug approvals. The FDA was also dissatisfied with its patchwork authority, left by the various generations of drug law reform. For instance, it could require batch-certification for antibiotics and insulin, but for no other drugs, and drugs approved before 1938 or 1962 were subject to much less restrictive regulation than newer products.

Sen. Kennedy's Labor and Human Resources Health Subcommittee and the House Commerce Health Subcommittee, then chaired by Paul G. Rogers, D-Fla. (1955-1979), spent months in intermittent hearings, issues-debates and drafting sessions on the 1978 administration bill. But neither subcommittee was able to bring out a bill, because of industry objections and because dealing with very technical issues that are also very controversial takes a great deal of time in Congress.

1979 Committee Action

Early in 1979 Sen. Kennedy introduced S 1075, which dropped the monograph system entirely, including the raw-data disclosure, but retained other features of the administration bill.

Markup sessions in subcommittee and in the full Labor and Human Resources Committee were difficult to follow because members tended to make major decisions "in principle" and then instruct the staff to draft language — not an unusual procedure for technical legislation. The subcommittee agreed to the measure unanimously on June 25, and the full committee voted to report it July 27. The committee report was not filed until Sept. 18.

A series of industry-backed amendments offered by Schweiker affected the tone but not the basic thrust of the bill, according to Kennedy aide David Riemer. A typical change narrowed the bill's definition of drug safety. In Kennedy's version, regulators were to consider not only the safety of a drug in its intended use, but also its potential for abuse, and other factors that Schweiker felt were too vague. The final version restricted safety judgments to use of the drug by patients and for purposes intended by the manufacurer.

Schweiker's amendments also added new requirements for FDA consultation with advisory committees, and set time limits on the new post-approval conditions such as limited distribution.

Schweiker's proposals also:
- Deleted new FDA authority to impose civil fines for drug-law violations.
- Eliminated proposed new independent litigating authority for the agency.
- Authorized the FDA to delegate its authority to approve preliminary human tests of drugs to medical school, hospital and other health facilities meeting certain standards.

Committee Report

In its report (S Rept 96-321), the Labor and Human Resources Committee argued that changes in federal drug regulation were needed because the process was "too unpredictable" during the research stage before approval for marketing, and "too rigid" after a drug was on the market. The report cited as particular problems the existing law's massive data requirements (30 volumes or more of data on safety and efficacy tests for a single new drug approval application) and lengthy approval time (a median of 23 months after submission of data on a drug's safety and effectiveness).

Despite the "voluminous" data requirements, there was a "lack of understanding" of how approved drugs were actually used and "inadequate information ... on adverse reactions, long-term risks, unanticipated benefits and potential new uses," the committee said.

FDA approval procedures were essentially those in use since 1938, the committee noted, although in the past four decades there had been "dramatic growth and change in how Americans use drugs." Ninety percent of today's prescription drugs were unknown in 1938, and Americans' spending on drugs had gone from $300 million a year then to $16 billion a year in 1979, the committee said. In 1977, doctors wrote 1.5 billion prescriptions, which averaged out to almost seven for every man, woman and child in the nation, it said.

1979 Floor Action

The Senate passed S 1075 Sept. 26 by voice vote, with only a few members present. Discussion and voting on the bill and three amendments lasted less than two hours.

Floor action came so soon after the printed committee report became available that many lobbyists were still digesting the committee amendments. Only a few hours before the vote, Kennedy aides assured Senate staffers, lobbyists and reporters that action would not take place that day.

The rush to passage apparently protected the compromise bill from any attempts to reopen troublesome issues that had stalled drug law revision for almost two years in Kennedy's subcommittee. "It was smooth," said AMA counsel John Lawrence. "It caught us by surprise."

But the smoothness also reflected the fact that Kennedy had worked out agreements within the committee on the most thorny issues, and that no committee members voted against the measure. Kennedy and Schweiker had "a triumph of negotiaton and diplomacy," said Jacob K. Javits, R-N.Y.

Two Nader associates, Dr. Sidney Wolfe of the Health Research Group and Caroline Brickey of Congress Watch, circulated a harshly worded critique of the bill on the day of the vote, but no other opposition surfaced then, despite the controversial nature of many of the bill's provisions.

Kennedy's handling of the bill prompted both industry and consumer lobbyists to speculate that presidential politics had spurred his determination to chalk up a win on a major "Kennedy health bill" in 1979. The Senate vote came the day after President Carter told a Queens, N.Y., "town meeting" that Kennedy had labored 16 years on national health insurance without success. "He has never gotten a comprehensive national health bill out of his subcommittee," Carter said, adding, "It's not easy."

But both majority and minority committee staff maintained that Kennedy's move was simply the end point of lengthy committee work on the drug issues, plus shrewd Senate politics. "You take your floor time when you can get it, and anyway, we dealt with all the amendments that senators brought to our attention. There was no reason to wait any longer," said one minority aide.

"Every group with an interest in this legislation has had many opportunities to be heard," Kennedy noted.

Floor Amendments

The Senate adopted three amendments to the bill.

Generic Drugs. An amendment by Orrin G. Hatch, R-Utah, placed new limits on makers of so-called "lookalike" drugs — copies of brand-name drugs generally retailed under a generic name at lower cost than the originals. However, some confusion over the meaning of the amendment was created because of a colloquy on the floor involving Hatch, Kennedy and Javits.

The amendment declared a drug to be "counterfeit" (illegal) if it was composed of the same active ingredients,

in the same strength, as the original drug, and looked so much like the original that it would probably confuse consumers. That appeared to mean that a manufacturer could copy the chemical composition of a drug as long as he made it look different from the original. The amendment replaced committee language that simply required copies of brand-name drugs to bear the trademark of the manufacturer.

Advocates of cheaper generic drugs, such as the AARP, argued that unless generics look like the originals, patients won't take them.

Manufacturers of the originals complained that generic manufacturers get a "free ride" on the reputation of the original, brand-name drug.

If Hatch's amendment meant that generic drugs had to be different colors or sizes than the original, it would affect the marketability of generic drugs, undermining state drug "substitution" programs. New York, for instance, required pharmacists to fill prescriptions with generic versions of drugs unless a doctor specified the brand-name version. Forty-five other states had similar laws, either requiring or permitting substitution.

The confusion came when Kennedy and Javits both declared, for the record, that Hatch's amendment would not affect the New York statute. "If two products have different marks on them, even though they are the same color, size and shape, they are not affected," Kennedy said. Hatch concurred — thereby creating a legislative record that baffled both industry and FDA officials. Hatch aide Ron Docksai said later that Hatch had not intended to bar copies that were the same size, color and shape as the original, but only wanted to require clearly distinguishable trademarks.

Drug Science Center. An amendment offered by Schweiker for Henry Bellmon, R-Okla., eliminated the training functions of a proposed new National Center for Drug Science, along with a $34.8 million, three-year authorization for those functions. The amendment also changed the name of the remaining research facility to the Office for Drug Science.

The committee had intended the new facility to support and conduct research on new drugs and on drug policy questions and to conduct training programs in clinical pharmacology for medical and other health students, researchers and practitioners.

Schweiker's brief floor explanation of the amendment was that the new office was "not intended to overlap with any existing programs." Staff sources later said Bellmon thought the new center would duplicate education functions of the Health, Education and Welfare (HEW, now Health and Human Services) Department's health manpower bureau, which supported medical and other health professions training. The National Institutes of Health, the federal medical research facility, had also sought to downgrade the status of the "center" to "office" — apparently permitting the new facility to be located within NIH.

The third amendment, by Kennedy, made minor technical changes in the bill.

Provisions

As passed by the Senate, S 1075:

● Eliminated the statutory distinction between "interstate" and "intrastate" activity for purposes of drug regulation, except for drugs explicitly authorized by state laws.

This extended FDA jurisdiction to all drug manufacturing, marketing and related activities carried on within individual states, except for those drugs specifically permitted by state statutes. Existing law authorized regulation only of drug-related activities which crossed state borders.

● Broadened the definition of "counterfeit" (illegal) drugs to include any prescription drug with active ingredients in the same strength as a comparable approved drug and which was so similar in appearance to the original that consumers would be confused.

● Dropped the statutory distinctions between drugs that had been "grandfathered" (exempted from provisions of earlier drug laws) or otherwise designated for special treatment. The effect was to make all drugs equally subject to all FDA regulatory powers.

● Prohibited submission of false or misleading statements to the FDA in applications and other materials.

● Authorized the FDA to hold off the market, for up to 30 days, a drug that appeared to be adulterated.

Criminal Liability. Reversed the "Park rule," that individual drug company executives were criminally liable for all violations of the drug law by their company regardless of whether they knew of the specific violation. Required instead that an executive be proved "negligent" in order to be found guilty of a violation of the drug laws.

(FDA attorney Robert Steeves said this provision did not change existing FDA enforcement procedures. Since the 1975 Park ruling, the agency had routinely served notice to the chief executive officer of a drug company, thereby establishing that he "must have known or should have known" of the alleged violation, Steeves said.)

● Raised criminal penalties for violations of the Food, Drug and Cosmetics Act to $50,000 for individuals and established a new $100,000 fine for businesses. Existing law did not distinguish between individuals and corporations. Existing fines were $1,000 for a misdemeanor, $10,000 for a felony. Existing imprisonment penalties continued in effect.

● Added three new standards — "identity," "stability" and "bioavailability" — to the existing standards ("strength," "quality" and "purity") that a drug must meet to be approved for marketing. ("Bioavailability" refers to how a drug acts within the body — for example, how quickly and how accurately active ingredients take effect.)

Drug labeling, advertising. Required prescription drug labels to show the name and address of both the manufacturer and the distributor of the drug. Under existing law, only one had to be identified.

● Required a drug manufacturer to prepare "patient labeling" (information about a drug's benefits and risks) and required a physician or pharmacist, in most cases, to make sure a patient got the information with the prescription drug. Also required pharmacies to make available to consumers a book containing the patient labeling for the pharmacy's 100 most frequently sold drugs.

● Permitted patient labeling to be withheld in three instances: if the FDA authorized physicians to withhold the information on the basis that it might be harmful to a patient; if the drug was dispensed by a hospital or similar facility that provided some alternative form of information; if the drug was used in an emergency.

● Required the secretary of HEW to consult with consumer, pharmacist and other interested health groups before establishing patient labeling regulations.

● Empowered the FDA to require pharmacies to post the prices of their 50 most frequently sold drugs.

● Required drug companies to provide doctors with "objective and balanced" drug information, in writing, during visits by company "detail men."

● Required publication and distribution to practitioners of a federal drug index listing all approved drugs, along with their risks, benefits and other appropriate information.

● Empowered the FDA to notify patients, physicians and others if a drug presented "substantial risk of illness or injury." This replaced an existing standard that the FDA must demonstrate "imminent danger" or "gross deception" to justify a warning against a drug.

● Explicitly authorized the FDA to provide general public information about drug use and drug products.

● Required that drug advertising ("promotional labeling") summarize side-effects and other information relating to a drug. Empowered the FDA, in certain circumstances, to review drug ads before publication. Explicitly authorized the FDA to require corrective advertising.

● Prohibited gifts from drug companies worth more than $10, or free samples of drugs, to doctors, other health professionals or members of their families. Permitted gifts of drugs only in these instances: from a pharmacy to a patient on the written request of a doctor; from a drug company to a doctor on the specific, written request of the doctor; to a charitable organization, if the drug was to be used for charitable purposes; in a medical emergency.

● Required sponsors of seminars or other educational activities on drugs to disclose their sponsorship.

● Limited access to a pharmacy's prescription records to doctors, patients, pharmacists, law enforcement officers, individuals seeking verification for payments and researchers meeting standards set by FDA. Prohibited drug manufacturers or distributors from inspecting prescription records. Prohibited individuals with access to the records from copying or disclosing information that could identify an individual patient except in certain circumstances, such as refilling a prescription. This provision was intended to end "prescription surveys," in which manufacturers checked to see whether individual physicians were prescribing their drugs.

● Required all labeling on drugs used by children, pregnant women or the elderly to include a statement as to whether the drug had been tested on that population group.

Drug approval procedures. Required any marketer of a drug to apply for and receive FDA approval before marketing any drug. This provision was intended to overrule a judicial interpretation that existing law did not require the maker of a generic drug to "even notify . . . [the] FDA that it is marketing a drug product," according to the Senate committee report.

● Exempted three categories of drugs from the mandatory application provision: over-the-counter (non-prescription) drugs which had been found safe and effective by the FDA within five years after enactment of the new drug law; homeopathic drugs; drugs that had been "grandfathered" (exempted from new requirements) by the 1938 drug law. For the grandfathered drugs, manufacturers would not have to submit applications for approval, but the drugs themselves would be subject to all FDA regulatory powers. Homeopathic drugs are substances, mostly herbal in origin, used in minute amounts to stimulate certain reactions in the body. The dosage levels are so small that the FDA considered many of these drugs to have no therapeutic effect. The FDA could revoke this exemption for any homeopathic drug that it found to have a risk or illness or injury.

● Replaced a requirement that manufacturers submit to FDA "full reports of investigations" on a drug's safety and effectiveness as part of an application for marketing approval. Instead, permitted drug companies to submit, and FDA to require, a comprehensive summary of investigators' reports. Required manufacturers to provide FDA access to the raw data on which the summaries were based. Barred release to the public of the comprehensive summaries.

● Required drug manufacturers to include in their applications for approval a second, shorter summary of safety and effectiveness tests. This summary, for public disclosure, would be comparable to an article in a respected scientific journal, and could exclude trade secrets.

● Specified certain mandatory administrative procedures for the FDA to follow in processing applications for approval. These included: a 45-day deadline for FDA determination on whether an application for drug approval met filing requirements, with automatic filing if the FDA did not meet the deadline; written explanations and hearings for persons whose applications were refused; a notice and public comment period on applications; a 30-day deadline for announcing the names of an application's reviewers, and a ban on changing reviewers on an individual application.

● Empowered the FDA to suspend approval of any drug found to present "an unreasonable risk of illness or injury to any segment of the population." This standard replaced a stiffer statutory requirement that the FDA must show a drug to be an "imminent hazard to the public health" in order to suspend approval. ("Suspension" means withdrawing approval without public notice and hearing; revocation of approval requires the more lengthy notice and hearing procedure.)

● Permitted the secretary of HEW to delegate his authority to suspend approval of a drug to the commissioner of FDA.

● Empowered the FDA to revoke approval for a drug if the manufacturer failed to comply with any of the new post-marketing requirements (continued surveillance for adverse reactions, for example), after having been warned in writing.

● Permitted a manufacturer to submit an abbreviated new drug application (ANDA) to market an approved drug after the original, approved drug had been on the market for seven years. The ANDA could omit both raw and comprehensive data.

● Required researchers to inform individuals participating in drug tests of the risks and benefits expected from the drug, and, except in unusual circumstances, to obtain their consent in writing.

● Required researchers to protect the health, privacy and rights of research subjects, and to keep a test drug from being promoted or advertised.

Expedited pre-market human testing. Authorized certain expedited procedures for the early phase of pre-market testing of drugs, involving small numbers of human subjects. The most important change was permitting the FDA to delegate its authority to approve this early-phase testing to medical schools or other entities doing health-related research, teaching or delivery of services. Delegation to entities that manufactured or distributed drugs was prohibited; however, an entity controlled by a drug manufacturer or distributor could be delegated if the research reviews were made by an independent "institutional review board"(IRB).

● Required the FDA to publish research guidelines; authorized it to advise informally researchers on proposed investigations; authorized an informal procedure for resolving disputes between the FDA and drug researchers.

Approval of non-investigational drugs. Required the FDA to permit, by regulation, the use of unapproved, non-investigational drugs for small numbers of patients with serious diseases or injuries, for which there were no "adequate" alternative methods of diagnosis or cure. Such drugs should not have an "unreasonable risk of illness or injury," and FDA regulations on patient privacy and informed consent must be observed. The approval was limited to three years, but could be renewed. The FDA now authorizes this use of drugs on a case-by-case basis. The effect of the provision would be to make such drugs available to patients not participating in research projects.

● Established statutory definitions for the two standards for FDA approval of drugs as follows: A "safe" drug was one

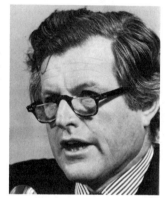

"Every group with an interest in this legislation has had many opportunities to be heard."

—Sen. Edward M. Kennedy, D-Mass.

whose health benefits outweighed its risks, when used by the designated patient population for the designated purposes. An "effective" drug was one which would have the effect claimed by a manufacturer, if used according to directions.

Breakthrough drugs. Authorized the FDA to approve for marketing new "breakthrough" drugs that met the statutory safety standard but had not met the full effectiveness requirement. Such a drug could be approved for prescription distribution only if early human tests provided some evidence of effectiveness, if it was for a very serious illness and was "definitely superior" to other available drugs, and if the patient's risk in taking the drug was less than the risk of not taking it while more tests were completed. This type of approval would run three years, could be renewed, could require limited distribution of the drug and would usually require a drug company to complete full effectiveness testing with a large patient population.

Post-marketing powers. Empowered the FDA to require limited distribution, continued surveillance, further scientific studies or batch certification as a condition for approving a drug for marketing. Each of these post-marketing conditions could run for only a few years, as specified in the bill, but could be renewed.

To impose post-marketing conditions, FDA would have to consult with advisory committees. For new drugs, the requirements could be imposed without notice. For already approved drugs, FDA would have to provide notice and an informal hearing before acting.

"Limited distribution" could mean approving a drug only for use in a hospital or only by specially qualified physicians. "Surveillance" would be monitoring for adverse side effects, abuse or other problems. "Batch certification" means testing each batch of a drug for stability, purity or other qualities.

● Permitted FDA to exempt from mandatory batch certification individual manufacturers or facilities that could produce a drug "in a consistently satisfactory manner."

● Required FDA to consult with consumer, health professions, science, manufacturer and other groups on the membership of advisory committees; required that at least one-third of each committee be members "reflecting interests of patients and consumers."

● Authorized subpoena powers for the FDA for matters relating to false or misleading information or articles that were unapproved, adulterated or otherwise prohibited, but not for a broad range of compliance issues such as good marketing practices.

● Authorized FDA to reimburse persons participating in drug regulation proceedings for attorney's fees or other related costs.

● Permitted the export of drugs not approved for domestic use, if the importing country approved the drug and if the secretary of HEW found that the drug was not "contrary to the public health" of the importing country. Established a task force with representatives from HEW, Commerce and the State Department and the Special U.S. Trade Representative to recommend regulations for these decisions.

This provision was more restrictive than the administration proposal, which would have permitted drug exports

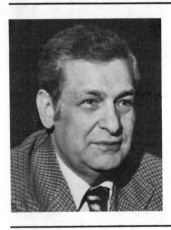

The bill is "one of those damn pieces of legislation where the intent is noble, and everybody agrees that there are some problems, but...."

—William F. Apple, president, American Pharmaceutical Association

approved by the importing nation unless the HEW secretary explicitly vetoed the drug. Existing law required exported drugs to meet U.S. safety and efficacy standards.

● Pre-empted new state drug labeling and packaging laws passed after enactment, but permitted the secretary of HEW to exempt a new state law, on request of the state, if the law "enhanced" the public health within the state and would not overburden interstate commerce.

Office for Drug Science. Established a new Office for Drug Science within HEW; authorized it to conduct or support studies in three general areas: developing new drugs, use of drugs, and the impact of drug regulation. The office would study the safety and effectiveness of approved drugs and could develop "orphan drugs" (those for rare diseases that don't appear to be highly profitable) or "breakthrough" drugs that were not being investigated elsewhere.

It would be barred from commenting on any matter before the FDA, except on the request of the FDA, or on matters relating to drug research supported by the office.

● Authorized $5 million for fiscal 1981, $7 million for fiscal 1982 and $9 million for fiscal 1983 for drug office activities.

● Established statutory authority for the existence of the FDA, and required presidential appointment and Senate approval of the FDA commissioner.

Reactions

The range of reactions to the Senate bill pointed out the controversies that would be debated when the House took up drug law revision.

Following the Senate action, Pharmaceutical Manufacturers Association (PMA) Washington officials declined to discuss specific objections to the Senate bill beyond a general statement from President Lewis Engman that S 1075 "fails to provide meaningful regulatory reform" and "will adversely affect the American consumer." Earlier PMA testimony showed strong opposition to the new post-marketing powers, patient information and certain other features of the bill.

One reason for PMA's apparent discretion was that the drug industry itself was divided on some key provisions, including how much drug-risk data to provide the public, and the new drug export standards. Jack Wood, director of public affairs at Hoffman-LaRoche, called the bill "an improvement over existing law."

Ben Gordon of the Health Research Group, a former Senate staff aide who worked on Sen. Gaylord Nelson's, D-Wis., drug hearings in the late 1960s, called S 1075 "a lousy bill." He and Brickey of Congress Watch were particularly critical of proposed changes on "breakthrough" drugs, export laws and criminal liability standards for drug company executives.

The other consumer-oriented group that followed the bill closely was not so critical. The American Association of Retired Persons' Wegner said he shared Gordon's worries about proposed changes on "breakthrough" drugs — "any way you slice it, it's a lowering of standards that now protect us," he said. Like the Nader officials, Wegner also thought Congress should not jettison the stricter criminal liability standard for drug company executives that was in effect "because it has a useful deterrent effect." But, he added, there was a lot in the bill to benefit consumers, and "we would be marginally better off under the Kennedy bill than under existing law."

The American Medical Association, according to its testimony, found the new information provisions, particularly those on patient package information (PPI), and the post-marketing powers objectionable because it feared they would interfere with individual judgments by doctors about the best drug therapy for patients.

The pharmacists' association, according to President William F. Apple, regarded S 1075 as "one of those damn pieces of legislation where the intent is noble, and everybody agrees that there are some problems, but...." The association found the PPI and certain other information provisions too costly and too untested. The American Pharmaceutical Association (APhA) estimated the information inserts would add almost $1.5 billion to drug costs in five years, and "I've never known any new cost that wasn't ultimately passed on to the consumer," Apple said.

Protecting Privacy of Medical Records

Should a patient have the right to read his doctor's notes on his diagnosis and treatment?

Should the sensitive, personal information in medical records be open to employers, credit bureaus, insurance companies, law enforcement officials, as it often has been?

Should the patient's permission be required?

Congress was considering questions such as these as it began work on landmark legislation that would entitle patients to see their own hospital records and set rules under which others could examine them.

The bill (HR 5935), reported by the House Government Operations Committee March 19, 1980 (H Rept 96-832, Part I), was developed in response to the 1977 report of the presidentially appointed Privacy Protection Study Commission, which found that medical records were more widely circulated than many patients imagined.

"And there are so many abuses, so many errors, so many offhand observations by a doctor" in these records that might haunt a person for a lifetime, said David F. Linowes, who chaired the commission.

Whether an individual was hired, promoted, insured or licensed to practice a profession, drive a car or marry could be influenced by evidence of cancer treatments, heart conditions, psychotherapy, epilepsy, sexually transmitted diseases and other ailments, the commission found.

Despite the potential impact of this information, the patient often was not allowed to look at his own medical record, according to the commission, which found few legal sanctions either to compel disclosure to a patient or to stop breaches of confidentiality.

As reported by the House Government Operations Committee, HR 5935 delicately balanced patient privacy against the information needs of public officials and others — and against political realities. For instance, it would apply only to hospitals and other medical facilities — not to private doctors' offices, which had been stiffly protected by the American Medical Association (AMA). And, in deference to the anti-regulatory mood of Congress, a Carter administration plan to enforce its provisions through Medicare and Medicaid was dropped.

On June 26, the House Commerce Committee — the second of four panels with jurisdiction over the measure, agreed to its version of the bill. The main difference between the two versions was that the commerce bill would apply solely to records kept by hospitals, federal outpatient clinics and similar facilities.

Other provisions of HR 5935 would prohibit hospital employees and others from releasing medical record information unless they had a patient's permission, in writing, to do so.

Exceptions. While the bill would bar employers, insurers and others from examining a person's records without his consent, it contained more than a dozen exceptions that would allow the Central Intelligence Agency (CIA) and medical researchers, among others, to look at them without a patient's permission — and, in some instances, without his knowledge.

Many of these exceptions would codify existing practices. For instance, Secret Service Director H. Stuart Knight said the service routinely depended on doctors and hospital officials "for bringing ... potentially dangerous persons to our attention."

The American Civil Liberties Union (ACLU) objected strongly to most of these exceptions and wanted stiffer legal barriers to non-medical uses of patient records. The American Psychiatric Association (APA) also insisted that the special stigma of mental health problems required tighter safeguards for psychiatric records than the House bill provided.

The Justice Department, on the other hand, was pressing hard for freer access to medical records for grand juries and other law enforcement purposes.

The AMA and the American Hospital Association (AHA) disliked the bill on general principles, though neither was fighting it very strenuously.

Because opposition was relatively mild, or limited to specific provisions, sponsors were optimistic that the bill would be enacted, perhaps even in 1980. The Carter administration, which submitted its own medical records privacy bill (HR 3444, S 865) in 1979, and the American Medical Records Association (AMRA) backed the legislation. The APA and ACLU also supported it, with some adjustments.

The bill's biggest hazard in mid-1980 appeared to be the time-short election-year schedule of Congress. Moreover, in addition to the House Government Operations Committee and the Ways and Means Committee, two

---

"There are so many abuses, so many errors, so many offhand observations by a doctor" in medical records that might haunt a person for a lifetime.

—David F. Linowes, chairman, Privacy Protection Study Commission

---

other panels — Commerce and Judiciary — also claimed jurisdiction over the legislation.

In the Senate, S 865 and S 503, introduced by Jacob K. Javits, R-N.Y., did not have to run a multi-committee gauntlet because other panels had waived jurisdiction to the Governmental Affairs Committee.

Changing Times

The centuries-old tradition of confidential doctor-patient communication was cracking under pressures from public and private health insurance plans, researchers and public health programs, and changing practices in medicine itself.

New medical school graduates were still taking the Hippocratic oath, promising that, "Whatever, in connection with my professional practice, or not in connection with it, I see or hear in the life of men, which ought not to be spoken abroad, I will not divulge, as reckoning that all such should be kept secret. . . ." But "determining what can or cannot be spoken abroad has become a complicated task," said Rep. Richardson Preyer, D-N.C., sponsor of HR 5935.

Fifty years ago, most medical treatment took place in a physician's office. A typical medical record simply noted dates of patient visits, medications prescribed and fees charged, according to the 1977 privacy panel report, *Personal Privacy in an Information Society.*

The modern physician working in a hospital, clinic or group practice has shared patient responsibility — and medical charts — with consulting specialists, medical students, nurses, social workers and others. And the doctor who might have to defend his professional decisions against a malpractice suit was more likely to keep detailed records than to entrust medical notes and impressions to what one writer called the "safe crevices of his mind," as doctors often used to do.

Sophisticated concepts of disease causation and prevention prompted doctors to question patients on their personal habits, occupations and family relationships. "A complete medical record [today] may contain more intimate details about an individual than could be found in any other single document," an AMRA official told the privacy commission.

Medical records have also been opened to public and private health insurance plans, which have insisted on knowing what they were paying for, and to quality control programs such as Professional Standards Review Organizations.

"Social needs . . . and epidemiological research," the commission found, had generated mandatory reporting of "death, birth, communicable diseases . . . drug addiction, gunshot wounds and child abuse," as well as registries of individuals with cancer or other diseases that might be related to environmental or occupational factors.

Other avenues into medical records have included reviews by employers, educational institutions or licensing agencies. Computerization has enhanced opportunities for data-sharing.

The volume of information was enormous, and growing. John H. F. Shattuck, director of the ACLU's Washington office, estimated that 190 million Americans were enrolled in public or private health insurance programs, 75 million in private disability plans and 60 million in the workers' compensation program, while about 3 million received Social Security disability payments — all with attendant demands for medical records.

An official of a 600-bed hospital told the commission that in a single month he received 2,700 requests for medical record information — about a third from insurers, a third from other physicians, and the remaining third from subpoenas, queries from other hospitals and attorneys, and miscellaneous requests.

Existing Protections. The rights of individuals to have access to records on them, and to correct them if necessary, mandated by the 1974 federal Privacy Act (PL 93-579) have applied, in general, only to records kept by the federal government. That bill created the privacy commission to recommend further privacy safeguards.

In 1977, the year the commission published its report, 19 states had "regulations, statutes or case law recognizing medical records as confidential and limiting access to them." Twenty-one states authorized revocation of a doctor's license for breaches of professional confidence. But, the commission noted, these legal sanctions applied only to physicians, not to other health professionals or to nonprofessionals who handled medical data. Patient rights were not foremost in the statutory prohibitions on disclosure, which usually focused on protecting doctors from being forced to testify on confidential matters. The commission was unable to find a single case "in which a physician or hospital had to compensate a patient for an injury resulting from breach of confidentiality."

Need for Legislation

Individuals were not in a position to protect their own medical records because "usually the choice is between signing [a consent form] and foregoing a job or some indispensable service or benefit," such as health insurance, the privacy commission's report stated.

The Government Operations Committee, in its report, made these arguments on behalf of the bill:

● "Surreptitious trafficking in medical information is common," and apparently widespread. For example, a 1975 Colorado grand jury investigation uncovered a 25-year history of medical records theft by a private firm whose investigators posed as doctors to solicit information by telephone or paid hospital employees to smuggle out medical records. The firm's customers included more than 100 of "the most prominent insurance companies in the country." Similar findings from an investigation in Canada suggested to the committee that these practices were common in North America.

● Most states did not have comprehensive medical records laws, and the few that did typically applied them only to state institutions. Nor did these statutes usually address the question of patient access.

ACLU's Shattuck and Dr. Marcia Goin, who chaired the APA Committee on Confidentiality, stressed the harm caused by breaches of confidentiality. "There are communities in which teachers are not hired, tenured or promoted" if it becomes known that they have sought psychotherapy, Goin said. Other examples cited by Goin: An insurance investigator threatened a physician's credit record when he resisted her repeated queries about a patient. And San Francisco police officials sought photographs and fingerprints of narcotics addicts at local drug abuse clinics — although even a hint of such surveillance "would devastate any drug treatment program," she said.

In a federally funded abortion study in New York state, researchers matched fetal death certificates with personal, marital and medical records in various government agencies all over the country, Shattuck testified in 1979. None of the 48,000 women whose records were examined "had given their consent or even knew about the study," yet a preliminary report to the New York state legislature "inadvertently revealed the names of some of the subjects," Shattuck said.

Dissenting Views. Six Republican members of the House Government Operations Committee disagreed on the need for the legislation. In dissenting views to the committee report, the six contended that the entire bill was "unnecessary."

"There just isn't any widespread invasion of medical records privacy in America today," wrote John N. Erlenborn, Ill., John W. Wydler, N.Y., Clarence J. Brown, Ohio, Robert S. Walker, Pa., Arlan Stangeland, Minn., and Jim Jeffries, Kan.

Three liberal Democrats on the panel criticized the bill's treatment of unauthorized access by intelligence and law enforcement officials. Ted Weiss, N.Y., said the committee adopted a disturbingly "vague" standard for unauthorized disclosure of medical files to CIA and Federal Bureau of Investigation (FBI) agents.

The bill would allow unauthorized — and unannounced — access to files of individuals who might be potential sources of intelligence. Weiss claimed. This standard left "the door wide open for unlimited access [by the agencies] to personal files" — in effect encouraging "the abuses which the legislation is intended to prevent," Weiss said. Robert F. Drinan, Mass., and Peter H. Kostmayer, Pa., concurred.

Interest Group Positions

AMA. Dr. Frederick W. Ackerman, chairman of the AMA council on legislation, endorsed what he called "appropriate right of access" for patients to medical information. But, Ackerman warned the Ways and Means Health Subcommittee earlier in 1980, "unlimited right of access" could be harmful, prompting some persons to "treat themselves," or devastating those who found they had a terminal illness.

Ackerman urged that outpatient clinics and similar facilities be dropped from the bill, but he added that the entire bill was undesirable because it would "lead to less creativity in state laws . . . in an area too complex to be subject to any . . . single solution."

AHA. The American Hospital Association thought federal legislation would lead to regulatory overkill, duplicating existing state laws, licensing regulations and voluntary industry standards. "We don't think this is the proper remedy, even though we agree with the principle," said AHA official Michael Hash.

AMRA. The American Medical Records Association was generally pleased with the bill, said spokeswoman Myra Nyberg, but wanted it to explicitly state grounds on which a medical institution could refuse disclosure in those cases where it was not required. Without such language, record-keepers might experience excessive pressures for disclosure, she said. (Committee aides noted that the bill was essentially "permissive" — that is, in cases not covered by the exceptions, nothing required disclosure.)

APA. Psychiatric, psychological and mental health treatment notes were "private speculations" of the practitioner, belonging neither to his employer nor to a patient, in the view of the American Psychiatric Association. While the bill would permit withholding these notes from patients, it lacked special provisions affecting access by third parties. As such, "it is a disclosure bill, not a privacy bill," Goin told the Ways and Means panel.

Psychiatric data should have the same absolute protections that the bill accorded drug abuse and alcohol abuse information, she said. (HR 5935 would allow existing, stricter federal rules for these programs to override its provisions.)

ACLU. Patients should have "absolute right of access to their own records," while government agencies should

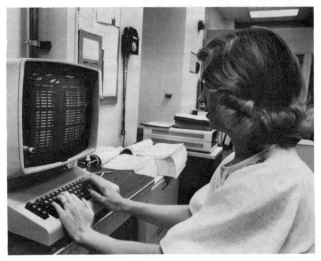
Medical Records Increasingly are Available on Computers

be barred from records unless the patient authorized access or a court found "a compelling law enforcement interest" in disclosure, Shattuck said. The ACLU shared many of the APA's concerns, he added.

Justice Department. The biggest threat to the bill's carefully crafted balance appeared to be Justice Department objections to a new judicial "balancing test." The bill would permit patients to challenge subpoenas or summonses for confidential medical information in court, where a judge could decide whether their "privacy interest" outweighed the law enforcement need for the material.

The ACLU and the APA were not entirely happy with this provision as reported by the House panel, while Justice Department lawyers warned that the test could be used to block federal investigations of fraud, grand jury inquiries and other essential law enforcement functions.

John C. Keeney, deputy assistant attorney general in the Justice Department's Criminal Division, said the department felt that patients should not be able to keep hospitals from reporting general admission and health status information. The bill would permit patients to block even this general information, and "obviously, those individuals about whom law enforcement authorities are most likely to inquire will exercise this opportunity," Keeney said.

Major Provisions

As reported by the Government Operations Committee, HR 5935:

● Would apply to the following types of institutions: federally operated medical facilities; hospitals and skilled nursing facilities; outpatient clinics and similar facilities receiving federal funds, at the discretion of the secretary of the Department of Health and Human Services (HHS, formerly Health, Education and Welfare); outpatient and intermediate care facilities operated by state governments, if those governments so decide. The protections for information compiled by a medical facility would continue for that information even if the institution ceased to function as a medical facility.

The bill would not cover medical information in private physicians' offices or occupational health information on workers that was maintained by employers or company physicians. It explicitly excluded records on inmates of correctional institutions.

● Would bar state or local laws from compelling disclosure of information protected by the bill. Would allow state laws that were stricter on disclosure, or stricter statutes on privacy of drug abuse, alcohol abuse or mental health information to override the bill.

● Would bar use of information disclosed under the bill for any purpose other than that for which it was disclosed.

● Would allow an incompetent patient's next of kin to authorize disclosure for that patient, if needed for medical treatment or for payment of medical charges; authorized persons aged 18 and older to exercise the patient rights spelled out by the bill; authorized parents or legal guardians of children under age 14 to exercise these rights; authorized individuals aged 14 to 17 or their parents to exercise these rights.

Patient Rights. Would require medical facilities to permit a patient to inspect and have a copy of any medical information they had on him.

● Would permit medical facilities to deny patient requests for: psychiatric or mental health treatment notes; information that could cause more harm to the patient than withholding it might; data that could identify confidential sources of information about a patient; information being collected only for civil actions. If information was withheld because disclosure was judged to be potentially harmful, the patient could designate a third party to whom the information must be disclosed.

● Would require a facility to correct a medical record, if requested in writing by a patient to do so, or inform the patient of its reason for refusal. If the correction was denied, the correction request must become part of the patient's record.

● Would require medical facilities to inform patients of their rights regarding medical records.

● Would permit a patient to authorize disclosure of medical information about himself. Allowed the patient to revoke the authorization unless it already had been acted on or the information was needed by a government agency to confirm spending on medical procedures.

Exceptions. Would bar disclosures not authorized by patients except in certain specified circumstances. Nonauthorized disclosures would be permissible in these cases:

● To employees of the medical facility, for carrying out their professional duties, and to medical consultants.

In a very general way, indicating only that an individual was a patient and his general condition, if the patient did not object.

● For health research projects that met specified standards and protected the identity of individual patients; for public health surveys, audits or evaluations; to identify a dead person; in emergency situations that might affect the health or safety of a person or the safety of property; to comply with legal standards, including child abuse reporting requirements, or in connection with a court-ordered examination of a patient.

● To the Secret Service or any federal agency with authority to conduct foreign intelligence or counterintelligence activities, if the information was needed to carry out such activities or for the protective functions of the Secret Service. Employees of the medical facility would be prohibited from informing the patient of the request.

To a patient's next of kin or persons with legal responsibility for him or a personal relationship with him.

To law enforcement agencies making specific written requests, if the information was to be used to investigate or prosecute criminal activities (such as fraud) in public health or disability programs; to help identify a suspect, fugitive or witness in an investigation; in connection with crimes committed at medical facilities or against their personnel; or simply to determine if a crime has been committed.

For requests in connection with court or administrative agency proceedings in which the patient was a party, or in response to subpoenas, summonses, warrants and search warrants, copies of which would become part of an individual's medical record. The bill stated that its provisions could not be interpreted as grounds for a facility to refuse to comply with valid subpoenas, warrants and summonses.

By federal medical facilities, for determining eligibility for military service-related benefits, promotion, assignment and similar matters, or to support claims for payment from a private insurance company or other carrier. Patients must be notified in advance of such disclosures.

Legal Procedures. Government agencies seeking medical information with summonses, subpoenas, warrants or search warrants would be required to meet certain conditions. They must have "reasonable grounds" to believe the information sought was relevant to their inquiry, and wait 10 days after serving the summons or subpoena before taking the information (14 days if the summons was mailed).

The bill would require agencies obtaining information by administrative or search warrant to provide patients with a copy of the warrant within 90 days unless an extension was granted by a court.

Patients receiving summonses or subpoenas could challenge them in court, and a decision must be made within seven days after the challenged agency had filed its response. If the court found that a patient's privacy interests were stronger than the agency's case, the challenge would stand; the court could deny the challenge if it found that the inquiry was legitimate, the medical information sought was relevant, and that the law enforcement need outweighed the privacy need. The bill explicitly placed the burden of proving his privacy interests on the patient.

Enforcement. The bill would provide criminal penalties as follows: fines up to $10,000 or imprisonment up to six months, or both, for fraudulently seeking or obtaining medical information from a medical facility or an authorization to disclose information; fines up to $30,000 or imprisonment up to 18 months, or both, for stealing or selling improperly acquired information.

The bill would authorize civil suits by patients against public officials or employees, medical facilities, health researchers and others for violations of patient rights. In most cases, complaints had to be filed within three years of the alleged violation. The following could not be sued: members of an institutional review board who determined "in good faith" that a research project outweighed privacy interests; medical facilities acting "in good faith" on certified requests from government agencies for information; medical facilities deciding "in good faith" that a patient's condition rendered him unable to act on his own behalf. ∎

Appendix

Chronology of Action on Health Programs, 1973-79

Health Legislation, 1973-79

1973

In the health area, the 93rd Congress spent its first session getting ready for things to come and fighting off Nixon administration proposals to end some federal health activities.

Legislators reopened debate over national health insurance, but insurance plans remained lodged in committee while the administration reworked its proposal. Congress also moved to give itself another year to come up with three bills addressing health services, health planning and health manpower needs by simply extending 12 health programs without change.

But the simple extension was a setback to President Nixon's budget makers, who had hoped to end five of the programs. And Congress rejected administration plans to end federal hospital services for the Merchant Marine and to taper off federal support for the training of medical researchers.

Only one major health bill won final approval in 1973. It gave federal aid for the first time to alternative medical groups called health maintenance organizations (HMOs) in the hope that they could hold down medical costs. Congress also considered other health bills dealing with issues ranging from medical emergencies to alcoholism.

National Health Insurance

National health insurance legislation did not make it out of the congressional starting gate in 1973, setting a pattern that was to prevail through 1976.

The four years of debate ended up producing little agreement about whether the country needed a national health insurance system to guarantee Americans good medical care at an affordable price. And there were deep divisions among health insurance supporters about the outlines of any proposed national scheme.

A health insurance bill came closest to making it out of committee in 1974, when the Ford administration was looking for a compromise. The 94th Congress basically decided to ignore the health insurance issue in 1975 and 1976, steered away by the price tag of a new social program, President Ford's increasingly adamant opposition to a comprehensive health program and a jurisdictional dispute between two House committees. But health insurance sup-

porters felt that Jimmy Carter's election as President in 1976 elevated the chances of legislative action in the 95th Congress.

Background

National health insurance proposals—once condemned as "socialized medicine"—had earned an air of respectability during the first four years of the Nixon administration. The Republican administration, as well as the American Medical Association (AMA), had come up with health insurance plans of their own by 1972. House and Senate committees held extensive hearings in 1970 and 1971, but took no further action.

The nation's mounting medical bill accounted for much of the continued interest in national health insurance. By fiscal 1975, the United States was spending $118.5-billion a year, or about $547 per person, on health care. Health spending had almost doubled since fiscal 1970 and more than quadrupled since fiscal 1960.

Experts attributed the dramatic growth in health spending to inflation, expensive advances in medicine and increased demand for health care fanned by expanded public and private insurance coverage. Others contended that there was no competition in the health profession to hold down medical charges.

Despite growth in private insurance coverage, there also were gaps in protection. Policies often did not cover services such as dental care or nursing home care. Payments for other services were limited or policies required patients to pick up some costs first. Critics also complained that private insurance placed too much emphasis on costly hospital care and too little on preventive care to catch health problems early.

A survey for the Social Security Administration also estimated that 22 million persons had no coverage at all under private or public plans in 1974.

Advocates of national health insurance contended that piecemeal changes in the nation's medical system would not get a handle on these problems. They promoted a national program as the best way to control skyrocketing costs, to guarantee everyone the same coverage for comprehensive benefits and to correct the slant toward hospital care.

1973 Action

Congressional committees, preoccupied by other issues, sidestepped action on health insurance in 1973 while the

Nixon administration sent its 1972 proposal back to the Department of Health, Education and Welfare (HEW) for redrafting. The revised administration proposal was not sent to Congress until 1974.

The House Interstate and Foreign Commerce Subcommittee on Health and the Environment held four days of hearings in December, but they were devoted to background issues rather than legislative proposals.

With the exception of the administration proposals, health insurance plans previously sponsored by various interest groups were reintroduced in 1973. They included the far-reaching proposal supported by organized labor and other, less drastic plans backed by the AMA, hospitals and commercial health insurers.

The only new proposal was offered by Sens. Russell B. Long (D La.), chairman of the Finance Committee, and Abraham Ribicoff (D Conn.). It proposed to cover all persons against the "catastrophic" costs of a long-term illness, replace the Medicaid program for the poor with a new federally funded program and give private insurers incentives to write standard benefit plans for others. *(Details of proposals, p. 16-A)*

Those backing the various proposals continued to criticize each other's plans. The administration and the AMA contended that the labor proposal, sponsored by Sen. Edward M. Kennedy (D Mass.), was too expensive and would give the federal government too much power over the practice of medicine. Those in the Kennedy camp complained that the other proposals would leave the system in the hands of private insurers who had no incentives to hold down medical costs. *(Details of national health insurance debate, pp. 12-A, 29-A, 45-A)*

Health Maintenance Organizations

The only major health bill (S 14—PL 93-222) approved by Congress during the year offered aid over a trial period to alternative medical groups called health maintenance organizations (HMOs).

HMOs were medical organizations offering comprehensive health services at a fixed monthly price that did not vary according to actual use of services. They were considered the principal alternative to traditional medical practices, which charged a fee for each service actually provided.

The final version of S 14 authorized $375-million in fiscal 1974-78 to aid HMO development. To give another boost to HMOs, the bill required certain employers to offer their workers the option of joining an HMO if they provided regular health insurance coverage.

While happy with the new federal aid, HMOs later claimed that the 1973 law asked them to meet utopian requirements that made their plans much more expensive than regular health insurance. They sought amendments to the law, which Congress eventually approved in 1976. *(p. 48-A)*

Background

Rising medical costs in the 1970s stimulated interest in HMOs. HMO prototypes had existed since the early 1900s and had enrolled seven million members, but their supporters argued that financing problems and resistance by organized medicine made it hard to start new HMOs.

The proponents maintained that HMOs could hold down costs through increased operating efficiency and their emphasis on "maintaining" health. The prepayment system, proponents argued, gave HMOs incentives to catch health problems before they required costly hospital care.

Numerous proposals to provide aid to HMOs were introduced in the 92nd Congress. The Senate passed a $5.1-billion HMO aid bill in 1972, but the House did not act.

In 1971, President Nixon endorsed a far-ranging federal aid program for HMOs, but the administration backed away from this endorsement later. By 1973, the administration favored only an experimental HMO aid program.

HMO legislation came under vigorous fire by the American Medical Association (AMA). The AMA claimed that the proposal would subsidize prepaid group practice over the traditional kind practiced by most of its members.

Senate Action

The Senate passed S 14 on May 15 after Republican objections forced Edward M. Kennedy (D Mass.), sponsor of the bill, to retreat from the more ambitious HMO aid plan he favored.

As reported (S Rept 93-129) by the Labor and Public Welfare Committee, the Senate version would have authorized $1.5-billion over three years to support HMO development. The bill also included special subsidies to help HMOs take care of the poor and those with health problems. Patients with poor health records often could not obtain regular health insurance.

Republicans argued on the floor in favor of the more limited aid proposal backed by the administration. "Before we even have a chance to get the test models off the ground, it is now proposed to fly with a whole fleet of HMOs...," complained Robert Taft Jr. (R Ohio). "We should adopt a fly-before-you-buy approach."

A series of test votes revealed that the committee bill might not pass the Senate. Rather than risk this public defeat, Kennedy managed to work out a compromise on the floor lowering the total authorization to $805-million.

House Action

House sponsors, led by Paul G. Rogers (D Fla.), were generally more willing to accept the experimental aid approach backed by the administration. The House Sept. 12 went along with the administration's views by passing a version of the bill authorizing only $240-million over a five-year period.

The House bill, reported (H Rept 93-451) by the Interstate and Foreign Commerce Committee, was a compromise drafted by William R. Roy (D Kan.) and James F. Hastings (R N.Y.). Roy, the principal architect of HMO legislation in the House, wanted the strongest bill he could get; Hastings was acting to meet some of the administration's objections.

Under the compromise, Hastings gave up a provision explicitly limiting the number of HMOs that could receive federal aid to 100. In return, however, Roy agreed to drop provisions offering special subsidies for HMOs taking care of medically risky patients and one overriding state laws restricting HMO development. The Senate version included an override provision.

A key feature of the legislation added by the House required employers offering health insurance plans to provide the HMO option.

President Nixon endorsed the House bill Sept. 10, arguing that it would provide a "fiscally responsible demonstration effort."

Conference Action

In their report (H Rept 93-714), House-Senate conferees made it clear that they had opted for the experimental, one-shot approach to HMO aid preferred by the House. The conference version lowered the Senate authorization to $375-million. Conferees also decided that this funding should last for five years instead of three, as provided in the Senate bill.

Conferees also dropped Senate provisions giving special subsidies to HMOs taking care of those with health problems, but they decided to require HMOs to undertake such special responsibilities anyway. HMO groups later complained that decisions like this one made their plans uncompetitive with regular health insurance. Congress wanted them to help meet problems plaguing the country's medical delivery system, HMO groups argued, but did not give them special financial support to offset the cost of doing so.

While the final bill ended up closer to the House version, conferees did accept a modified version of the Senate provision overriding state laws restricting HMO development. The state laws, often enacted because of pressure from organized medicine, were regarded as a major reason why HMO development had been so slow in some parts of the country. In other major decisions, conferees kept the House provision requiring employers to offer the HMO option.

Congress cleared the bill Dec. 19.

Provisions

As signed into law, S 14:

Authorizations

	Fiscal 1974	Fiscal 1975	Fiscal 1976	Fiscal 1977	Fiscal 1978
	(in millions of dollars)				
Grants and contracts for feasibility studies, planning and initial development	$25	$55	$85	—	—
Grants and contracts for initial development	—	—	—	$85	—
Capitalization of loan fund for initial operation costs	(-----$75-----)		—	—	—
Independent study of quality care assurance	(--------$10--------)		—	—	—
HEW research and evaluation of quality assurance	$ 4	$ 8	$ 9	$ 9	$10

Requirements for HMOs

• Required HMOs to offer certain basic health services and to provide supplemental services if a member of an HMO contracted for them at additional costs; prohibited any limit on the use or cost of such services after an HMO member had paid an enrollment fee on a pre-set, periodic basis, unless use of a service specifically was restricted under the act.

• Allowed an HMO to charge members "nominal" payments in addition to the enrollment fee for basic services unless the additional payments posed a barrier to the attainment of care by an HMO member.

• Required prepaid enrollment fees for basic and supplemental health services to be fixed uniformly without regard for an individual's or family's medical history.

How an HMO Works

Mr. Joe Patient's hypothetical medical ailment illustrates how a model group-practice HMO might work, according to the Group Health Association of America. Joe pays the HMO a monthly premium, which covers provision of a broad range of services without limits on cost or duration.

Assume Joe develops severe leg pains. He goes to his HMO medical center for an appointment with his doctor, one of several staff internists. His doctor suspects an inflamed spinal disc and refers Joe to an orthopedic surgeon on the staff. The surgeon puts Joe in a local hospital for traction to try to relieve the inflammation. The treatment does not work.

Next, Joe is referred to a staff neurosurgeon. He makes some laboratory tests and recommends surgery to remove what he has diagnosed as a ruptured disc. After the operation and several sessions with the HMO's physical therapist, Joe recovers completely.

Without HMO coverage, Joe might get separate bills from several doctors or surgeons, the hospital, a physical therapist and a laboratory department. His private hea'th insurance might cover all, part or none of the bills, depending on his policy. Under a liberal HMO coverage plan, the HMO would pick up the entire cost of Joe's illness.

• Allowed HMOs eligible for aid to be organized on a group- or individual-practice basis; required individual-practice associations to share equipment and staff where possible.

• Required an HMO to make basic and supplemental services available within its service area 24 hours a day, seven days a week; required an HMO to reimburse an HMO member for medical care by another source if the HMO could not provide such care first.

• Required an HMO to assure that at least one-third of its policy-making body would be made up of members of the HMO and to assure members from medically underserved populations "equitable" representation on the body.

• Required an HMO to set up a program ensuring continuous quality of care.

• Required an HMO to assume full financial risk for the cost of providing care to its members but allowed an HMO to carry reinsurance for costs above certain amounts.

• Required HMOs to have an open enrollment period of at least 30 days a year unless the Secretary of Health, Education and Welfare (HEW) waived the open enrollment requirement; except in rural areas, limited enrollment of individuals from a medically underserved population to no more than 75 per cent of the total enrollment.

• Barred an HMO from expelling a member because of his health status and from refusing a member continuous re-enrollment.

Aid to HMOs

• Authorized grants and contracts to public or private nonprofit entities to study the feasibility of establishing, planning or initially developing HMOs; authorized loan guarantees to private, profit-making entities serving the medically underserved for the same purposes.

- Required groups planning an HMO to notify the appropriate medical society of their intentions.
- Required the Secretary of HEW to give priority to applicants for initial development aid who gave assurances that at least 30 per cent of the HMO's enrollment would be from medically underserved populations.
- Authorized loans to public or private nonprofit HMOs for initial operating assistance; authorized loan guarantees to private, profit-making HMOs serving the medically underserved for the same purpose.
- Allowed initial operating assistance only to HMOs which had made all reasonable attempts to secure funds from other sources.
- Set aside 20 per cent of appropriated funds for assistance to HMOs serving non-urban areas; authorized general use of such funds if they were carried over to a following fiscal year.
- Authorized the HEW Secretary to contract with HMOs for the care of Indians and migrant workers.
- Required the HEW Secretary to give priority to applicants he determined to be the most economically viable, in conjunction with priority consideration to applicants intending to enroll the medically underserved.

General Provisions

- Authorized the HEW Secretary to bring civil suits against HMOs aided under the act which did not comply with its provisions.
- Pre-empted restrictive state laws hindering the development of HMOs assisted under the act.
- Required employers of 25 or more workers to offer an HMO option if they offered a traditional health benefits plan; stipulated that the employer would not be required to bear any more cost for the HMO option than he did for a traditional health plan.

Expiring Health Programs

Congress rejected Nixon administration efforts to ax several popular health programs and extended 12 expiring programs for one year without change.

Legislation (S 1136—PL 93-45) cleared June 5 authorized a total of $1.27-billion in fiscal 1974 for the programs—five of which President Nixon wanted to end or phase out. The 12 programs had been scheduled to expire June 30.

In most cases, congressional sponsors of the extension bill sidestepped debate over the merits of the individual programs. Instead, they stressed that Congress needed more time to evaluate the programs and draft appropriate revisions. This approach won Republican support for the legislation.

Budget Proposals

In his fiscal 1974 budget submitted to Congress in January, Nixon mounted a general attack on social welfare programs launched under Democratic Presidents. In the health field, the President proposed to end or phase out federal support for five programs:

- Hill-Burton hospital construction, a grant program that began in 1946. The budget said the supply of hospital beds was adequate on a national basis and additional federally backed construction would only increase the excess capacity and drive up hospitalization costs.

- Regional medical programs. The administration contended that the programs had failed to establish regional health care systems and duplicated existing programs. The original program, set up in 1965, was a Great Society measure to improve regional health care for heart disease, cancer and stroke.
- Community mental health centers. The administration argued that Congress did not intend to provide permanent federal funding for the program when it passed the original legislation in 1963.
- Public health training programs. The budget contended that other sources of funding could replace federal money spent on training.
- Allied health training programs.

The administration also proposed funding categorical family planning and migrant health programs under a general health services formula grant to the states. Under legislation proposed by the administration, the other five programs—health services research, health statistics, comprehensive health planning, medical libraries and developmental disabilities (such as mental retardation)—would have been extended or made permanent without substantial change.

The budget-cutting proposals bore the imprint of Caspar W. Weinberger, who became Secretary of Health, Education and Welfare (HEW) in February 1973 after serving as director of the Office of Management and Budget.

Mental Health Controversy. Weinberger and congressional liberals clashed most openly over the proposed phase-out of federal funding for community mental health centers. Weinberger argued that Congress only intended that the program "demonstrate" the effectiveness of treating the mentally ill in community-based settings instead of in institutions. Since that effectiveness had been demonstrated, the HEW Secretary maintained, state, local and private money should replace federal funding.

The program's supporters in Congress especially resented Weinberger's move to instruct them on their own legislative intent. They argued that the program was meant to support a national network of community mental health centers, and many areas still had no centers. They also insisted that state and local governments did not have the money to replace federal funding, so some centers would close.

Legislative Action

The Senate March 27 passed its version of the bill, which authorized $2.2-billion for the 12 expiring programs. The Senate made no changes in the funding recommended by the Labor and Public Welfare Committee in its report (S Rept 93-87) on the measure.

The House Interstate and Foreign Commerce Committee tried to broaden support for the extension by lowering the total authorization to $1.27-billion when it reported the bill in May (H Rept 93-227).

A last-minute drive by the administration to whip up Republican opposition in the House came too late; the House passed the bill May 31 with only one dissenting vote.

House sponsors stressed that committees needed more time to rework the programs. Even Minority Leader Gerald R. Ford (R Mich.) argued that there was a rationale for a one-year extension.

The Senate cleared the bill for the President by accepting the lower price tag on the House version by a unanimous vote. In the face of the overwhelming support for the measure, President Nixon discarded any ideas he might have had about a veto and signed the measure into law June 18.

Provisions

As signed into law, the bill authorized the following amounts in fiscal 1974:

- $42,617,000 for health services research and development.
- $14,518,000 for national health surveys and studies.
- $23,300,000 for public health training.
- $26,750,000 for migrant health services.
- $360,500,000 for comprehensive health planning services.
- $8,442,000 for assistance to medical libraries.
- $197,200,000 for hospital construction and renovation under the Hill-Burton Act.
- $159-million for regional medical programs.
- $44,345,000 for training in allied health professions.
- $118,024,000 for family planning and population research.
- $234,120,000 for community mental health centers and special community programs in drug abuse, alcoholism and children's services.
- $41,750,000 for services and construction projects to aid the developmentally disabled such as the mentally retarded and persons suffering neurological diseases from childhood.

Impoundment

Meanwhile, several health groups went to court to seek the release of fiscal 1973 health appropriations impounded by the administration. In the face of legal pressure, the administration reversed itself in December and announced that it would release most of the impounded health money.

Emergency Care, PHS Hospitals

President Nixon lost his bid to close eight Public Health Service hospitals, and Congress insisted on new federal support for medical emergency services. For a time, the two unrelated issues were intertwined in complicated legislative action.

Background

PHS Hospitals. The Public Health Service (PHS) hospitals provided care primarily for members of the Merchant Marine and the Coast Guard, military personnel and other federal beneficiaries.

The hospitals were located in Boston, Baltimore, Galveston, New Orleans, Norfolk, San Francisco, Seattle and Staten Island, N.Y.

The Nixon administration first proposed to end inpatient services at the hospitals in 1971, arguing that it would cost too much to modernize the aging facilities. Congress insisted that the hospitals should remain open.

In 1973, the administration again argued that it would save money to close the hospitals. Health, Education and Welfare (HEW) Secretary Caspar W. Weinberger also maintained that it was unfair for the federal government to provide direct medical care for some people and not for others.

Opponents of the closings, led by House and Senate members representing the affected cities, insisted that it would cost the federal government more over the long run to contract for the care of PHS beneficiaries at other hospitals than to modernize the PHS hospitals. The hospitals' supporters also pointed out that the PHS facilities offered their communities unusual services such as bone marrow transplants and special cancer treatments.

Emergency Medical Care. Both the House and Senate had passed legislation beefing up federal support for emergency medical services in 1972, but did not reconcile differences between the two versions.

Supporters of new federal support argued that proper emergency care could save an estimated 60,000 lives a year. They also stressed that only 5 per cent of ambulance personnel had completed the recommended training course and only 10 per cent of acute-care hospitals could handle all kinds of emergencies.

Legislative Action on S 504

President Nixon vetoed the first bill (S 504) passed by Congress in 1973 addressing these two issues, and the House could not come up with the votes needed to override the veto. But Congress eventually got its way on both matters in other legislation.

Senate Action. As passed by the Senate May 15, S 504 authorized federal grants to state and local governments to modernize emergency rooms and equipment, train ambulance personnel and other professionals in emergency medicine and improve other components of an emergency medical care system. The bill, reported (S Rept 93-135) May 3 by the Labor and Public Welfare Committee, authorized $240-million in fiscal 1974-76 and reserved 15 per cent of available funds for emergency medical systems in rural areas.

The PHS hospital issue got bound up with the legislation when the Senate accepted a rider proposed by Warren G. Magnuson (D Wash.) barring HEW from suspending operations at the hospitals without congressional approval.

House Action. Legislative action in the House followed the same pattern. The House passed an emergency medical services bill on May 31 after adding the PHS hospital closure rider on the floor. House sponsors said they were shocked by the poor quality of emergency care, but some Republicans questioned whether the situation called for another new federal health program.

The House version, as reported (H Rept 93-149) by the Interstate and Foreign Commerce Committee, authorized $145-million in federal grants to emergency medical systems in fiscal 1974-76. The House bill did not contain the earmarked funding for rural areas.

Conference Action. House-Senate conferees compromised in a version reported July 10 (H Rept 93-370). The bill authorized $185-million in fiscal 1974-76 and kept the Senate earmark for rural emergency medical care programs. Sponsors envisioned a network of about 300 emergency medical systems across the country.

Congress cleared the bill July 19.

Veto, Override Attempt

Congress sustained President Nixon's veto of S 504. In his Aug. 1 veto message, Nixon argued that the PHS hospitals had "outlived their usefulness." He also called the emergency medical service program too expensive and unnecessary.

The Senate easily overrode the veto Aug. 2 by a 77-16 vote. Senators voting to override included Republicans active in health matters.

After intensive lobbying by both sides, the House sustained the veto on Sept. 12 by a 273-144 vote—five votes short of the two-thirds majority needed for an override. The vote represented the President's narrowest victory in his 1973 veto battle with Congress. The vote had taken on major political significance as a test of the President's strength among Republicans despite his Watergate troubles.

Lobbying. Major civic, health, labor and veterans' groups had mounted intensive lobbying efforts for a successful override. But the Republican strategy of promising future presidential support for the emergency medical services provisions while concentrating objections on the PHS hospital rider worked well enough.

The strategy culminated the day before the House vote when Republicans introduced legislation identical to the vetoed bill minus the PHS hospital rider. House Minority Leader Gerald R. Ford (R Mich.) promised to convince President Nixon to sign the stripped-down version.

Second Legislative Effort

Emergency Medical Services. A second version (S 2410—PL 93-154) of the emergency medical services bill did win the President's approval. The new bill was virtually identical to S 504 except for its deletion of the PHS hospital rider.

The Senate passed S 2410, reported (S Rept 93-397) by the Labor and Public Welfare Committee, on Sept. 19. The House passed similar legislation, reported (H Rept 93-601) by the Commerce Committee, on Oct. 25. After passing the legislation back and forth between the two houses to reconcile minor differences, Congress cleared the bill on Oct. 31. Congress again extended the program in 1976. *(p. 54-A)*

Provisions. As signed into law, S 2410:

● Authorized $30-million in fiscal 1974 and $60-million in fiscal 1975 for grants and contracts to plan, establish, initially operate or expand area systems of emergency medical care.

● Authorized $70-million in fiscal 1976 for grants and contracts for all of the above purposes except planning.

● Provided that grants and contracts could be awarded to a state or local government, regional government entity or private non-profit agency which developed a plan for a system which would include adequately trained personnel, a communications system, transportation facilities, treatment facilities accessible to all persons in a given area, educational programs and contingency programs to handle natural disasters and mass casualties.

● Authorized $5-million in each of fiscal 1974-76 for grants and contracts to conduct research in emergency medicine.

● Authorized $10-million in fiscal 1974 for grants and contracts to medical and related health schools for training programs in emergency medical care.

PHS Hospitals. Congress also got its way on the PHS hospital issue by adding the anti-closure language to a $21.3-billion weapons procurement bill (PL 93-155). The defense procurement bill was too important for the President to veto because of a comparatively minor disagreement.

The hospital rider, added by the Senate Sept. 28, directed the HEW Secretary to take all steps necessary to continue the operation of the eight PHS hospitals.

Biomedical Research

Congress put the Nixon administration on notice that it would not tolerate cutbacks in federal support for biomedical research training programs.

While Congress did not complete action on the legislation, both houses passed a bill (HR 7724) guaranteeing the continuation of federal grants for the training of young medical scientists. The Senate approved a heavily amended version that also set up a commission to write guidelines for the use of humans in research testing.

Administration Proposal. In January, the administration proposed to stop awarding new research grants. It wanted to spend $275-million for training programs in fiscal 1974-75, only enough to honor commitments for previously awarded research fellowships and traineeships.

The administration argued that there was no longer any pressing need for new research scientists. It also maintained that a scientist's income expectations enabled him to obtain educational support from other sources.

House Response. The House insisted on increasing the proposed funding for research training to $416-million in fiscal 1974-75, passing HR 7724 on May 31.

Sponsors of the bill suggested that the administration proposal could spell disaster for the nation's medical research efforts. The Interstate and Foreign Commerce Committee, which reported the bill May 23 (H Rept 93-224), also noted that a Department of Health, Education and Welfare (HEW) study found a need for 7,100 new medical scientists by 1975.

The committee did respond to the administration's argument that researchers supported by federal funds often went into private practice of medicine rather than research or education. The House bill required a student to spend two years in research or education for every year of federal support he received.

Administration Shift. In the face of congressional criticism and united opposition by the medical community, the administration revised its proposal on July 9. It proposed a smaller program providing $90-million in fiscal 1974-76 for new fellowships awarded for postdoctoral researchers.

Senate Action. The Senate Labor and Public Welfare Committee flatly rejected the administration's new proposal, voting to authorize $208-million for training in fiscal 1974. Its version of HR 7724, reported Aug. 3 (S Rept 93-381), set up a new, unified program of national research service awards. Those receiving awards would be required to spend one year in research or education for every year of support. The Senate passed the bill Sept. 11.

The Senate version also responded to reports that humans—particularly prisoners, children and the mentally retarded—often faced grave risks from research testing without being fully informed of the hazards they might encounter. The Senate bill set up a new national commission appointed by the President to develop regulations to protect the rights of humans in research.

Controversial Research. The House and Senate also used the legislation as a vehicle to impose curbs on controversial kinds of medical experimentation.

The House adopted an amendment prohibiting HEW from funding any research using live human fetuses. Some sponsors of the bill suggested that the House ran the risk of implying that it approved of other kinds of equally unethical research by only banning one type of testing. But, with the discussion tinged by abortion-related debate, the amendment passed 354-9.

After Edward M. Kennedy (D Mass.), floor manager of the bill intervened with a compromise, the Senate also banned fetal research, but only until the new commission could draw up guidelines.

The Senate also adopted an amendment outlawing HEW funding of psychosurgery—a controversial type of brain surgery generally performed to control violent or hostile behavior.

The bill did become law in 1974.

Abortion

The Supreme Court touched off a highly emotional debate Jan. 22 when it set guidelines strictly limiting the power of the states to regulate abortion. The court ruled, 7-2, that the decision to have an abortion during the first three months of pregnancy should be left entirely to a woman and her doctor.

Proposed constitutional amendments to overturn the decision were introduced immediately in Congress. In general, the proposals fell into two categories. The first type would have outlawed abortion completely or except under extreme circumstances, such as to save the life of the mother. The second type would have left regulation of abortion up to the states.

A highly visible "pro-life" lobby began to organize to campaign for the amendments, choosing red roses as its symbol. But the right-to-life groups had little legislative success in 1973.

Most members of Congress were anxious to remain neutral on the explosive issue, and the proposed amendments remained buried in committee in 1973. In July, Rep. Lawrence J. Hogan (R Md.) tried to get the anti-abortion proposals to the floor directly by moving to discharge the Judiciary Committee from further consideration of them. But Hogan did not get enough support for his move. Rep. Don Edwards (D Calif.), chairman of the Judiciary subcommittee with jurisdiction over the proposals, argued that there was not enough backing for them in committee to justify hearings.

Legislative Amendments. Congress did approve two abortion-related amendments. The first, added to legislation (PL 93-45) extending 12 health programs, let institutions receiving federal funds refuse to perform abortion procedures. The amendment, named after its Senate sponsor, Frank Church (D Idaho), also outlawed discrimination against hospital staff members who either performed abortions or refused to do so because of religious or moral beliefs.

The second amendment, attached to the 1973 foreign aid act (PL 93-189), prohibited the use of U.S. funds overseas to pay for or encourage abortions.

Child Abuse

Congress approved legislation (S 1191—PL 93-247) providing federal aid for the prevention and treatment of abused and neglected children.

The bill authorized $85-million in fiscal 1974-77 to aid the estimated 60,000 children who were beaten, burned, poisoned or neglected by their parents each year. Congress expected the funds to support demonstration programs.

The administration opposed the Senate version of the bill, passed July 14 after it was reported (S Rept 93-308) by the Labor and Public Welfare Committee. The Senate version provided for a five-year, $90-million program emphasizing regional child abuse prevention programs. The administration called the separate program unnecessary because other funding was available for child abuse prevention programs.

The administration then worked with the House Education and Labor Committee to tailor the bill more to its liking. The committee reported a new version Nov. 30 (H Rept 93-685) that shortened the funding period to three years and placed more emphasis on state programs. The House version, passed Dec. 3, also cut total funding to $60-million.

But further Senate amendments incorporated in the final bill brought funding back close to the Senate total and restricted grants to states to 20 per cent of available funds. Congress cleared the measure Dec. 21.

Provisions

As signed into law, S 1191:

● Authorized $15-million in fiscal 1974, $20-million in fiscal 1975 and $25-million in each of fiscal 1976 and 1977 for federal aid to programs for the prevention, identification and treatment of child abuse.

● Earmarked at least 5 per cent, but no more than 20 per cent, of appropriated funds for grants to states with child abuse programs providing for the confidential reporting of child abuse incidents, the prompt investigation of reported incidents and the cooperation of legal and social services agencies.

● Earmarked at least 50 per cent of appropriated funds for demonstration programs for the prevention and treatment of child abuse.

● Established a National Center on Child Abuse and Neglect within the Department of Health, Education and Welfare to study the incidence of child abuse.

Lead-Based Paint Poisoning

Congress approved a two-year extension of the Lead-Based Paint Poisoning Prevention Act of 1970. A key feature of the extension legislation (S 607—PL 93-151) set a limit on the allowable lead content of interior paints.

Authorities estimated that 400,000 children in the United States suffered from lead poisoning. Many were poisoned by eating paint chips peeling from the walls of older housing.

The Senate version, passed May 9 after it was reported (S Rept 93-130) by the Labor and Public Welfare Committee, provided for a four-year extension and a restrictive lead content limit for paints. The House, acting Sept. 5, voted for a two-year extension and a less stringent content limit. The House Banking and Currency Committee reported the revised bill on July 12 (H Rept 93-373).

The final version, drafted by House-Senate conferees (H Rept 93-522), was closer to the House bill. Congress cleared the measure Oct. 24. President Nixon signed the bill Nov. 9 although the administration had opposed extension of the program on a categorical basis.

Congress extended the program again in 1976 in a section of a disease control bill. *(p. 50-A)*

Provisions

As signed into law, S 607:

● Authorized $25-million in each of fiscal 1974-75 for grants by the Department of Health, Education and Welfare (HEW) to local government agencies and private nonprofit agencies to detect and treat lead-based paint poisoning; increased the maximum federal share of such programs to 90 per cent from 75 per cent.

● Authorized $35-million in each of fiscal 1974-75 for grants by the Department of Housing and Urban Development (HUD) to local government agencies and private non-profit agencies to eliminate lead-based paint hazards in old housing.

● Authorized $3-million in each of fiscal 1974-75 to conduct research on the extent of lead-based paint hazards in the United States; required the chairman of the Consumer Product Safety Commission to study safe lead-content levels in paint by Dec. 31, 1974.

● Authorized grants to state agencies if they served local communities directly or if local government agencies were barred by state law from carrying out the grant programs.

● Required the HEW Secretary and the HUD Secretary to take steps to prohibit the use of lead-based paint in residential buildings constructed or renovated with federal assistance or in any toy, drinking or eating utensil or piece of furniture distributed or manufactured after enactment of the bill.

● Defined lead-based paint as paint containing more than 0.5 per cent lead by weight before Dec. 31, 1974, or more than 0.06 per cent after that date; provided that the chairman of the Consumer Product Safety Commission could propose, if warranted by a commission study, a level other than 0.06 per cent, but no higher than 0.5 per cent.

● Pre-empted all state and local laws governing allowable lead content in paint.

Alcoholism Programs

Rejecting administration proposals, the Senate passed a bill (S 1125) June 21 continuing the basic structure of existing federal alcoholism prevention programs through fiscal 1976. The legislation, extending a 1970 act, was not considered by the House in 1973.

The Nixon administration had proposed phasing out project funding for community alcohol treatment programs and had not funded any new projects since June 1972. It argued that state and local governments could pay more for alcoholism prevention and treatment projects.

Supporters of the projects attacked the proposal. "I'm not just a little concerned, I'm damn angry," said Harold E. Hughes (D Iowa), a reformed alcoholic who was chief sponsor of S 1125.

The Labor and Public Welfare Committee, reporting the bill June 13 (S Rept 93-208), provided $300-million in fiscal 1974-76 for grants to alcoholism prevention projects. The measure also authorized $160-million in fiscal 1975-76 for formula grants to the states and open-ended funding for special grants to states that had adopted laws treating alcoholism as a disease instead of criminal behavior.

Drug Industry Investigation

The Senate Labor and Public Welfare Subcommittee on Health kicked off a major series of hearings on the drug industry in December. Subcommittee Chairman Edward M. Kennedy (D Mass.) viewed the hearings as the first step toward updating drug regulatory laws last revised in 1962.

Criticism. Consumer advocate Ralph Nader and Sen. Gaylord Nelson (D Wis.), chairman of a select subcommittee that had investigated the drug industry for six years, led the attack on prescription drug costs and promotion practices.

They blamed the drug industry and organized medicine for restrictions on the prescription of generic drugs, those known by their chemical names. Generic drugs generally cost less than brand-name equivalents.

Nader also blamed high drug prices on 17-year exclusive patents granted for particular drugs. The patents gave one drug firm exclusive rights to market a drug even if another company could produce it at a lower cost.

The two critics also indicted drug advertising and promotional techniques. Nelson charged that the drug industry spent about $5,000 on each U.S. doctor in 1971 trying to persuade him to prescribe certain drugs.

"In my judgment, drug advertising by its very nature cannot provide unbiased information to physicians," Nelson told the subcommittee.

Defense. C. Joseph Stetler of the Pharmaceutical Manufacturers Association refuted the charges. In particular, Stetler argued that reduction of patent rights would encourage lower industry productivity and higher prices.

Stetler also maintained that medical advertising was screened carefully by the Food and Drug Administration. He insisted that doctors were well equipped to judge the accuracy of claims made by drug companies.

Proposals. Health, Education and Welfare Secretary Caspar W. Weinberger stole the spotlight during the hearings by announcing that the government would limit Medicare and Medicaid payments for prescription drugs to "the lowest cost at which the drug is generally available." This policy was expected to promote prescription of the lower-priced generic drugs.

Nader and Nelson also supported increased use of generic drugs. They also proposed shortening the period a drug firm could hold exclusive marketing rights and curtailment of prescription drug advertising.

VA Medical Programs

Congress July 19 cleared for the President legislation (S 59—PL 93-82) expanding Veterans Administration (VA) medical programs.

President Nixon had vetoed similar legislation in 1972.

S 59 broke new ground in the VA medical program by ensuring that veterans and their dependents would be eligible for out-patient care and by providing hospital and medical care to the wife or widow and the dependents of veterans who were totally disabled from service-connected causes or who died as a result of a service-connected disability.

A key provision of the final bill extended regular out-patient care privileges to veterans eligible for hospital care, peacetime veterans and veterans with 80 per cent disabilities as a result of a service-connected injury. Under existing law, outpatient care had to be related to hospitalization.

The VA was authorized to enter into contracts for the medical care of dependents and survivors who were not eligible for care under the regular military medical insurance program (CHAMPUS).

Reacting to charges that VA facilities were not adequate to serve all veterans in need of care, the earlier legislation also had manadated certain minimums for the number of beds to be maintained in VA hospitals and for staff-to-patient rations. In his veto message, President Nixon had said that these provisions could lower the quality of care available.

The compromise version directed the VA to maintain enough beds to ensure immediate acceptance of all seeking care and required the National Academy of Sciences to study staff-patient rations.

Background. S 59 differed only slightly from the legislation (HR 10880) vetoed by Nixon Oct. 27, 1972. Nixon had said that version ran counter to his administration's health policy, which was "to sharply reduce the federal government's role in the direct provision of services." The bill also would have "unnecessarily added hundreds of million of dollars to the federal budget."

S 59 was reported by the Senate Veterans' Affairs Committee (S Rept 93-54) and passed by the Senate March 6, 1973.

The House Veterans' Affairs Committee reported a compromise version (HR 9058—H Rept 93-368) that met some of the administration's main objections to S 59. The House committee version then was passed by the House without amendment July 17 and sent to the Senate. The Senate July 19 agreed to the House changes, completing congressional action.

Provisions. As signed into law, S 59 (PL 93-82):

● Extended outpatient care privileges to veterans currently eligible for hospital care, peacetime veterans and those 80 per cent or more disabled because of service-related causes.

● Authorized the VA to contract for care of dependents of veterans with total and permanent service-connected disabilities and survivors of veterans who died as a result of service-connected injuries if they were not eligible for care under the military insurance program.

● Authorized, under limited circumstances, the VA to reimburse certain veterans for hospital and medical services not normally furnished by the VA.

● Required the VA to staff and maintain enough hospital beds to admit all eligible veterans in need for care and to double the number of VA nursing home beds to 8,000.

● Increased per diem reimbursements for care of veterans in state soldiers' homes and increased to 65 from 50 per cent the maximum federal share of building or renovating costs of such homes.

School Lunch Payments

Congress Oct. 24 completed action on a bill (HR 9639—PL 93-150) to increase federal payments to school nutrition programs pinched by rising food costs.

As cleared, the bill contained a House-approved, two-cent increase in the basic federal payment per school lunch served, raising it to 10 cents from eight cents.

Other key provisions were designed to reduce the financial burden on both the states and the students participating in the various feeding programs, including free and reduced-price lunches served to needy students and school breakfasts. The additional cost of all the increases in federal payments was estimated at $146-million a year.

The Nixon administration had opposed even a two-cent increase in the federal school lunch payment as inflationary. But rapidly rising food costs were creating hardships for school food administrators who termed the situation an "emergency." A study by the Senate Select Committee on Nutrition had estimated that school lunch prices might rise five cents to 10 cents without increased federal reimbursements, which could result in a drop in the number of schools participating and in the number of students able to afford the full price of a school lunch. Increases in the basic school lunch reimbursement rate had been approved in 1971 and 1972.

House Action

The bill easily passed the House Sept. 13 by a 389-4 vote. The only issue both in the Education and Labor Committee (H Rept 93-458) and on the House floor was the two-cent increase, which the Agriculture Department estimated would cost an additional $84-million a year. A Republican-sponsored amendment to kill the increase was easily rejected, 127-272.

Senate Action

The Senate responded even more generously to reports of a financial emergency in the federal school nutrition program in its version passed Sept. 24 by a vote of 83-4.

While the Agriculture Committee had approved a version close to the House bill in order to hasten final action (S Rept 93-404), floor amendments offered by Hubert H. Humphrey (D Minn.) substantially increased the cost by raising the basic federal reimbursement to 12 cents, escalating the reimbursement rates automatically and expanding eligibility for reduced-price lunches. Opponents argued the amendments would jeopardize presidential acceptance of any school lunch legislation.

Final Action

With the exception of their insistence on the 10-cent reimbursement level for school lunches, House conferees accepted major Senate provisions not contained in the House-passed version (H Rept 93-540).

Final action hit a snag, however, when the House rejected 145-218 a Senate amendment to one item technically in disagreement that would have guaranteed New York, New Jersey, Rhode Island and Maryland payments no less than they received in fiscal 1973 for the free and reduced price lunch programs. It was modified to apply only to fiscal 1974 and subsequently was approved by both houses.

Commodity Payments. The bill also made permanent the provisions of a bill passed earlier in the year that had applied only to fiscal 1973. The measure cleared on March 15 (HR 4278—PL 93-13) had required that federal commodity supplies for child nutrition programs be maintained at their budgeted levels. If supplies fell below 90 per cent of the value of the commodities originally programmed, the Agriculture Secretary would be required to pay the difference in cash. The measure had stemmed from a decrease in the volume and variety of federal food donations to child nutrition programs because of rising prices and commodity shortages. It passed the House March 5 by a vote of 352-7 (H Rept 93-36) and the Senate March 14 (S Rept 93-59).

Major Provisions

As signed into law, HR 9639 (PL 93-150):

• Increased the basic federal payment for every school lunch served to 10 cents, from eight cents under existing law; increased the additional minimum federal payment per free lunch to 45 cents, from 40 cents, and the minimum payment per reduced-price lunch to 35 cents, from 30 cents.

• Established the basic federal payment for every school breakfast served at eight cents; set the federal payment per free school breakfast at a minimum of 20 cents and a maximum of 45 cents; set the minimum federal payment per reduced-price breakfast at 15 cents.

• Required that federal reimbursement rates be adjusted semiannually beginning Jan. 1, 1974, to reflect automatically changes in the consumer price index for food served away from home.

• Expanded eligibility in fiscal 1974 for reduced-price lunches to children of families whose income was as much as 75 per cent over the applicable poverty guidelines prescribed by the Secretary of Agriculture.

• Required school lunch funds to be allocated to the states by a formula based on the number of free and reduced-price lunches served, rather than on the number of children classified as coming from poor families; stipulated that no state would receive smaller payments under the programs in fiscal 1974 than it did in fiscal 1973.

• Required the Secretary to determine by Feb. 15 of each year the estimated value of all school lunch commodities which would be delivered by the end of the fiscal year; if the value was less than 90 per cent of the value initially programmed for the year, the Secretary would be required to pay states the difference in cash by March 15.

• Extended through fiscal 1975 a special supplemental feeding program for new mothers and their infants; authorized $40-million for the program in fiscal 1975; made agencies of Indian tribes eligible to administer the program.

• Authorized the Secretary to use Section 32 funds if necessary to pay the states cash in lieu of commodities by March 15, or to fund the supplemental feeding program in the absence of regular appropriations.

• Required that the special school milk programs be available to any school or nonprofit child care institution requesting it; required that children eligible for the free lunch program also be eligible for the free milk program.

1974

Congress looked at ways in 1974 to ready the country's medical care system for a national health insurance program, but again adjourned without acting on health insurance proposals.

Much time was spent on trying to assure that families would have access to good medical care once a health insurance program paid the bills. The most important piece of legislation enacted during the year established a network of local groups to improve the distribution of treatment facilities and to curb unneeded development adding to health care costs. Congress also considered but did not finish work on a bill designed to ease urgent doctor shortages in many rural and inner-city areas.

Other proposals were written to tighten up guidelines for existing federal programs. Congress passed a bill making major changes in health services programs for the mentally ill, migrant workers and the poor, but President Ford pocket vetoed it on spending grounds. Historic legislation setting up a commission to draft guidelines for the use of humans in medical research did become law.

A host of other bills dealing with specific health problems also won congressional approval.

National Health Insurance

Policy disagreements halted the first serious negotiations over national health insurance legislation, and the 93rd Congress adjourned at the end of the year without acting on the issue.

The legislative outlook had seesawed during the session.

Early in 1974, it appeared that the right combination of forces might break the stalemate that had prevented enactment of comprehensive health insurance legislation for 30 years. The administration was pushing for action and willing to talk compromise. Key congressional Democrats also agreed that the time had come to act and indicated that they would compromise, too. The House Ways and Means Committee and Senate Finance Committee opened the first legislative hearings on health insurance in three years.

New Administration Proposal

On Feb. 6, President Nixon formally unveiled a revised version of the administration's health insurance proposal.

The three-part proposal would have required employers to offer their workers insurance plans covering standard health benefits, provided federally subsidized coverage of the poor and restructured the Medicare program for the aged. A major new feature limited the amount any family would have to pay out of its own pocket for medical care to $1,500 a year. *(Details, box, p. 16-A)*

The administration kept up a steady push for congressional action. President Nixon went on national radio May 20 to stress that health insurance remained his number one domestic priority and to pledge the administration's willingness to compromise with Congress on some aspects of the legislation.

Mills-Kennedy Compromise

Introduction of a new Democratic compromise proposal sponsored by Sen. Edward M. Kennedy (D Mass.) and House Ways and Means Committee Chairman Wilbur D. Mills (D Ark.) also temporarily brightened prospects for action. The compromise was somewhat like organized labor's comprehensive plan, but allowed a larger role for private insurers and required patients to share some costs.

But labor groups viewed the compromise as a retreat and took the position during 1974 that no bill was better than a compromise altering key features of their plan. Health, Education and Welfare (HEW) Secretary Caspar W. Weinberger and other administration officials condemned labor's stance. "We firmly reject the view of those few who counsel that no action be taken until some vague future time when they believe that the plan that they personally favor could be enacted without change," Weinberger said.

Policy Differences

Hearings held by the Ways and Means Committee revealed that there still were plenty of disagreements despite the talk of compromise. *(Highlights of testimony, box, p. 14-A)*

Key disagreements focused on the following two areas:

● Financing method. The labor and Kennedy-Mills plans relied on new payroll taxes, thus making participation in the program mandatory; the administration, private insurers and medical groups wanted a voluntary program financed through privately paid premiums or tax credits.

● Federal role. The labor and Kennedy-Mills plans envisioned a large federal role in the administration of the program with only limited participation, if any, by the states and private insurers; other groups wanted a larger role for the states and private insurers.

Pressure for Long-Ribicoff

The pressure to do something in 1974 and the complexity of comprehensive proposals heightened congressional interest for a while in a plan promoted by Sens. Russell B. Long (D La.) and Abraham Ribicoff (D Conn.). It would have covered all families for the costs of a "catastrophic" illness, federalized the Medicaid health program for the poor and encouraged private insurers to standardize their benefits.

Ribicoff, a former HEW Secretary himself, argued that a giant new health program run by the federal government would be a "bureaucratic nightmare."

But the administration, labor groups and almost every other outside organization denounced the "catastrophic" approach. They argued that it would leave too many basic health needs unmet.

Attempt at Negotiations

By the time the Ways and Means Committee completed its hearings in early July, the momentum for action had weakened. Impeachment proceedings against President Nixon were expected to tie up the House.

But following Nixon's resignation Aug. 8, key members of Congress revived the drive to enact health insurance legislation. They were strongly supported by President Ford, who asked Congress just a few days after taking office to write "a good health bill" before adjournment.

At Mills' direction, the Ways and Means Committee staff drew up a compromise draft bill. It most closely resembled the administration plan, but included elements of other major bills. It set up a compulsory basic program financed through private insurance premiums paid by employers and employees. A state-run program would have covered the poor and another new program, financed through payroll tax increases, would have covered all families for "catastrophic" illness.

Mills rushed the committee through approval of the less controversial features of the compromise, but on Aug. 20 the committee broke sharply over the compulsory aspect of the plan and its financing provisions. After other very close votes, the committee tentatively approved a key section of the staff compromise by 12-11 vote.

The squabbling—dubbed a legislative wake by some—went on for an hour Aug. 21 and then Mills called a halt. He was not, Mills said, going to the floor with any bill approved by such a narrow margin in committee. "I think the members of the committee will agree with me that we've done everything we can to bring about a consensus," he said. "We don't have that consensus."

There was some talk about returning to the health insurance issue during a post-election session, but such a move never materialized. Liberals were content to wait until 1975, given the election of 75 new Democrats to the House in November. Mills, hospitalized by alcoholism after several bizarre public appearances with a strip-tease dancer, was in no shape to lead the search for a compromise. He lost the Ways and Means chairmanship in December.

Health Planning

Acknowledging that poor planning was partly responsible for the nation's mounting medical bill, Congress approved new efforts to make sure that costly health facilities and services were developed only where and when needed.

Legislation (S 2994—PL 93-641) cleared Dec. 20 charged a new national network of local planning agencies—called health systems agencies—with preventing unnecessary development, establishing priorities for development of services and facilities that were needed and monitoring uses of federal health funds in their particular areas. New state planning and development agencies were asked to carry out the same responsibilities on a statewide level.

Need

Changes in the nation's health planning systems were considered essential before enactment of national health insurance legislation. Existing planning programs had failed to correct oversupplies of hospital beds and health professionals in some parts of the country and shortages in other areas. Extra beds in underused hospitals alone were costing the country more than $1-billion a year to maintain.

Existing planning programs lodged authority for health decisions in overlapping state and local agencies, which often found their proposals unenforceable in the face of political opposition. The agencies, for instance, found it hard to convince a community that its hospital did not need some expensive new piece of medical equipment if it were available in another hospital nearby.

S 2994 replaced three of the programs that were supposed to exert some control over the development of new health facilities and services:

● The comprehensive health planning program set up in 1966. In 1974, 218 area-wide agencies covering 79 per cent of the nation's population were in operation under this program.

● Regional medical programs authorized in 1965 to encourage regional arrangements between medical schools and research and health care institutions to bring to local areas national advances in the treatment of heart disease, cancer and stroke.

● The Hill-Burton hospital construction program set up in 1946 to provide federal aid to help correct severe shortages of hospital beds in many parts of the country. The program had helped finance construction of almost 500,000 hospital beds through mid-1974.

Controversy

Much of the controversy over the legislation focused on what role it would provide for governors, mayors and other local elected officials.

While the final version allowed a local public agency to serve as the local health planning group, state and local governments continued to argue that the measure lodged

Who Stood Where and For What on Proposals...

A seemingly endless procession of spokesmen for every group with at least some tangential interest in health legislation moved through the Ways and Means Committee's hearing room in the Longworth House Office Building to present positions on national health insurance between April and July 1974.

Some committee members suggested that the hearings had not brought out much new information because the positions of major groups had been well defined for a long time. *(Proposals, box, p. 16-A)*

The highlights of testimony by groups with different interests in the health care field included:

National Physician Groups

The American Medical Association (AMA) reaffirmed its support for its "Medicredit" bill and formally opposed all other proposals. At the same time, AMA witnesses suggested that there was no public demand for major changes in the health care system.

The AMA particularly opposed financing health insurance through payroll taxes and creation of a new federal bureaucracy to run the program. The group suggested that the Long-Ribicoff "catastrophic" proposal was unacceptable because it did not cover basic benefits. The American Dental Association generally took the same positions and backed Medicredit also.

The conservative Association of American Physicians and Surgeons opposed all proposals for "politicized medicine" and urged the committee to heed the lessons of Medicare. More public spending for medical care would only fan inflation, the group said.

Providers of Health Care

The American Hospital Association also re-endorsed its own proposal (HR 1). The hospital group called for a strong federal role symbolized by a Cabinet-level Department of Health or independent agency, but recommended that regulation of the program be left to the states. The group also criticized financing through payroll taxes and recommended that any program be phased in over a period of time.

The hospital association also insisted that catastrophic coverage, such as that provided under the Long-Ribicoff bill, should be part of a comprehensive program. A separate federal program for catastrophic illness would duplicate and complicate coverage already provided under private insurance, it said.

The Group Health Association of America testified that the administration bill would best guarantee equal treatment for health maintenance organizations (HMOs) in a national health insurance program. The group did not endorse the general provisions of any bill.

Speaking for the nation's medical schools, the Association of American Medical Colleges called for a compulsory program not requiring patient cost-sharing, but endorsed no single bill. To assure enough future providers of health care, the group said that a national health insurance program should be integrated with development of health manpower resources.

Health Insurers

The nation's private health insurers generally opposed a separate catastrophic program run by the federal government, which the Long-Ribicoff bill included. The Blue Cross Association argued that catastrophic coverage should be integrated with basic coverage so that a patient would not have to deal with two different insurers for the same illness. Private insurers should provide both basic and catastrophic coverage for everyone except those covered by Medicare and a federalized Medicaid program, the association suggested.

The National Association of Blue Shield Plans agreed that a catastrophic program should not stand by itself and called the Long-Ribicoff bill "another national health insurance proposal...with a $2,000 deductible." Both of the nonprofit "Blues," which handled the largest single portion of the health insurance business, generally endorsed a plan requiring employers to offer basic and catastrophic benefits and a similar federal plan for the poor.

Representing the commercial health insurers, the Health Insurance Association of America promoted its own proposal (HR 5200) and opposed any government takeover of the private health insurance business. The association also argued that the Long-Ribicoff bill would destroy the existing private system of catastrophic coverage, which would be more efficient than a federal program.

While arguing that they had done a good job responding to the nation's health insurance needs and controlling costs, the groups also recommended that any proposed new regulation under health insurance remain at the state level. The National Association of Insurance Commissioners, representing state insurance com-

---

too much authority in private groups. After the overwhelming majority of health planning agencies designated under the law turned out to be private groups, state and regional governmental groups went to court in 1976 to challenge the law.

The American Medical Association (AMA) also opposed the bill, contending that it gave too much decision-making power to the federal government as well. The AMA also filed suit against the law in 1976.

The measure had the general support of the administration, although it objected to the bill's authorization of $1-billion in fiscal 1975-77.

House Action

The House Interstate and Foreign Commerce Committee reported its version of the bill Sept. 26 (H Rept 93-1382). It resisted the efforts of some state medical societies and state and local governments to alter provisions requir-

...To Adopt National Health Care Insurance

missioners, also argued that there was no evidence that state regulation was so poor that it should be replaced by federal control.

Organized Labor Groups

Organized labor groups stood fast in their support of the original Kennedy-Griffiths proposal (HR 22) and attacked the Kennedy-Mills "compromise." "If Mills-Kennedy is this committee's idea of 'compromise,' then I must say, in all candor, we will oppose it," said Andrew J. Biemiller of the AFL-CIO. Instead of rushing into a compromise designed to get by a presidential veto, he said, Congress should wait until 1975 and devise a better program.

Leonard Woodcock of the United Auto Workers also contended that Kennedy-Mills went "too far in satisfying those elements in the system who are opposed to basic, necessary change" and particularly criticized the bill's requirement for patient cost-sharing.

Woodcock also attacked the Long-Ribicoff proposal, which he said did not make sense. Private insurers were good at providing protection for catastrophes, but did a poor job of covering basic health care costs, he said. The Long-Ribicoff proposal, he argued, would provide for a government takeover of "what private insurance does best" while leaving basic coverage unaltered.

Woodcock also predicted that "there will be no next year for national health insurance if catastrophic—and only catastrophic—is enacted this year."

Business Groups

Major business groups, including the National Association of Manufacturers (NAM) and U.S. Chamber of Commerce, argued that national health insurance should build on the existing private system and strongly opposed financing any plan with new payroll taxes. Instead, both groups said, joint employer-employee contributions for premiums should finance the basic program with federal general revenues financing coverage for the poor.

The NAM opposed requiring employers to pay any specific percentage of premium costs by law. In line with legislation (S 3343) it had proposed, the Chamber recommended limiting the employer share to 50 per cent.

The two groups split over whether a program should be compulsory. The NAM said that individual employees should have the right not to participate in employer plans, but the Chamber argued that "if

employers are obligated to offer a comprehensive health insurance plan, their employees should be required to avail themselves of it." The voluntary aspect of the administration plan was unsatisfactory, the Chamber suggested.

The Chamber was critical of the Long-Ribicoff proposal because it would supplant, not supplement, private efforts and establish the principle of payroll tax financing. Congress also would be under continuing pressure to expand the program, argued Roger C. Sonnemann of the Chamber. "Over a period of time, the initial free-standing catastrophic program would be a program paying virtually all health and medical care services for the entire population," he said.

The business groups, however, reserved most of their criticism for the Kennedy-Mills approach because of its payroll tax financing and proposed role for the federal government.

Consumer, Senior Citizens Groups

The Consumer Federation of America and National Council of Senior Citizens endorsed the original Kennedy-Griffiths bill (HR 22), dismissing all other proposals, including the Kennedy-Mills plan, as inadequate.

Elizabeth Langer of the Federation called HR 22 the most progressive financing plan because general tax revenues would cover 50 per cent of the program's cost. She argued that the administration and Kennedy-Mills plans were regressive because they relied primarily on payroll taxes on income up to a given ceiling or fixed premium contributions.

The National Retired Teachers Association and American Association of Retired Persons also criticized the Long-Ribicoff, Kennedy-Mills and administration bills, but supported no general health insurance plan. Instead they backed legislation (HR 13385) to reform the Medicare program, sponsored by Hugh L. Carey (D N.Y.), a Ways and Means Committee member.

Other Groups

Groups concerned with special benefits covered by many of the proposals generally testified that all of the plans placed too many limitations on these benefits. The groups included those in the mental health, alcoholism and pharmaceutical fields. They found proposed limitations on the use of certain services too strict and questioned patient cost-sharing for these services or prescription drugs required under most of the proposals.

ing all the new planning agencies to be private groups independent of local political control.

On the floor Dec. 13, however, the House added provisions pushed by John E. Moss (D Calif.) that allowed the local planning agencies to be public units. The amendment also stipulated that local governments would control the governing body of a public agency.

William R. Roy (D Kan.), a key sponsor of the bill, opposed the Moss amendments but suggested that they would

have little effect because HEW did not want to name public units as planning agencies.

Senate Action

The Labor and Public Welfare Committee, reporting its bill Nov. 12 (S Rept 93-1285), decided to let public bodies serve as local planning agencies. But it did not guarantee local governments operating control over a public planning group.

Brief Descriptions of 7 Major Health Insurance...

Brief descriptions of the key features of the major health insurance proposals pending in Congress in 1974 follow.

● Comprehensive Health Insurance Act (HR 12684—Nixon-Ford administration bill). The plan would require employers to offer insurance plans with standard benefits to their employees, but employee participation would be voluntary. After three years, employers would pay 75 per cent of required premiums. The same benefits would be available to the poor in a new federal program and to the elderly under Medicare.

States would administer all but the Medicare program and private insurers would provide policies subject to state regulation. Employers and employees would pay premiums for their plans and the federal government would finance care of the poor and aged from general revenues and the Medicare Trust Fund.

Each family would pay a maximum deductible of $450 before payments began and then 25 per cent of all covered services. After a family had spent $1,500 out of its own pocket, the plan would cover all further "catastrophic" expenses. For families with income under $5,000, required deductible and copayments would be related to income.

● Comprehensive National Health Insurance Act (S 3286, HR 13870—Kennedy-Mills bill). The bill would require all employers and employees to participate in a new national program with standard benefits and provide the same coverage to the poor and Medicare participants. Employers would pay a new 3 per cent and employees a new 1 per cent payroll tax on the first $20,000 of income. Unearned income and federal welfare payments also would be taxed.

An independent Social Security Administration would run the program and private insurers would act as financial intermediaries, but not pay claims.

Each family would pay a maximum deductible of $300 before payments began and then pay 25 per cent of all covered services. After a family with income above $8,800 had spent $1,000 out of its own pocket, the plan would provide catastrophic coverage. Maximum cost-sharing for the poor would be related to income.

● Catastrophic Health Insurance and Medical Assistance Reform Act (S 2513, HR 14079—Long-Ribicoff bill). The plan would provide catastrophic coverage for most families after the 60th day of hospitalization or when they had incurred $2,000 in medical bills. Families would pay a maximum copayment of $1,000 for catastrophic care.

A new federal program would cover most services for the poor before catastrophic benefits took effect. Private insurers would be encouraged by financial incentives to offer federally approved plans with standard benefits to the non-poor.

HEW would administer the catastrophic and medical assistance programs while private insurers would continue to operate programs for the non-poor. Employers and employees eventually would pay a new .4 per cent payroll tax on income taxed for Social Security purposes to finance the catastrophic program; state and federal general revenues would finance the assistance program.

● Health Care Insurance Act (S 444, HR 2222—American Medical Association's "Medicredit"

The Senate committee also endorsed a controversial administration proposal providing special grants to states that set rates for insurance reimbursement of medical bills. Such regulation, in effect, limited medical fees. The AMA strongly opposed the proposal—killed by the House committee.

The Senate passed the measure without changing the rate regulation proposal Nov. 25.

Conference Action

There were few major differences between the two versions of the bill, and House-Senate conferees filed a report (H Rept 93-1640) on Dec. 19.

Their key decision was to keep Senate provisions that did not assure local governments automatic control of a public health planning agency. The tough Senate provision for regulation of medical payments was turned into a demonstration program in six states.

The Senate agreed to the conference report the same day, the House Dec. 20.

Provisions

As signed into law, S 2994:

● Required governors to designate boundaries for health systems agency areas in their states; generally required the areas to include a population of from 500,000 to 3 million persons; allowed the HEW Secretary to revise boundaries.

● Within 18 months of enactment, required the Secretary to designate a nonprofit private organization, unit of local government or public regional planning body as the health systems agency for each area; allowed the Secretary to designate the agencies on a conditional basis for two years; required the Secretary to consult governors before designating health systems agencies.

● Required health systems agencies to employ at least five staff members.

● Required the agencies to be governed by a body including a majority (but no more than 60 per cent) of health care consumers; required the remaining members of the governing board to be health care providers (one-third of whom must be "direct" providers rather than insurers); allowed local government officials to serve as either consumer or provider members of the board.

● Required health systems agencies to: 1) develop general and annual plans establishing priorities for health services and facilities needed in their areas; 2) make grants for the development of needed resources; 3) review and approve or disapprove each proposed use of federal health funds in their areas (the Secretary could make the funds available even if the agency disapproved proposed uses if he stated his reasons for overruling the agency); 4) review the need for

...Programs Considered By Congress in 1974

bill). In a voluntary program, each family would receive a tax credit to cover premiums for standard plans. The credits would be given on a sliding scale depending on income, with the very poor receiving federal vouchers to cover premiums.

The program would be administered by a federal advisory board and private insurers would continue to provide all coverage. In effect, the plan would be financed by federal income tax revenues, with states financing a portion of coverage for the poor.

Families would pay 20 per cent of the first $500 for hospital care, first $500 of physician services and $500 of dental care. Catastrophic benefits would be provided after a family had spent 10 per cent of its combined taxable income minus out-of-pocket expenses for basic benefits.

● Health Security Act (S 3, HR 22—Griffiths-Corman bill supported by organized labor). The plan would provide comprehensive benefits under a compulsory program for all Americans without deductibles or copayments.

A new board within HEW would administer the program and the federal government would act as insurer. The program would be financed by federal general revenues and new payroll taxes of 1 per cent of an employee's first $15,000 of income and 3.5 per cent of an employer's entire payroll. Unearned income would be taxed at 1 per cent.

● National Health Care Services Reorganization and Financing Act (HR 1—American Hospital Association bill). The bill would require employers to offer plans with standard benefits, but leave employee participation

voluntary. The federal government would cover the aged and poor using Social Security and general tax revenues. Employers would pay at least 75 per cent of required premiums.

A Cabinet-level Department of Health would administer the program and private insurers would act as principal carriers. The bill would require creation of local health care corporations to provide services paid for by an annual enrollment fee within five years. Employers, employees and individuals would finance the basic system with premiums and fees.

Families would pay no deductibles for covered services but copayments for each service. Catastrophic benefits would be provided after expenditure of amounts based on income.

● National Health Care Act (S 1100, HR 5200—Health Insurance Association of America bill). Under a voluntary program, employers and individuals would be offered tax incentives to purchase plans with standard benefits. The federal government would provide state grants to subsidize coverage of the poor, near poor and uninsurable.

A new council within the Executive Office of the President would administer the program and private insurers would provide all policies. The plan would be financed through various federal income tax deductions and general federal revenues to fund state grants for coverage of the poor.

Benefits would be phased in fully within 10 years, with copayments required for most services. After expenditure of $5,000 in out-of-pocket costs, catastrophic benefits would be provided.

---

new institutional health services and hospital modernization, and 5) at least every five years, review health facilities and inform state planning agencies whether they were appropriate for their areas.

● Authorized planning grants to health systems agencies equal to the population of the area times 50 cents; limited the maximum planning grant to $3.75-million and the minimum grant to $175,000; authorized bonus grants to agencies collecting additional funds from nonfederal sources.

● Authorized governors to select state planning and development agencies; beginning in fiscal 1980, barred federal payments for development of health resources to states which had not designated a state planning agency meeting the Secretary's satisfaction.

● Required state planning and development agencies to: 1) prepare state health plans; 2) administer a program certifying the need for each new health facility and 3) at least every five years, review the appropriateness of all institutional health services.

● Established statewide health coordinating councils to assist state planning agencies; required at least one half of the members of the council to be health care consumers; allowed governors to appoint up to 40 per cent of the total membership of the council; required a majority of a governor's appointees to be health care consumers.

● Required the councils to review and approve or disapprove state plans submitted to HEW for federal formula grants for health programs.

● Authorized grants equal to up to 75 per cent of operational costs to state planning agencies.

● Authorized grants to up to six states which regulated or planned to regulate medical payment rates to demonstrate whether rate regulation was effective.

● Required state planning agencies to draw up plans detailing the number and type of hospital beds needed in their states, plans for distribution of those beds and plans describing which hospitals were in need of modernization.

● Required states to determine that a hospital was needed before a hospital could apply for modernization assistance.

● Allotted hospital construction and modernization funds to each state on the basis of population, financial need and need for medical facilities; allowed states to use the funds for modernization, construction of new outpatient facilities, conversion of existing facilities and construction of new inpatient facilities in areas of recent population growth.

● Required states to use at least 25 per cent of their allotments for outpatient facilities in medically underserved areas; barred states from using more than 20 per cent of their allotments for construction of new inpatient facilities.

PL 93-641 Authorizations

	Fiscal 1975	Fiscal 1976 (millions)	Fiscal 1977
Health systems agency planning grants	$ 60	$ 90	$125
State planning and development agency grants	25	30	35
Demonstration grants for state rate regulation	4	5	6
Centers assisting planning agencies	5	8	10
Construction and modernization grants	125	130	135
Area health services development grants	25	75	120
Total	**$244**	**$338**	**$431**

● Authorized loans and loan guarantees for modernization and construction projects.

● Earmarked 22 per cent of funds appropriated for state modernization and construction allotments for special project grants made by the HEW Secretary; allowed the Secretary to use the grants for modernization needed to eliminate imminent safety hazards or to assure compliance with licensure or accreditation standards.

● Authorized maximum annual grants to health systems agencies equal to $1 times the population of a health systems area for development of health resources.

Biomedical Research

Congress took a historic first step toward greater protection of the rights of human beings used in medical and behavioral experiments, rights that scientific researchers had not always observed or interpreted with any uniformity.

Legislation (HR 7724—PL 93-348) cleared June 28 created a two-year commission to come up with guidelines for the use of human subjects in biomedical testing. The measure was the first ever to address ethical questions posed by medical research.

Congress asked the commission to pay special attention to controversial research, including research on children, prisoners and the mentally ill and research using live human fetuses. The commission also was charged with looking into the practice of psychosurgery—removal of part of the brain to control behavior.

The commission had no power to enforce its recommendations, but the Secretary of Health, Education and Welfare (HEW) was required to publish his reasons for rejecting them if he decided that proposed regulations were inappropriate. While the commission's guidelines were to apply only to research funded by HEW, such policies generally influenced standards used by other researchers in the United States and abroad.

The legislation called for a permanent advisory council to replace the commission at the end of 1976, but Congress agreed in 1976 to extend the commission's life for another year. *(1976 emergency medical services bill, p. 54-A)*

A second major section of the bill created a national program of awards for young scientists and doctors in research training activities. Those receiving awards were required to pay back their support with service in research, teaching or medical practice fields. This program was renewed in 1976 by a biomedical research bill (HR 7988). *(p. 51-A)*

Legislative Background

Both the House and Senate passed HR 7724 in 1973. The House limited its version to the new research training program, responding to a since-discarded proposal by the administration to phase out research training support. The Senate expanded the House bill, adding provisions creating a permanent commission to monitor medical research involving humans. *(p. 8-A)*

The administration supported the intent of the Senate bill and backed creation of a special panel to look into research issues. But it suggested that regulations addressing the research questions could be developed better by internal HEW procedures.

Conference Action

House-Senate conferees filed a report (H Rept 93-1148) on June 25 after months of negotiations over the widely differing versions of the bill.

The conferees' major disagreement focused on the new research commission proposed by the Senate. Edward M. Kennedy (D Mass.), chief Senate sponsor, wanted a permanent commission, while Paul G. Rogers (D Fla.), leading House conferee, wanted a temporary body.

The compromise accepted by conferees provided for the temporary commission and the permanent advisory council. In line with action in both houses, the bill imposed an immediate ban on fetal research, pending development of commission guidelines.

Conferees combined provisions of the House and Senate bills dealing with the new research training program, but adopted the Senate requirements for repayment of support with service. The Senate bill asked for one year of service from researchers for each year of support, while the House wanted two years of service for each year of support.

Provisions

As signed into law, HR 7724:

● Created a national program of biomedical and behavioral research training awards within HEW.

● Authorized HEW to make awards to individuals for research training at the National Institutes of Health (NIH) and other HEW agencies, nonfederal public institutions and nonprofit private institutions; earmarked at least 25 per cent of appropriated funds for awards to individuals.

● Authorized HEW to make grants to nonfederal public institutions and nonprofit private institutions for research training awards to individuals selected by the institutions.

● Authorized $207,947,000 in fiscal 1975 for research training awards and grants.

● Limited the period of awards to any one individual to three years except under special circumstances approved by the HEW Secretary.

● Required each award to cover travel and subsistence expenses for individuals and the cost of supportive services provided by an institution.

● Required each individual receiving an award to repay each year of support with one year of research or teaching in the health field; if approved by the Secretary, also allowed individuals trained in health care professions to repay each year of support with 1) one year in the National Health Service Corps, 2) 20 months in a geographic area lacking adequate health professionals in his specialty, or 3) 20 months of service in a health maintenance organization eligible for Medicare payments and located in a medically underserved area.

● Allowed individuals not trained in a health profession to repay each year of support with 20 months of service in a health-related activity if the Secretary determined that there were no suitable research or teaching positions available.

● Required individuals who failed to meet their service requirements to repay the amount of their awards plus interest to the federal government; allowed partial credit for partial service.

● Established an 11-member National Commission for the Protection of Human Subjects of Biomedical and Behavioral Research; required the Secretary to appoint the commission's members within 60 days of enactment; required five members (but no more than five) to have engaged in biomedical or behavioral research involving human subjects.

● Limited the life of the commission to two years after enactment.

● Required the commission to conduct a study to identify the basic ethical principles which should guide research involving human subjects, to develop guidelines reflecting these principles and to recommend appropriate regulations for HEW-funded research involving human subjects.

● Required the commission to devote special attention to research involving children, prisoners and the institutionalized mentally infirm.

● Required the commission to determine the need for a mechanism to protect the rights of human subjects in research not funded by HEW and to recommend such a mechanism to Congress if necessary.

● Within four months of the members' appointment, required the commission to recommend policies for research involving live human fetuses; until the commission made the recommendations, barred HEW from funding any fetal research except to save the life of the infant.

● Required the commission to study the use of psychosurgery in the United States in 1968-72 and recommend policies for such procedures.

● Required the commission to study the ethical, social and legal implications of advances in medical and behavioral sciences.

● Required the Secretary to publish any of the commission's recommendations in the *Federal Register* for comment within 60 days of receipt; after publication, required the Secretary to determine, within 180 days, the appropriateness of recommended regulations; if the Secretary disapproved the recommendations, required him to publish his reasons for doing so in the *Register*.

● On July 1, 1976, created a permanent National Advisory Council for the Protection of Subjects of Biomedical and Behavioral Research to advise the Secretary and review HEW policies.

● Required all entities seeking HEW research grants or contracts to provide assurances that they had established institutional review boards to monitor research involving human subjects sponsored by them.

● Stipulated that no individual could be forced to perform or assist in performing in any health service or research program funded by HEW if it would violate his religious or moral beliefs; barred institutions receiving HEW research funds from discriminating against such individuals.

● Authorized medical schools to apply for federal grants for special projects and programs designed to emphasize the implications of medical advances on individual and societal rights.

Cancer Funding

Extending a research campaign launched in 1971, Congress approved a dramatic expansion of funding for the National Cancer Institute. It passed legislation (S 2893—PL 93-352) authorizing a total of $2.8-billion in fiscal 1975-77 for cancer research—a $1.2-billion boost in the previous three-year authorization.

Another key provision of the bill set up a temporary presidential panel to review the balance of funding allotted to various kinds of research conducted by the National Institutes of Health (NIH).

Background

Congress had boosted funding for the cancer institute substantially in a 1971 act, responding in part to President Nixon's call for an increased effort to find a cure for cancer. The debate over the 1971 act focused on whether the cancer institute should operate independently of NIH. Congress eventually sided with those who opposed isolation of the cancer program.

Scientists had another concern by 1973. They charged that the Nixon administration was beefing up the budgets of the highly visible research programs for cancer and heart disease by starving other research programs.

"Instead of advances over the broad front of NIH research activities, the NIH generally has stood still while the National Cancer Institute and National Heart and Lung Institute have surged ahead," the Senate Labor and Public Welfare Committee said of the direction of NIH research programs since 1971.

Legislative Action

The Senate committee, reporting the measure March 20 (S Rept 93-736), decided to use the highly popular cancer authorization bill as a means of setting up a panel to oversee Nixon administration policy on all medical research programs. The committee envisioned a permanent panel that would report any misgivings about administration policy directly to the President and congressional committees.

While the administration strongly supported an extension of the cancer program, HEW officials threatened a veto unless the provision for the special panel was killed. They argued that the panel would undercut HEW's authority.

Benno C. Schmidt, chairman of the President's Cancer Panel on which the Senate committee wanted to pattern the new research committee, also argued against creation of the special panel. He argued that the new panel was unlikely to influence the President if Nixon had not asked for its creation.

The bill sailed through the Senate by a unanimous vote on March 26, however.

The House dropped the provision for the special panel in its version of the bill, passed overwhelmingly May 2. The Interstate and Foreign Commerce Committee reported the measure March 27 (H Rept 93-954).

The committee had added one provision not in the Senate bill. It gave the force of law to internal NIH procedures for peer review by scientists of all NIH research grant and contract applications.

Following their approach on other bills, House-Senate conferees compromised by turning the permanent panel in the Senate version into a temporary council with primarily advisory responsibilities. The final version, set out in a conference report (H Rept 93-1164), also kept the House provisions for NIH peer review. Congress cleared the measure July 10.

Provisions

As signed into law, S 2893:

● Authorized $750-million in fiscal 1975, $830-million in fiscal 1976 and $985-million in fiscal 1977 for cancer research programs.

● Authorized an additional $53.5-million in fiscal 1975, $68.5-million in fiscal 1976 and $88.5-million in fiscal 1977 for cancer detection and treatment programs.

● Repealed a 1971 law limiting to 15 the number of new regional centers HEW could establish to demonstrate for physicians advanced methods of diagnosing and treating cancer.

● Required Senate confirmation of all future directors of NIH.

● Extended permanently the general authority of NIH to enter into contracts for research.

● Required, by law, peer review by scientists of applications for research grants and contracts to NIH, the National Institute of Mental Health, the National Institute on Alcohol Abuse and Alcoholism and the National Institute on Drug Abuse.

● Established a President's Biomedical Research Panel made up of the chairman of the President's Cancer Panel and six members appointed by the President; required at least five members of the panel to be physicians or scientists; allowed the President to select the chairman of the panel.

Cancer Funding, 1972-1977

The following chart details the growth of federal spending for the National Cancer Institute since passage of a 1971 act expanding cancer research programs:

	Authorized Amount	Budget Request	Appropriated Amount
		(in millions)	
Fiscal 1972	$420	$374	$378
Fiscal 1973	530	426[1]	485[2]
Fiscal 1974	640	500	524[3]
Fiscal 1975	803.5	600	691.7
Fiscal 1976	898.5	586.8	743.6
Fiscal 1977	1,073.5	687.7	815

[1] As amended, 1973.
[2] Under continuing resolution.
[3] Includes authorized reduction of 5 per cent of the final appropriation.

Source: Appropriations Acts

● Required the panel to review and make recommendations for research programs conducted by NIH and the National Institute of Mental Health.

● Terminated the panel 18 months after all its members were appointed; required the panel to report its findings to Congress and the President within 15 months of the members' appointment.

Health Wage-Price Controls

Cost controls came off the health care industry for the first time since 1971.

The administration, while proposing an end to general wage and price controls, asked Congress to continue health care controls beyond their April 30 expiration date. Administration officials argued that they still expected inflationary increases in the cost of health care and petroleum products, the only other area in which they proposed to extend controls.

Both the Senate Banking, Housing and Urban Affairs Committee and the House Banking and Currency Committee voted to table the administration's request, thus letting the health controls expire April 30.

While extremely concerned by the rise in health care costs, the administration then gave up thoughts of reimposing cost controls and turned to other cost containment ideas.

Health Services

A bill (HR 14214) revising five major health services programs fell victim to a presidential pocket veto at the end of the year.

President Ford vetoed the bill after congressional adjournment, opposed to its $1-billion increase in the funding recommended by the administration. Ford also complained about the measure's creation of several new programs that he said "would result in an unjustified expenditure of federal taxpayers' funds."

Congress eventually succeeded in enacting similar legislation in 1975 over a second Ford veto. *(p. 27-A)*

Basic Provisions

As cleared by Congress Dec. 10, the vetoed bill would have authorized a total of $1.9-billion in fiscal 1975-76, most of it for five programs:

● Community mental health centers.
● Health services formula grants to the states.
● Family planning.
● Migrant health centers.
● Community health centers for the needy in rural or inner-city areas.

The measure also created several other new programs and set up a national center to look into the medical, legal and social aspects of rape.

To meet criticism that guidelines for community mental health centers had been unfocused, the bill would have required them—as well as migrant and community health centers seeking federal aid—to provide a number of specific services, encourage more consumer participation in their affairs and take steps to collect all available funds from outside sources.

All five of the basic programs expired June 30. In 1973, they had been extended without change for one year while Congress studied proposed revisions.

Administration Proposal

As it did in 1973, the administration proposed to phase out federal support for community mental health centers. The administration continued to argue that the program was successful so it was time to turn its operation over to state and local governments.

The administration also wanted to end separate categorical programs for family planning, migrant health care and neighborhood health centers for the poor, a program formerly run by the Office of Economic Opportunity. The administration proposed to lump the three programs together under a single funding authority.

Congressional Attitudes

Congress again wanted nothing to do with the administration's proposal to end federal support for community mental health centers. Supporters of the program maintained that the proposal would force some of the 626 existing centers to close, as well as jeopardize the start-up of an additional 870 centers needed to serve the entire country.

Members of Congress also expressed qualms about ending the categorical status of the family planning and other programs. "When we don't pinpoint programs, they have a way of disappearing," noted Rep. Richardson Preyer (D N.C.).

Administration officials continued to argue, however, that a program combining funding for several categorical activities would give state and local officials more flexibility. The 1974 proposal was a modest version of a health block grant plan pushed unsuccessfully by the Ford administration in 1976. *(p. 55-A)*

Legislative Action

The House Interstate and Foreign Commerce Committee, reporting the bill June 27 (H Rept 93-1161), rejected the administration's proposals, but agreed to tighten requirements governing the operation of various health service centers. The House approved the bill Aug. 12 without change.

The Senate passed its version of the bill, reported (S Rept 93-1137) by the Labor and Public Welfare Committee, on Sept. 10. The Senate added a number of provisions setting up new programs.

House-Senate conferees worked out differences between the two versions and Congress cleared the conference report (H Rept 93-1524) on the measure Dec. 10.

Nurse Training

Legislation (HR 17085) extending funding for nurse training programs was also pocket vetoed by President Ford after adjournment of the 93rd Congress. As cleared Dec. 20, the bill authorized $654-million in fiscal 1975-77 for general assistance programs for nursing schools and students. The programs had expired June 30.

The bill also would have created new programs designed to train nurses in advanced medical treatment techniques and in skills needed to provide certain kinds of physician care. Many experts believed that more highly trained nurses could help reduce the need for more doctors in some parts of the country.

Ford, vetoing the bill Jan. 4, 1975, said it was too expensive and failed to emphasize the kind of training programs the country most needed.

The bill had been reported Nov. 30 by the House Interstate and Foreign Commerce Committee (H Rept 93-1510) and passed by the House Dec. 12. The Senate approved the bill Dec. 19 without sending it to committee, making one minor change in the House version. The change was accepted by the House the following day.

Legislation similar to HR 17085 was enacted as part of a health services bill over another Ford veto in 1975.

Health Manpower

A bill (S 3585) to extend expiring health manpower programs died in conference at session's end when House-Senate conferees failed to agree on provisions designed to alleviate doctor shortages in many rural and inner-city areas of the country. Other provisions of the legislation would have addressed such major health manpower problems as the shortages of doctors in primary care specialties and the increasing U.S. reliance on graduates of foreign medical schools at a time when qualified Americans could not get into crowded U.S. medical schools.

While the legislation did not get through Congress, its provisions became a model for many features of a health manpower bill cleared in 1976. *(p. 41-A)*

Background

When Congress last rewrote health manpower legislation in 1971, its major concern was an overall shortage of doctors and other health professionals. The 1971 law gave schools incentives to increase enrollment, but did not address other health manpower problems that had become more apparent since then. Experts concluded that "more was not necessarily better."

Despite an increased supply of doctors, rural and inner-city areas continued to experience physician shortages. The number of doctors compared to population remained disproportionately high in the Northeast and West and disproportionately low in the South and North Central states. And the doctor-to-population ratio in metropolitan areas was more than twice that in rural areas.

Another major concern was maldistribution of doctors by medical specialty. Evidence pointed to possible surpluses of surgeons and other highly trained "super specialists" and generally undisputed shortages of doctors in fields such as family practice, internal medicine and general pediatrics.

A third concern was U.S. reliance on foreign-trained doctors. Experts had questioned whether graduates of foreign medical schools were as well-trained as their U.S. counterparts and deplored the "brain drain" of medical resources from developing countries. Older municipal hospitals and state mental institutions in particular were highly reliant on the foreign medical graduates.

All the parties involved with the health manpower legislation agreed on the problems, but promoted different remedies.

Some legislators wanted to force medical schools and medical students to address these problems in exchange for continued federal support; others were more friendly to the medical schools' campaign for continued federal funding, but wanted some show of cooperation in return. Medical schools and organized medicine sought ways to assure continued federal support with the least expansion of federal requirements. The administration backed a decrease in support for medical schools coupled with an expansion of programs supporting students and giving them incentives to meet the manpower needs on a voluntary basis.

Senate Bill

As originally reported (S Rept 93-1133) Sept. 3 by the Labor and Public Welfare Committee, S 3585 embodied a proposal sponsored by Edward M. Kennedy (D Mass.) and Jacob K. Javits (R N.Y.) making drastic changes in existing health manpower programs.

In order to aid areas with doctor shortages, the committee bill would have required all students entering medical school—including those receiving no federal student assistance—to agree to practice in the medically underserved areas for at least two years after graduation. Medical schools whose students did not agree to the service requirement would lose federal grants awarded to subsidize the education of each student. These "capitation" grants constituted the most direct form of federal aid to medical schools.

The Health, Education and Welfare (HEW) Secretary would have selected the students actually needed for service by lottery. Students failing to complete required service would have owed the federal government the amount of their capitation support.

Republican critics labeled the bill a "doctor draft," but Kennedy disagreed. "There is nothing in the Constitution which either requires or guarantees to any young person that he will become a doctor," Kennedy argued. "If he wants to become a doctor..., with the kind of support that he will receive from the American taxpayers, he should be willing to serve for two years."

The Senate Democratic leadership told Kennedy the committee bill was doomed when it reached the floor Sept. 23, and he tried to backpedal to a milder substitute. But the Senate instead adopted a substitute sponsored by J. Glenn Beall Jr. (R Md.) and Robert Taft Jr. (R Ohio).

Their substitute, passed Sept. 24, would have required medical schools to guarantee that 25 per cent of their incoming students had volunteered to practice in physician-shortage areas after graduation. These students, who would have received scholarships in exchange for service, could have elected to join the federal government's National Health Service Corps or establish private practice in primary care in a medically underserved area.

To enforce the requirement, the Senate bill would have cut off basic federal grants to schools where 25 per cent of the incoming class did not volunteer to serve.

The substitute proposal also killed provisions of the committee bill which would have established federal regulation of medical licensing and postgraduate training (hospital residency) programs for physicians. In order to correct shortages of specialists in primary care, the committee bill would have given the HEW Secretary authority to allocate residency positions by specialty.

House Bill

The House version of the bill took a different approach to the problem of doctor maldistribution by creating new incentives for young physicians to practice in doctor shortage areas. The House passed the measure Dec. 12 without making any changes in the version reported by the Interstate and Foreign Commerce Committee (H Rept 93-1509).

Under the House bill, all medical students seeking federal scholarship assistance would have had to agree to practice in doctor shortage areas after graduation. For each year of scholarship support, the student would have been required to practice for a year in the National Health Service Corps, Indian Health Service or in private practice in a medically underserved area.

The bill also would have required all medical students—regardless of whether they received federal student aid—to repay the federal government the amount of capitation support paid on their behalf to medical schools. Students could have owed the federal government up to $8,-400 after four school years, but the bill waived up to $2,100 in repayments for each year a medical school graduate practiced in a medically underserved area. The bill, in effect, required medical schools to enforce the repayment requirement by cutting off capitation support to any school whose students did not agree to the condition.

Conference Dispute

Meeting just before adjournment Dec. 20, House-Senate conferees deadlocked. Kennedy tried to revive some of the controversial features of his original committee bill—which was entirely unacceptable to House conferees. Time ran out for further negotiations.

Even if the bill had been cleared for the President, there was no certainty that Ford would have signed it. Both the House and Senate versions differed substantially from proposals advanced by the administration. The administration favored a phase-out of capitation support and supported greater reliance on forms of student assistance encouraging practice in doctor shortage areas. The administration also opposed the cost of the bills. The House bill authorized a total of $1.6-billion in fiscal 1975-77; the Senate version authorized $2.1-billion over the same period.

Legislative authority for most of the programs covered by the bill had expired June 30. But the health training programs continued to receive funding under continuing resolutions.

Loans for Health Students

With the fate of the comprehensive health manpower bill up in the air, Congress acted in August to make new funding available for assistance programs for students in the health professions. The legislation (S 3782—PL 93-385), cleared Aug. 8, was a repudiation of an administration proposal to curtail student loan aid.

The administration had proposed to rule out loans to students entering medical, dental, nursing and other health professions schools in the fall of 1974 by limiting loans to students who had already received them. Administration officials argued that special loan programs for students in the health professions were no longer needed.

S 3782 was an emergency measure passed by the Senate July 23 without being sent to committee. The House Interstate and Foreign Commerce Committee reported the bill July 31 (H Rept 93-1240). House action followed Aug. 5, and the Senate cleared the bill Aug. 8 by agreeing to a House amendment.

As cleared, S 3782 made no substantive changes in student aid programs. It authorized $60-million for health professions loans and $35-million for nursing loans in fiscal 1975, the same amounts authorized in fiscal 1974. The bill also authorized $40-million for scholarships for students who agreed to serve in the National Health Service Corps after graduation. Members of the corps practiced in areas with health manpower shortages.

Congress extended the programs again in 1976 in a biomedical research bill (HR 7988). *(p. 51-A)*

Health Services Research

Three expiring health programs won routine renewal. Legislation (HR 11385—PL 93-353) cleared July 11 extended funding for research in health services delivery, compilation of medical statistics and assistance to medical libraries. The programs expired June 30.

A key provision of HR 11385 directed the Department of Health, Education and Welfare (HEW) to set up separate centers for health services research and health statistics.

The House, acting Jan. 21 on the bill as reported by the Interstate and Foreign Commerce Committee (H Rept 93-757), had settled on a single agency. But the Senate version passed May 2 (S Rept 93-764) provided for two separate agencies. House-Senate conferees agreed in their report (H Rept 93-1170) on the Senate's approach.

The administration supported extension of the three programs, but questioned establishing the two new agencies by law. An administration-backed proposal eliminating construction aid for medical libraries was accepted by Congress.

Provisions

As signed into law, HR 11385:

● Established a National Center for Health Services Research in HEW to undertake research, evaluations and demonstrations dealing with health services, health manpower and health facilities.

● Required the HEW Secretary to develop at least six independent health services research centers; required one of the new centers to focus on technology related to health care delivery and another to focus on improvement of management and administration in the health care field.

● Authorized $65.2-million in fiscal 1975 and $80-million in fiscal 1976 for health services research programs; authorized an additional $80-million in fiscal 1977 if Congress did not formally extend the program before that time; required the Secretary to use at least 25 per cent of appropriated funds for projects undertaken directly by HEW.

● Established a National Center for Health Statistics in HEW.

● Authorized $30-million in each of fiscal 1975-76 for health statistics programs; authorized an additional $30-million in fiscal 1977 if Congress did not formally extend the program before that time.

● Authorized $17.5-million in fiscal 1975 and $20-million in fiscal 1976 for assistance to medical libraries; authorized an additional $20-million in fiscal 1977 if Congress did not formally extend the program before that time.

● Repealed authority for construction assistance to medical libraries.

Abortion

The continuing abortion controversy brought large numbers of right-to-life lobbyists to the Capitol in 1974, but those seeking to overturn the 1973 Supreme Court decision striking down state restrictions on abortion made little legislative headway. Abortion opponents also lost a bid to outlaw federally funded abortions under the Medicaid health program for the poor.

The Senate Judiciary Subcommittee on Constitutional Rights held hearings throughout 1974 on a number of proposals to restrict or prohibit abortion under the Constitution, but took no action. The comparable subcommittee in the House continued to show no interest in holding hearings.

Anti-abortion forces suffered a major setback June 27 when the House voted 123-247 against an amendment to the fiscal 1975 Labor-Health, Education and Welfare (HEW) appropriations bill (HR 15580—PL 93-517) that would have barred use of HEW funds to pay for abortions or abortion-causing drugs. The Senate adopted an abortion funding ban amendment to the bill, but it was dropped in conference.

Highlights of Hearings

The hearings underscored the sharp differences of opinion about the abortion issue.

Sen. James L. Buckley (Cons-R N.Y.), a leading abortion opponent, flatly maintained that a fetus had a constitutionally protected right to life. Rep. Bella S. Abzug (D N.Y.), a leader of pro-abortion forces, argued just as strongly that Congress could not impose any particular moral ethic on the entire country. At several points, witnesses questioned whether a male-dominated legislature was qualified to make any decisions about abortion for women.

Religious leaders were equally divided. John Cardinal Krol, archbishop of Philadelphia and president of the U.S. Catholic Conference, maintained that abortion was not just a "Catholic" issue.

"The right to life is not an invention of the Catholic church or any other church," he said. "It is a basic human right which must undergird any civilized society."

But Methodist Bishop James Armstrong, appearing on behalf of the Religious Coalition for Abortion Rights, opposed the amendments outlawing abortion. "Our belief in the sanctity of unborn human life makes us reluctant to approve abortion," he said. "But we are equally bound to respect the sacredness of the life and well-being of the mother, for whom devastating damage may result from an unacceptable pregnancy."

Doctors and scientists also disagreed over the question of when life begins, and squabbled about the medical risks of abortion.

Medical Peer Review

Some organized medical groups and state medical societies continued to press in 1974 for repeal of a provision in a 1972 law (PL 92-603) requiring establishment of local peer review organizations to monitor the quality of care given Medicare and Medicaid patients. The law gave professional medical groups until Jan. 1, 1976, to set up local organizations, called professional standards review organizations (PSROs), to police themselves.

The Senate Finance Committee held hearings on the PSRO program in May, but had no desire to repeal the program or amend it in 1974. Some amendments were approved in 1975 after Sen. Wallace F. Bennett (R Utah), chief sponsor of the program, retired. *(p. 34-A)*

Opposition

Medical groups opposing the program expressed three fears, suggesting that it would 1) interfere with the doctor-patient relationship if there were not enough protection of confidential medical records, 2) give the Health, Education and Welfare (HEW) Secretary the ultimate power to set norms for quality medical practice, and 3) lead to the practice of "cookbook medicine," with doctors following safe but not necessarily appropriate procedures in order to avoid peer review. Opposition to the PSRO program was strongest in states like Texas and Louisiana and among conservative doctors.

The American Medical Association's (AMA) position on PSROs was so confused in 1974 that it had to send three witnesses to testify on various aspects of its views. In late 1973, the AMA's House of Delegates had endorsed a policy calling for repeal of the law, but also directed the group's leadership to seek amendments to the statute. In June 1974, however, the AMA cleared up the confusion and voted to cooperate in the implementation of the program.

A conservative medical group, the Association of American Physicians and Surgeons, filed suit challenging the law. The Supreme Court in late 1975 upheld the constitutionality of the law.

Drug Industry Investigation

The Senate Labor and Public Welfare Health Subcommittee continued a major investigation of the prescription drug industry in 1974 in order to ready reform proposals for action later. The series of hearings began in December 1973.

In early 1974 the subcommittee focused its attention on prescription drug promotion and marketing practices. Former drug salesmen told the subcommittee that they had tended to downplay the side effects of drugs they were promoting and had given away expensive gifts in hopes of influencing doctors to prescribe certain drugs. Hearings held later in the year evoked charges that the Food and Drug Administration (FDA) had harassed scientists reporting negative findings in drug research studies. The subcommittee also investigated industry complaints that excessive FDA regulation had slowed introduction of new drugs in the United States.

Alcoholism, Drug Abuse Programs

Congress passed three bills in 1974 addressing the problems of alcoholism and drug abuse.

Alcoholism Prevention

Ignoring administration objections, Congress approved legislation (S 1125—PL 93-282) continuing a full-scale federal effort to help the nation's estimated nine million alcoholics and problem drinkers.

House and Senate sponsors of the bill came up with a final version without a formal conference.

The Senate had approved S 1125 on June 21, 1973, providing a total authorization of $460-million through fiscal 1976 for alcoholism prevention and treatment.

The House version, passed Jan. 21, 1974, without formal committee action, reduced this amount to $294-million. *(Senate action, p. 10-A)*

The final bill authorized $374-million in fiscal 1975-77, including funds for special grants to states that had adopted model laws dealing with the treatment of alcoholics. The final version also created a new agency within the Department of Health, Education and Welfare (HEW) to supervise alcoholism, drug abuse and mental health programs.

The administration wanted to spend less on the alcoholism-related programs, arguing that federal money should be used to test treatment methods while state and local agencies carried out the major share of alcoholism prevention and treatment activities.

The program was extended again in 1976. *(1976 action, p. 53-A)*

Provisions. As signed into law, S 1125:

● Extended the 1970 Comprehensive Alcohol Abuse and Alcoholism Prevention, Treatment and Rehabilitation Act of 1970 through fiscal 1976.

● Authorized $80-million in each of fiscal 1975-76 for formula grants to states for the prevention and treatment of alcoholism.

● Authorized $80-million in fiscal 1975 and $95-million in fiscal 1976 for grants to projects for the prevention and treatment of alcoholism.

● Authorized $13-million in each of fiscal 1975-77 for special grants to states which adopted a model statute designed to treat alcoholism as a disease, not a criminal offense; limited the maximum annual grant to $100,000 plus 10 per cent of a state's basic formula grant.

● Prohibited hospitals receiving federal funds from discriminating in admission policies or treatment services against any person solely because of his problems with alcohol; required medical records of those treated for alcoholism to be kept confidential except under specific conditions.

● Established an Alcohol, Drug Abuse and Mental Health Administration within HEW to supervise the activities of the National Institute of Mental Health, National Institute on Alcohol Abuse and Alcoholism and National Institute on Drug Abuse.

Education Programs

Congress Sept. 4 renewed funding for a 1970 act providing federal grants for educational programs addressing the dangers of drug abuse. The bill (HR 9456—PL 93-422) authorized $90-million in fiscal 1975-77 for the programs.

The legislation also placed new emphasis on educational programs conducted in schools as opposed to other community settings. Congress also insisted on continuing the programs on a categorical basis instead of combining them with other federal drug abuse and alcoholism activities.

The House had passed the bill (H Rept 93-605) on Oct. 30, 1973, after adopting an amendment making it clear that the measure specifically covered educational programs directed at alcohol—considered the country's most abused drug by many experts.

The Senate approved its version June 25, 1974; the Labor and Public Welfare Committee stressed in its report (S Rept 93-954) that it wanted the programs to educate, not to scare or confuse, students.

Sponsors drafted a final version without a formal conference.

Provisions. As signed into law, HR 9456:

● Authorized $26-million in fiscal 1975, $30-million in fiscal 1976 and $34-million in fiscal 1977 for drug and alcohol abuse education programs.

● Reserved at least 60 per cent of appropriated funds for programs in elementary and secondary schools; authorized use of up to 10 per cent of appropriated funds for grants to state education programs.

Narcotic Treatment Programs

Legislation (S 1115—PL 93-281) tightening federal controls on the distribution of methadone and other narcotics used in treatment programs cleared May 1. The bill was an effort to stem the illegal diversion of such drugs to street traffic.

Basic provisions of the bill required those dispensing drugs in narcotic maintenance or detoxification programs to register each year with the Attorney General. The bill also required such persons to comply with federal standards for security, record-keeping and the unsupervised use of narcotics by patients in treatment programs.

The number of patients in legal methadone programs had shot up to 73,000 by 1973, compared to fewer than 400 in 1968. At the same time, the number of arrests involving diversion of synthetic narcotics, especially methadone, had increased nearly 900 per cent in the seven-year period ending in 1971. Deaths involving methadone misuse also had increased.

Federal narcotics officials blamed part of the situation on careless administration of treatment programs and thefts of treatment center supplies.

The Senate originally passed S 1115 (S Rept 93-192) on June 8, 1973. On March 19, 1974, the House approved a virtually identical bill that was not formally reported from committee. The Senate accepted the House version. The Justice Department backed the bill.

Nutrition Programs

Congress enacted three measures designed to improve nutritional programs for diverse groups of the population—the elderly, children, the needy, disaster victims, institutions, summer camps, some Indian reservations and needy women, infants and children through supplemental feeding programs.

A common thread in all the legislation was the supplying of food commodities by the Agriculture Secretary. While these commodities generally had been bought at surplus prices as a form of price support, there were few surpluses in 1974 and the Nixon administration proposed that the Agriculture Department pay cash to the programs instead of buying commodities at non-surplus, market prices under authority that was to expire June 30, 1974. Congress opposed that proposal, extending the purchasing authority and requiring commodity assistance.

School Lunch

Congress June 18 cleared for the President's signature HR 14354 (PL 93-326), to extend through fiscal 1975 the Agriculture Secretary's authority to purchase food commodities for school lunch programs at non-surplus prices.

The legislation guaranteed that school lunch programs would continue to receive donated food commodities through fiscal 1975 even if the government had to purchase them at market prices. But the bill did not rule out the possibility that the administration could put into effect its controversial proposal to replace school lunch commodities with cash payments after fiscal 1975.

The Nixon administration's intention was revealed Feb. 12 when Sen. George McGovern (D S.D.) released a confidential memo to Agriculture Secretary Earl L. Butz from Clayton K. Yeutter, assistant agriculture secretary for marketing and consumer services. It contended that replacing commodities with cash payments would reduce the federal cost of aiding school nutrition programs at a time when crop surpluses were not available for government purchase. Opponents of the administration plan argued that individual school districts had less buying power than the federal government and that surplus crops could reappear.

The bill simply required the Agriculture Secretary to use his commodity procurement authority in fiscal 1975 only, a compromise between the House and Senate versions of the legislation. The House version would have left use of the authority in fiscal 1975 up to the Secretary's discretion. The Senate passed a stronger bill to make use of the authority mandatory and permanent.

The Secretary's authority to buy commodities at market prices, provided under the 1973 farm act (PL 93-86), would have expired June 30 without congressional action. The administration had proposed to use the authority in fiscal 1975, but argued that the procurement level should be left up to the Secretary.

Legislative Action

The House May 7 passed the bill by a 359-38 vote, making no changes in the version reported by the Education and Labor Committee (H Rept 93-1022).

The Senate passed its companion measure by voice vote May 21, with no change in the bill reported by the Agriculture and Forestry Committee (S Rept 93-380).

Conferees filed their report June 13 (H Rept 93-1104). The House adopted it June 17 by a 345-15 vote and the Senate on June 18 by voice vote.

Provisions

As signed into law, HR 14354 (PL 93-326):
● Required the Agriculture Secretary to purchase, at levels programmed by the Agriculture Department, food commodities for distribution to school lunch and other child nutrition programs and to feeding programs for the elderly in fiscal 1975.
● Required the average commodity donation to school lunch programs to have a value of 10 cents per meal (or an equivalent, adjusted for inflation) in fiscal 1975 and all following years.
● Required the Secretary to emphasize donation of high protein food commodities to school lunch programs.
● Made permanent the authority of the states to serve reduced-price school lunches to children from families with incomes up to 75 per cent above those in the Agriculture Secretary's poverty income guidelines.
● Increased the authorization after fiscal 1975 for purchase of school food service equipment to $40-million from $20-million.
● Increased the fiscal 1975 authorization for the supplemental feeding program for women, infants and children to $100-million from $40-million.

Nutrition for Elderly

Congress June 27 cleared for the President's signature HR 11105 (PL 93-351), to authorize $600-million in fiscal 1975-77 for nutrition programs for the elderly.

The popular nutrition programs, first authorized in 1972 as Title VII of the Older Americans Act, were set up to provide persons age 60 and older with one hot meal a day, five days a week.

As cleared, the most controversial provision of the bill, added by the Senate, would require all programs under the Older Americans Act to be carried out by the commissioner on aging within the Department of Health, Education and Welfare (HEW) or officials directly responsible to him. The provision was a response to a proposal by HEW to delegate certain responsibilities for these programs to HEW regional officials.

The administration supported extension of the nutrition programs, but recommended an open-ended authorization and only a one-year extension.

Legislative Action

House Action. The Education and Labor Committee reported its bill March 18 (H Rept 93-914). The House passed it March 19 by a 380-6 vote under suspension of the rules without debate.

Senate Action. The Labor and Public Welfare Committee reported the bill June 13 (S Rept 93-932) with amendments to block the delegation of responsibility to regional officials, to add a new transportation program for the elderly, and to limit the amount local agencies would have to pay in shared costs for elderly programs. The Senate passed the bill June 19 by 90-0 after rejecting an amendment to drop the ban on delegation of responsibility.

Final Action. No formal conference was necessary. The House June 26 agreed to the Senate changes with a slight modification. The Senate approved the final version June 27, completing action three days before the authorization was to expire.

Provisions

As signed into law, HR 11105 (PL 93-351):

• Authorized $150-million in fiscal 1975, $200-million in fiscal 1976 and $250-million in fiscal 1977 for nutrition programs for the elderly.

• Authorized $35-million in fiscal 1975 in formula grants to the states for transportation programs for the elderly, with emphasis on transportation needed in connection with the nutrition programs; required the states to give priority to areas with inadequate or no public transportation.

• Barred the commissioner on aging from delegating any of his responsibilities to officials directly responsible to him.

• Required the Secretary of Agriculture to provide food commodity assistance to the nutrition programs with a value of at least 10 cents per meal (adjusted annually for inflation).

• Limited the local share of costs for the Retired Senior Volunteer Program (RSVP) to 10 per cent the first year of assistance, 20 per cent the second year, 30 per cent the third year, 40 per cent the fourth year and no more than 50 per cent in all subsequent years.

Other Legislation

Congress cleared several other health bills during the year. It had begun to consider many of them in 1973.

Infant Death Syndrome

Legislation (S 1745—PL 93-270) authorizing $9-million in fiscal 1975-77 for educational and counseling programs dealing with the sudden infant death syndrome, a mysterious disease known as crib death, cleared April 10. Crib death killed at least 10,000 infants a year, but there was no definite known cause or cure for the disease. Because crib death occurred suddenly to apparently healthy infants, parents of children killed by it often suffered acute guilt feelings and needed counseling.

As cleared, the bill was much closer to the version passed by the House Jan. 21 after the Interstate and Foreign Commerce Committee was discharged from further consideration of the bill. The Senate version, passed Dec. 11, 1973 (S Rept 93-606), would have provided a separate authorization of $24-million for crib death research. The final bill, devised without formal conference, dropped the extra Senate funding for research.

Institute on Aging

President Nixon May 31 signed a bill (S 775—PL 93-296) similar to a measure that he pocket vetoed in 1972. The bill, which the administration still called unnecessary, established a National Institute on Aging within the National Institutes of Health (NIH). The bill's supporters argued that existing NIH research programs slighted the problems of the aged.

The Senate had passed S 775 (S Rept 93-299) on July 9, 1973. The House bill was reported (H Rept 93-906) by the Interstate and Foreign Commerce Committee on March 13, 1974, and passed by the House May 2. The Senate cleared the measure May 16 by accepting minor House amendments.

In addition to establishing the new institute, the bill created an advisory council on aging to make recommendations to the Department of Health, Education and Welfare (HEW).

Diabetes Research

Congress July 10 cleared legislation (S 2830—PL 93-354) authorizing $41-million in fiscal 1975-77 to set up new centers for diabetes research and to establish a national commission to formulate a long-range plan to fight diabetes. Diabetes afflicted as many as 10 million Americans.

The Senate passed the bill Dec. 20, 1973 (S Rept 93-653), and the House approved a less expensive version (H Rept 93-894) on March 19, 1974. House-Senate conferees compromised (H Rept 93-1147) on funding for the new centers and dropped a Senate provision providing funds for the prevention of diabetes.

The program was extended in 1976. *(p. 54-A)*

Arthritis Research

Similar legislation (S 2854—PL 93-640) dealing with arthritis was cleared Dec. 19. The bill authorized $50-million in fiscal 1975-77 for research, prevention and training programs addressed to arthritis. Final action on the noncontroversial measure came when the Senate agreed to accept the House version, passed Dec. 18 without formal committee action. The Senate version (S Rept 93-1251), approved Oct. 11, would have authorized a total of $76-million.

As cleared, the bill established a national commission to draw up a plan to attack arthritis, a blanket term covering more than 100 diseases attacking joints and connective tissues.

The legislation was extended in 1976. *(p. 54-A)*

1975

Congress completed one overhaul of the federal health machinery in 1975, reworking health services programs for the mentally ill, migrant workers and the poor. It again did not reach any final agreement on proposals to ease doctor shortages in many rural and inner-city areas. Economic and political conditions stalled action on national health insurance. And neither Congress nor the administration made any formal moves to deal with the rising cost of medical malpractice insurance, perhaps the most pressing problem faced by the medical profession in 1975.

The administration set the tone for its actions early in 1975 by proposing cutbacks in funding for many health programs and cost-saving but unpopular changes in the Medicare program for the aged and Medicaid program for the poor. Congress rejected or did not consider most of these proposals.

Many other bills got initial consideration in 1975, but did not win final approval until 1976.

Health Services

Congress July 29 decisively set aside President Ford's veto of a health services and nurse training bill (S 66—PL 94-63). Ford objected to the bill's cost and its extension of programs the administration wanted to end. He had pocket vetoed similar legislation at the end of the 93rd Congress. *(p. 20-A)*

The support for the veto override attested to the political popularity of the existing programs covered by the bill—family planning, community mental health centers, migrant health care, health centers for the poor, nurse training and state formula grants for health services. It was the first time Congress had overridden a Ford veto in 1975.

As cleared by Congress July 16, the bill authorized $553-million in fiscal 1976-78 for nurse training programs, $30-million in fiscal 1976 for the National Health Service Corps and $1.42-billion in fiscal 1976-77 for the other health services programs. Sponsors of the measure had hoped to avoid a veto by trimming more than $500-million from the funding contained in the pocket-vetoed legislation.

Continuing Dispute

Early in the year, Congress and the administration resumed their two-year-old dispute over major health services programs. Disagreements continued to stem from philosophical conceptions of the proper federal role in health care.

The administration believed that much federal support for the direct provision of health care should be replaced by funding from other sources. Sponsors of S 66 insisted that the federally supported programs addressed national problems that would be ignored by state and local governments strapped for funds.

In line with its beliefs, the administration proposed for the third year in a row to phase out support for the community mental health centers program. It also made a new proposal to end formula grants to the states for health services. The Department of Health, Education and Welfare (HEW) also announced plans to set regulations requiring state, local and private sources to pick up 20 per cent more of the costs for major health services programs covered by S 66.

Legislative Action

Congress wanted no part of the administration proposals, but it did approve steps designed to make health centers providing medical care more efficient.

Reporting S 66 on March 6 (S Rept 94-29), the Senate Labor and Public Welfare Committee called the administration's proposed cuts in health services programs unconscionable. The existing economic crisis would make it much harder for the various health services centers to collect outside funds, the committee argued.

The full Senate agreed, passing the bill by an overwhelming vote on April 10. The combined Senate authorization for the health services and nurse training programs was $2.5-billion.

Before approving a new health services bill (HR 4925—H Rept 94-192) June 5 and another nurse training bill (HR 4115—H Rept 94-143) May 7, the House substantially trimmed the authorization levels in the pocket-vetoed bills to a combined total of $2-billion.

The House May 7 also passed a third bill (HR 4114—H Rept 94-137) that eventually was added to S 66. It dealt with a funding extension of the National Health Service Corps, which sent government doctors to medically underserved areas.

In an effort to avoid another veto, Senate conferees readily accepted the lower funding levels contained in the House-passed legislation. The three House-passed bills were amalgamated into one (S 66). The conference report (H Rept 94-348) also resolved some other minor differences.

Veto and Override

Ford issued a veto message July 26. He conceded that S 66 did reduce the authorization levels in the pocket-vetoed bills, but argued that they were still excessive. Repeating earlier arguments, Ford also maintained that it was time to end federal support for some of the programs covered by the bill.

The Senate overrode the veto by a 67-15 vote on July 26 without really bothering to discuss it. No one spoke in favor of the veto.

The House followed suit July 29 by a 384-43 vote.

"It's just like voting against motherhood if you vote against health...," conceded Rep. Samuel L. Devine (Ohio), top Republican on the committee that wrote the bill. But Congress "can't continue to vote for bills that blow the budget."

But Republican leaders had trouble defending the President's assertion that the bill was too expensive because it was an authorization rather than an appropriations measure. Supporters argued that appropriations committees no doubt would reduce the authorization levels.

A coalition of health groups also lobbied heavily for an override. It included the American Nurses' Association, Planned Parenthood-World Population, National Association for Mental Health, National Council of Community Mental Health Centers and women's, environmental and labor groups.

Provisions

As enacted over the President's veto, S 66:

Health Services Programs

State Formula Grants

● Authorized formula grants based on population and financial need to the states for public health services programs; required states to use not less than 1) 15 per cent of the grants for mental health services and 2) 70 per cent of the remainder of the grants for services provided in communities.

● Authorized grants to the states for the detection, prevention and treatment of hypertension (high blood pressure).

Family Planning

● Authorized grants for projects, research, training programs and information activities dealing with family planning; required the HEW Secretary to report annually to Congress with five-year plans for federal family planning programs.

● Required, in general, federal grants to cover at least 90 per cent of the cost of a new project.

● Imposed maximum criminal penalties of $1,000 in fines and one year's imprisonment on persons running federally funded programs who coerced their clients into having abortions or sterilizations by threatening them with loss of services.

Community Mental Health Centers

● Required new and existing community mental health centers seeking federal grants for initial operation to provide the following services within two years of receipt of a grant: inpatient services, outpatient services, day care and partial hospitalization services, emergency services, specialized services for children and the elderly, consultation and education services including assistance to courts and other public agencies, and half-way house services for those discharged from a mental institution; required the centers to provide services for those abusing alcohol or drugs if the community needed such services.

● Required the centers to make medically necessary services available 24 hours a day, seven days a week; allowed the centers to arrange with other health professionals to provide services.

● Required centers receiving their first federal assistance under the bill to be governed by a board of community residents, of whom not more than half could be providers of health care.

● Required centers to maintain programs to assure the quality of care, to use an up-to-date medical records system and to establish a professional advisory board made up of staff members to assist the governing board.

● Authorized maximum grants of up to $75,000 to help public or nonprofit private groups plan community mental health center projects.

● Authorized grants to support a center's first eight years of operation; set the maximum annual federal grant at the lower of 1) the difference between a center's projected operational costs and the amount of funds collected from other sources and 2) a declining percentage of projected operational costs. (See next provision, below)

● Limited the maximum federal share of projected operational costs for centers not located in poverty areas to 80 per cent in the first grant year, 65 per cent in the second year, 50 per cent in the third year, 35 per cent in the fourth year, 30 per cent in the fifth and sixth years and 25 per cent in the seventh and eighth years; limited the maximum federal share for poverty centers to 90 per cent in the first two years and then lowered the federal share by 10 per cent in each of the following six years.

● Authorized special grants to centers for provision of consultation services, for conversion of centers that ·did not

Authorization Levels

As enacted into law over the President's veto, S 66 authorized the following amounts (in millions of dollars):

Health Services Programs[1]

	Fiscal 1976	Fiscal 1977
Formula grants to the states for health services[2]	$115.00	$125.00
Family Planning		
Project grants	115.00	115.00
Training	4.00	5.00
Research	55.00	60.00
Information	2.00	2.50
Subtotal	176.00	182.50
Community mental health centers		
Planning	3.75	3.75
Initial operation	50.00	55.00
Consultation and education	10.00	15.00
Conversion grants	20.00	20.00
Financial distress grants	15.00	15.00
Construction	5.00	5.00
Subtotal	103.75	113.75
Rape prevention and control	7.00	10.00
Migrant health centers		
Planning and development	4.00	4.00
Operation	30.00	35.00
Hospital care	5.00	5.00
Subtotal	39.00	44.00
Community health centers		
Planning and development	5.00	5.00
Operation	215.00	235.00
Subtotal	220.00	240.00
Control of diseases borne by rats	20.00	—
Home health services	10.00	—
Hemophilia treatment	7.00	9.00
Total	**$697.75**	**$724.25**

[1] The bill also extended the programs through fiscal 1975 at the fiscal 1974 authorization level of $663-million.
[2] Includes $15-million in each fiscal year for prevention and treatment of hypertension.

National Health Service Corps

	Fiscal 1975	Fiscal 1976
Basic operations	$ 16.00	$ 30.00

Nurse Training Programs [1]

	Fiscal 1976	Fiscal 1977	Fiscal 1978
Construction:			
Grants	$ 20.00	$ 20.00	$ 20.00
Interest subsidies	1.00	1.00	1.00
Capitation grants	50.00	55.00	55.00
Financial distress grants	5.00	5.00	5.00
Special projects	15.00	15.00	15.00
Advanced nurse training	15.00	20.00	25.00
Nurse practitioner programs	15.00	20.00	25.00
Traineeships	15.00	20.00	25.00
Student loans	25.00	30.00	35.00
Total	**$161.00**	**$186.00**	**$206.00**

[1] The bill also extended the programs through fiscal 1975 at the fiscal 1974 authorization level of $236-million.

offer required services prior to enactment, and for the renovation or leasing of facilities; authorized grants for new construction of facilities if at least 25 per cent of the community's residents were poor.

● Authorized continuation grants to existing centers previously funded by the federal government, but required such centers to meet the bill's new service requirements after receipt of two annual continuation grants; authorized no more than three additional annual grants to centers that were financially pressed after the end of their federal funding period.

Migrant Health Centers

● Authorized grants for the planning and operation of health centers serving migrant and seasonal agricultural workers; required the HEW Secretary to give priority for assistance to areas where at least 6,000 migrant workers and their family members lived for more than two months a year.

● Required federally assisted migrant health centers to provide or arrange to provide physician services, diagnostic services, preventive eye and ear care for children, family planning and prenatal services, emergency medical services and preventive dental services; if appropriate, required the centers to provide or arrange to provide hospital services, home health services, nursing home services, mental health care, physical therapy and other services.

● Required all assisted centers to provide or arrange to provide environmental health services and, if appropriate, screening for infectious and parasitic diseases and accident prevention programs.

● Required a majority of a center's governing board to be made up of individuals served by the center; required centers to make services available promptly, to maintain quality assurance programs, to demonstrate their financial responsibility, to set fees in accordance with a patient's ability to pay and to collect third-party reimbursements for patients eligible for Medicare or Medicaid.

● Authorized special federal grants to help cover the costs of hospital care for workers served by the centers.

Community Health Centers

● Authorized grants for the planning and operation of health centers located in medically underserved rural or inner-city areas; required the centers to provide services similar to those provided by migrant health centers.

Miscellaneous

● Established a National Center for the Prevention and Control of Rape within the National Institute of Mental Health to study the medical, legal and social aspects of rape and to serve as an information clearinghouse.

● Extended through fiscal 1976 programs to control diseases borne by rodents.

● Authorized grants to establish, operate or expand programs providing health care at home; gave priority for assistance to areas with large numbers of elderly or medically indigent residents.

● Established national commissions or committees to study and make recommendations dealing with Huntington's disease, a degenerative disorder of the nervous system; epilepsy and the mental health of the elderly.

● Authorized grants to establish centers for the treatment of hemophilia, a blood disorder, and to develop blood separation centers making available blood components hemophiliacs need to aid blood clotting.

National Health Service Corps

● Authorized a one-time grant of up to $25,000 to medically underserved communities to help them acquire equipment and facilities needed to open a practice for a member of the National Health Service Corps.

● Extended the National Health Service Corps program through fiscal 1976.

Nurse Training Programs

● Authorized grants, loan guarantees and interest subsidies for the construction or renovation of nursing educational facilities.

● Authorized annual per-student ("capitation") grants of 1) $400 to four-year nursing schools, 2) $275 to two-year nursing schools and 3) $250 to hospital-based nursing schools; barred capitation grants to schools that did not either 1) increase enrollment by 5 or 10 per cent, depending on the size of the school, or 2) carry out at least two of the following programs: a continuing education program, a recruitment program for students from disadvantaged backgrounds, a nurse practitioner program training nurses to give care usually provided by doctors, or a clinical training program at sites remote from the school's main campus.

● Authorized grants to nursing schools in financial distress, grants to establish programs for the advanced training of nurses in fields such as burn therapy, grants for the short-term training of nurse's aides and nursing home orderlies, and grants to establish nurse practitioner programs.

● Authorized federal loans and scholarships to nursing students; authorized traineeships for nurses wishing to enter teaching, administrative or advisory fields.

National Health Insurance

Despite some optimistic talk early in the year, economic and political realities made national health insurance a low-priority issue in 1975.

Leery of the budget impact of a new social program, the Ford administration reversed its policy and withdrew its support for health insurance legislation. Major lobby groups did not pressure Congress for speedy action.

And two powerful House committees—Interstate and Foreign Commerce and Ways and Means—claimed authority to write health insurance legislation and quickly found themselves locked in a hopeless jurisdictional struggle. Rather than aggravate the dispute, they contented themselves with holding some new hearings on health insurance. For the most part, the hearings covered familiar ground. *(See box, p. 14-A)*

Early Optimism

The 93rd Congress had closed with feelings high that the influx of newly elected liberal House members would help break the 30-year stalemate over health insurance legislation in 1975. The fact that the busy House Ways and Means Committee was required by a 1974 committee reform measure to establish subcommittees added to the favorable legislative outlook.

Like those before it, the 94th Congress opened Jan. 14 with renewed calls for action on health insurance. "I have assured the chairmen of the appropriate committees that national health insurance will be one of the first bills—if not the first — considered" House Speaker Carl Albert (D Okla.) told the opening session of the new Congress.

"I am personally persuaded...that the Congress can no longer postpone major decisions to assure the availability of health services to all persons in the United States," added Ways and Means Chairman Al Ullman (D Ore.) the same day. Ullman said he hoped his committee could draft a bill as early as the summer of 1975.

Ford Opposition

The optimistic timetable hit its first snag Jan. 15 when President Ford made it clear in his State of the Union message that he would veto any new spending legislation. The new spending moratorium applied to national health insurance legislation, and the administration declined to reintroduce its proposal in 1975.

Health, Education and Welfare (HEW) Secretary Caspar W. Weinberger initially said that the administration would resubmit a version of its bill in 1976 when it expected an improvement in the economy.

However, when Ford called for further spending cuts in October, the new HEW Secretary, David Mathews, said his department would not propose national health insurance.

The administration's decision came under attack in Congress and even provoked criticism by some ex-administration officials.

"The very fact that the administration has chosen not to resubmit its national health insurance proposal reflects a decision based on expediency, rather than careful planning," Charles C. Edwards, HEW assistant secretary for health until January 1975, wrote in the March 13 issue of the *New England Journal of Medicine*. While he questioned whether the country's medical delivery system was ready for national health insurance, Edwards suggested that the administration should try to work with Congress instead of encouraging a ""tug-of-war" over the issue.

Other Problems

But presidential opposition was not the only factor stalling action on health insurance in 1975.

While trying to write legislation to provide emergency health insurance for the unemployed, the Ways and Means and Commerce Committees quickly discovered that neither panel was likely to relinquish any authority over national health insurance. The dispute killed the emergency health insurance bill. *(Details, below)*

The Democratic leadership did not put heavy pressure on the two committees to resolve their dispute and it continued tacitly throughout the year. Energetic schedules for committee action fell by the wayside.

The Ways and Means Health Subcommittee decided to hold some more hearings on health insurance despite the fact that the committee had held months of hearings in 1974 on the issue. The hearings began in November and continued almost every day for a month. To keep its jurisdictional claims fresh too, the Commerce Subcommittee on Health and the Environment held some hearings in December.

Organized labor decided that 1975 had not turned out to be the best year for it to push for its comprehensive plan despite the election of the liberal House freshmen. Other outside interest flagged. The anti-Washington feeling apparent during the year also dampened desires to establish a major new social program run by the federal government.

Policy Shifts

The early days of the 94th Congress saw some policy shifts on the national health insurance issue.

The principal change was the American Medical Association's (AMA) shift to a plan requiring employers to offer standard health insurance plans, an approach similar to that of the administration's 1974 proposal. In the past, the AMA had supported only a strictly voluntary health insurance program.

In other actions, Edward M. Kennedy (D Mass) returned as the chief Senate sponsor of the comprehensive health insurance plan backed by the AFL-CIO, United Auto Workers (UAW) and other organized labor groups. In 1974, Kennedy had hoped to win support for a less broad bill that he cosponsored with Rep. Wilbur D. Mills (D Ark.). But the expected support, especially from labor, did not materialize.

Two other major proposals, those sponsored by the Health Insurance Association of America and the American Hospital Association, also were reintroduced. Senators Russell B. Long (D La.) and Abraham Ribicoff (D Conn.) in October revived their 1974 plan, which would revise insurance coverage for the poor and protect all Americans from the catastrophic costs of a long-term or serious illness.

Given the years of debate over national health insurance, however, it was clear by 1975 that the specifics of the major proposals were much less important than the principles they embodied.

The major conflict remained unchanged from earlier years:

Should the program rely primarily on the private sector, as the AMA, hospital and insurers' plans would, or on the public sector, as the labor plan would?

Emergency Health Insurance

Considered an emergency need in the early months of 1975, legislation providing health insurance for the unemployed got bogged down in jurisdictional disputes and never made it to the floor in either house.

Because its consideration was looked upon as a trial run for action on national health insurance, the emergency proposal locked two powerful House committees in a struggle over their jurisdictional claims. Basically, the struggle was over how much the Ways and Means Health Subcommittee, chaired by Dan Rostenkowski (D Ill.), and the Interstate and Foreign Commerce Subcommittee on Health and the Environment, chaired by Paul G. Rogers (D Fla.), each would have to say about the shape of a national health insurance bill.

A similar jurisdictional split developed between the Senate Finance and Senate Labor and Public Welfare Committees. But the Senate leadership kept the dispute from breaking out into the open.

Background

Support for an emergency health insurance program reflected a general concern that the growing number of workers losing their jobs might have to do without medical care.

But spokesmen for medical groups freely admitted that they also feared increases in bad debts as the recession deepened.

No one knew how many of the nation's 7.5 million unemployed workers in early 1975 had lost health insurance provided through their jobs. But those favoring an emergency program argued that most jobless workers would not be able to afford an individual policy, which cost roughly 20 per cent more than a group insurance plan. At the same time, they argued, unemployment benefits gave many jobless persons too high an income to qualify for the Medicaid program for the poor.

Supporters included major hospital, medical, insurance and labor groups. The administration emerged as the only major opponent of an emergency program, maintaining that it would be too expensive, inequitable and impossible to administer.

Senate Action

The Labor and Public Welfare Committee approved an emergency insurance proposal (S 625—S Rept 94-76) on March 17 that would have used general tax revenues to pay for whatever benefits an unemployed worker would have received had he kept his job. But because the Senate leadership wanted the House to act first, the bill never came up on the floor.

House Controversy

Both the Ways and Means Committee and Commerce Committee reported emergency health insurance bills in early 1975 (HR 5970—H Rept 94-171, Part I and Part II). But the jurisdictional conflict between the two panels kept the legislation from reaching the floor.

Committee members showed they were more concerned about preserving their committees' jurisdictional claims over national health insurance and about setting health insurance precedents they favored than they were about the legislation at hand. Provisions of bills were written specifically to make the legislation fit more snugly under each committee's jurisdiction.

"In both committees, we're striving mightily to carve out our own turf," observed William A. Steiger (R Wis.), a Ways and Means member.

Fears that major health insurance questions were being decided complicated the battle over the legislation. The Ways and Means Committee, for instance, fought for days over whether the federal government or private insurers should run a program designed to continue health insurance coverage for workers who lost their jobs in the future. James C. Corman (D Calif.), chief House sponsor of labor's health insurance plan, objected strongly to letting private insurers run this program. Labor forces favored federal control of health insurance.

The Commerce Committee argued less about health insurance precedents and worried more about getting its own proposal ready for floor action. It rushed through markup of an alternative measure amid talk about the need to fortify the committee's jurisdictional claims.

In the end, however, committee leaders decided they did not want to get into a full-scale confrontation on the floor. Instead, they just let the bills die.

In earlier years, the jurisdictional issue was more clear-cut. The Rogers subcommittee dealt with almost all other health legislation, while Ways and Means reserved primary claim on most national health insurance bills.

But in 1974, the House adopted a committee reform plan that virtually guaranteed the jurisdictional confusion that developed. The plan gave the Commerce Committee

authority over all health legislation except that financed through payroll taxes, but exactly how the change affected national health insurance legislation remained uncertain. In 1975, health insurance bills were referred to both committees, sometimes jointly.

Abortion

Abortion opponents suffered two major legislative setbacks in 1975.

On Sept. 17, the Senate Judiciary Subcommittee on Constitutional Amendments rejected a number of proposed amendments to overturn the 1973 Supreme Court decision striking down restrictions on abortion. The votes put an end to the Senate committee's consideration of the abortion issue in the 94th Congress.

In action on a health services bill (S 66), the Senate also voted 54-36 on April 10 to table an amendment barring federal funding of abortions under the Medicaid program for the poor except those needed to save the life of the mother. The vote reversed the Senate's position on a similar amendment in 1974. *(p. 23-A)*

Dewey F. Bartlett (R Okla.), sponsor of the amendment, argued that the federal government had no business paying for a procedure many taxpayers found highly repugnant. Senators attacking the amendment tried to steer clear of the emotional controversy surrounding abortion, arguing instead that the proposal was illegal and unfair to poor women unable to afford abortions without Medicaid.

After rejecting the Bartlett proposal, the Senate adopted an amendment imposing criminal penalties on persons running federally funded family planning programs who coerced their clients into having an abortion. This amendment became law as part of S 66. *(p. 27-A)*

[In 1976 Congress did adopt an amendment barring the use of federal funds for abortion except when the life of the mother were endangered. *(p. 45-A)*

Developmental Disabilities

Congress Sept. 23 approved legislation (HR 4005—PL 94-103) expanding federal efforts to help the mentally retarded and others suffering from health problems known as developmental disabilities. Developmental disabilities, including cerebral palsy and epilepsy, generally originate in childhood and continue indefinitely.

The bill authorized a total of $287-million in fiscal 1976-78, including $150-million for formula grants to the states for programs aiding the developmentally disabled. The bill also authorized funding of $65-million over the same period for special projects and $63-million to aid university-affiliated centers training personnel to care for the mentally retarded.

A second part of the legislation required the states to guarantee protection of the legal rights of the developmentally disabled and required the use of individual treatment plans for the mentally retarded and others in federally funded institutions. These requirements and a legislative statement of the rights of the developmentally disabled were a compromise replacement for Senate provisions that would have set very detailed requirements for such institutions.

The programs covered by the bill actually expired June 30, 1974. Both the House and Senate passed bills similar to HR 4005 in 1974, but conferees did not have time to work out a final version before the 93rd Congress ended.

The administration favored extension of the programs, but at lower funding levels. It also had objected to the Senate-passed provisions that would have set detailed standards for institutions caring for the disabled.

Legislative Action

The House Interstate and Foreign Commerce Committe, reporting (H Rept 94-58) the bill March 13, reduced the authorization in its 1974 bill to show its willingness to compromise with the administration. The House bill, passed April 10, dealt only with the extension of programs aiding the developmentally disabled.

The Senate, acting June 2, added the provisions requiring institutions caring for the disabled to meet detailed requirements for staffing, living conditions, medical and other services and admission and release policies, among other things. Institutions not meeting the requirements faced a cutoff of all federal funds. These provisions were added by the Labor and Public Welfare Committee (S Rept 94-160).

House-Senate conferees modified these provisions in their report (H Rept 94-473). The compromise required states to assure the Department of Health, Education and Welfare (HEW) that institutions receiving these funds would draw up individual treatment plans for the disabled by Sept. 30, 1976. To receive federal grants after Sept. 30, 1977, states were required to adopt a system to protect and advocate the legal and personal rights of the developmentally disabled.

Other key provisions drafted by conferees:

● Added those suffering from dyslexia, a reading disability, and autism, a severe emotional disturbance characterized by complete withdrawal, to persons eligible for federal aid under the programs.

● Required states to use at least 10 per cent of their formula grants to develop and implement plans to reduce inappropriate placement of the developmentally disabled in institutions. The House had pushed for this emphasis.

● Created a new program providing for grants to special projects aiding the developmentally disabled and reserved 25 per cent of the grant funds for projects with national significance.

Drug Regulation

The Senate voted in September to suspend the use of diethylstilbestrol (DES) as a growth stimulant in livestock until the government determined that the drug did not pose a serious cancer threat to humans. But the House never acted on the legislation (S 963), which also would have increased the independence of the Food and Drug Administration (FDA).

Background

The DES controversy had been simmering for several years. The synthetic female hormone was used as a growth stimulant in animal feed and in a "morning-after" contraceptive pill.

DES was first implicated as a cancer-causing drug in 1971 when evidence linked a rare form of vaginal cancer in young women to a drug containing DES that had been taken by their mothers during pregnancy. The drug also had been linked to sexual abnormalities, such as breast development, in sons of women who had taken DES.

The FDA issued a ban on DES in animal feed in 1972, but the order was overturned in 1974 by a federal court on grounds that the agency had not given manufacturers of the drug a full hearing.

After the Senate acted, the FDA again proposed to ban DES in animal feed in early 1976. But the drug still remained in use as an animal feed component in late 1976 because the manufacturers had requested a hearing. The FDA granted the hearing request in December 1976.

Senate Action

As reported (S Rept 94-264) July 3 by the Labor and Public Welfare Committee, S 963 would have banned the sale of the drug for feed for animals eaten by humans. The committee said it was approving the ban because the FDA had not moved against the drug at that time and DES traces showed up in the livers of cattle and sheep after slaughter.

The measure also established guidelines for the labeling and packaging of DES drugs, including warnings that the morning-after pill should be used only in emergency cases, such as rape or incest.

The second title of the committee bill, which attracted much less attention, established the FDA as a legal entity within the Department of Health, Education and Welfare (HEW). Provisions also gave the FDA commissioner sole responsibility for the administration of laws under his jurisdiction.

The committee argued that the agency's actions were so important to consumers that it should be made more accountable to Congress and the public and should be shielded from political interference by high-ranking HEW officials.

The Senate passed the bill Sept. 9 after agreeing to a substitute that would have suspended the use of DES in livestock feed until HEW determined it was a safe drug.

Farm-state senators, led by Carl T. Curtis (R Neb.), objected strongly to the ban proposed in the committee bill. They argued that Congress was poorly equipped to start passing judgment on individual drugs and contended that use of DES kept beef prices down. Supporters of the measure argued that eliminating the health hazard was worth any additional cost.

House Decision

Paul G. Rogers (D Fla.), chairman of the House Interstate and Foreign Commerce Subcommittee on Health and the Environment, decided that he did not want to act on legislation dealing with a single drug and only a few aspects of the FDA's authority. Instead, the subcommittee began to consider a broader revision of FDA's powers.

Health Maintenance Organizations

In an effort to make an alternative type of medical care easier to sell to the public, the House Nov. 7 passed legislation (HR 9019) easing requirements imposed under a 1973 law on health maintenance organizations (HMOs).

HMOs provided a range of health services for a set periodic fee.

The 1973 law was designed to help HMOs get a better foothold in the medical care market, long dominated by more traditional kinds of medical practice. But HMOs found that many of the act's ambitious requirements made their plans too expensive to sell when their cost was compared to regular health insurance premiums. To meet the requirements for federal aid, HMOs had to provide a comprehensive package of benefits, open their enrollment to the sickest of patients and charge uniform fees regardless of a family's health experience.

The House voted to repeal or delay the effective date of many of the requirements and to trim the list of required services. The Senate did not act in 1975, but a compromise version of the bill won final approval in 1976. *(p. 48-A)*

The amendments had the support of a coalition of private groups led by the Group Health Association of America. The coalition included insurance associations and HMO groups. Organized labor and the administration also supported a relaxation of some of the 1973 act's requirements.

The only protest came from the American Medical Association (AMA), which originally fought federal aid for HMOs. The AMA argued that the amendments would allow HMOs to collect federal funds without requiring them to do anything special to improve health care.

House Action

The House Interstate and Foreign Commerce Committee reported (H Rept 94-518) the bill on Sept. 26.

The committee agreed with findings that many fledgling HMOs were reluctant to apply for federal aid because of the somewhat utopian requirements of the 1973 act. But it also blamed the Department of Health, Education and Welfare (HEW) for slow implementation of the act.

The House passed the measure Nov. 7 over the objections of some the AMA's congressional allies.

Biomedical Research

The House and Senate in 1975 passed different versions of a catch-all bill (HR 7988) to extend funding authority for a number of health research programs that expired June 30, 1975. Final action on the bill came in 1976. *(p. 51-A)*

Major provisions of the bills extended research programs dealing with heart, lung and blood diseases and genetic diseases such as sickle cell anemia. The legislation also contained provisions continuing a biomedical research training program revised in 1974 and a loan program for students in the health professions, which was also renewed in 1974.

The research programs had bipartisan support.

House Action

The House Interstate and Foreign Commerce Committee reported (H Rept 94-498) its version of the bill Sept. 22 and the bill won routine approval on the floor Oct. 20.

As passed by the House, the bill authorized $715-million in fiscal 1976-77 to combat heart, lung and blood diseases. Congress had approved a major expansion of this program in 1972.

Rather than extend separate research programs for two genetic diseases, the House decided to create a new general program for research on diseases caused by hereditary factors. Congress had created categorical programs in 1972 to conduct research on sickle cell anemia, which caused genetic disorders in blacks, and Cooley's anemia, which primarily affected children of Italian and Greek descent.

The bill did not include any specific funding for the research program, but provided $45-million for testing and counseling programs for parents who suspected that they might carry a genetic disease. The administration called the new program unnecessary.

A third section of the House bill extended the 1974 research training program for young doctors and scientists.

Senate Action

The Senate, passing the bill (S Rept 94-509) Dec. 11, added several provisions to the House version.

It approved a $375-million authorization in fiscal 1976-78 to fight genetic diseases, and added a separate program to combat sickle cell anemia. The Senate version also included $60-million in fiscal 1976 for loans to students in the health professions because of a delay in action on a larger health manpower bill. *(Story below)*

Health Manpower

Congress postponed final decisions on key health manpower issues until 1976 as debate continued over controversial proposals conditioning federal aid to medical schools on efforts to ease doctor shortages in rural and inner-city areas.

Both the House and Senate had passed bills aimed at solving doctor maldistribution problems in 1974, but the bills died in conference at the end of the session. *(Background, p. 21-A)*

In 1975, the House repassed legislation (HR 5546) similar to its 1974 bill. The key feature of the measure required all medical students to repay some federal aid if they did not practice for a while after graduation in doctor-shortage areas.

In the Senate, health manpower proposals were still pending before the Labor and Public Welfare Committee at the end of the year. But a major administration policy shift cleared the way for senators to begin negotiations over a compromise acceptable to the President.

Controversy

As reported (H Rept 94-266) June 7 by the Interstate and Foreign Commerce Committee, HR 5546 contained two sections strongly opposed by medical schools, the American Medical Association (AMA) and the administration.

The first required all medical students to practice in a medically underserved area after graduation or repay basic per-student ("capitation") support paid by the federal government on their behalf to medical schools. Four years of service in a doctor-shortage area would cancel out the entire debt.

The second section limited the number of postgraduate residency training positions that would be available to young doctors beginning in 1978. The provision was an effort to control the influx of foreign doctors into the United States. Other provisions called for new regulations designed to get more residency training positions in primary care fields like internal medicine.

The Department of Health, Education and Welfare (HEW) initially opposed using the capitation lever to get doctors into underserved areas. It had proposed to cut aid to medical schools while expanding student assistance programs encouraging practice in doctor-shortage areas.

The AMA and medical schools attacked the repayment provision from another angle, arguing that it would discriminate against the health professions. They also argued that the repayment requirement would primarily hurt low-income students.

The administration, AMA and medical schools all agreed that the residency training section was too extreme and unwarranted, given voluntary efforts to increase the number of primary-care doctors.

But sponsors of the bill argued that medical schools and doctors should be required to take more effective steps to ease physician maldistribution in return for hefty federal support for medical education. "There is no other educational support by the federal government comparable to this given medical students," said Paul G. Rogers (D Fla.), pointing out that federal funds made up nearly half of medical schools' support.

House Floor Fight

The House passed the bill July 11 after a floor fight over the two controversial provisions. David E. Satterfield III (D Va.) was unsuccessful in his efforts to kill the repayment provision, but the residency training section was knocked out of the measure by a 207-146 vote.

Vigorous lobbying preceded the voting. The AMA, medical schools, students and their families mounted a heavy mail campaign against the capitation repayment requirement in particular.

On the floor, Satterfield and Tim Lee Carter (R Ky.) argued that the federal government could not tell doctors where to practice. "This will not work in America," Carter argued. "We cannot force students who really do not want to go to a certain area to go to the area, or we should not do it."

Rogers insisted that the bill would not force anyone to do anything. But if medical students were not going to meet national needs, he maintained, they should repay some of their federal support. The House sided with Rogers, voting 209-153 to keep the proposal.

As passed by the House, the bill authorized nearly $1.8-billion in fiscal 1976-78 to continue a host of health training programs. The measure also provided for an expansion of funding for National Health Service Corps scholarships, which required service in a doctor shortage area in exchange for support.

Administration Shift

In September, the administration agreed that the stick might prove more effective than the carrot in getting medical schools to address doctor maldistribution problems. HEW officials announced that the White House was willing to support proposals that would cut off capitation support to medical schools that did not try to solve these problems. President Ford personally approved the major policy shift.

The new administration proposal built on the 1974 Senate version of the health manpower bill. It proposed to deny capitation funds to schools that did not set aside an increasing percentage of their first-year slots for students accepting scholarships requiring service later in a doctor-shortage area. It also required schools to reserve residency positions in their affiliated hospitals for training in primary care fields.

Edward M. Kennedy (D Mass.), chairman of the Senate Labor and Public Welfare Subcommittee on Health, praised the administration's shift. The subcommittee began negotiations with HEW which led to final action on the health manpower bill in 1976. *(p. 41-A)*

Medical Peer Review

Congress agreed in 1975 to delay the operational date of a medical peer review program designed to save federal health dollars, but it ignored continued calls for repeal or extensive revision of the program.

Under a 1972 law, local physician groups were given until Jan. 1, 1976, to set up professional standards review organizations (PSROs) to police the quality and necessity of care given Medicare and Medicaid patients. The PSRO concept had been strongly opposed by some organized medical groups who charged that it would lead to the practice of "cookbook medicine," but the controversy had died down somewhat by 1975. *(Background, p. 23-A)*

An amendment included in a Medicare bill (HR 10284—PL 94-182) delayed the 1976 deadline until Jan. 1, 1978. The original law had given the Department of Health, Education and Welfare (HEW) the power to designate a group not controlled by doctors as the PSRO for a certain area if a physician group did not act by 1976. The two-year delay, however, did not apply in PSRO areas where the largest professional medical association had voted formally to oppose the program or had rejected a proposed PSRO.

Medical Malpractice Insurance

A Senate committee briefly held hearings in 1975 on proposals that would have established federal programs to help doctors cope with the rising cost and increasing unavailability of medical malpractice insurance. But after insurers, doctors and lawyers all agreed that the states should handle the problem, the committee dropped any ideas for federal action.

Background

Many doctors claimed that they could no longer afford the cost of malpractice insurance, which had reached $15,000 to $20,000 a year for physicians in high-risk specialties. And, claiming financial losses, insurers told doctors in many states that they planned to stop writing malpractice insurance policies.

The situation was serious because few doctors wanted to continue to treat patients without malpractice coverage.

Experts traced the malpractice problem to a number of intertwined causes. Insurance companies said they were getting out of the malpractice business because it was unpredictable and unprofitable, pointing to increases in the number of claims filed and the size of claims paid. Rising consumer awareness, the growing complexity of medicine, more impersonal doctor-patient relations and other reasons were cited to explain the growing number of claims.

Doctors liked to blame lawyers for the large sums sought in malpractice suits, but lawyers countered that it was their job to help patients claiming injury get the best deal possible.

All the developments meant higher malpractice insurance premiums. Doctors and hospitals freely conceded that the costs were passed on to patients. The medical profession also conceded that fear of malpractice suits increased the practice of "defensive" medicine—a tendency to order tests or X-rays that were not really necessary, but could provide protection in a malpractice suit. This practice also drove up health spending.

Proposed Solutions

The Senate Labor and Public Welfare Committee briefly considered ways to deal with the problem on a national basis. The proposed bills would have set up a national no-fault malpractice insurance program, set federal guidelines for state arbitration programs or allowed the federal government to reinsure private malpractice policies. Spokesmen for doctors, trial lawyers, hospitals and the Ford administration opposed the bills during April hearings.

Some 30 states adopted legislation during the year in order to make sure that malpractice insurance would remain available, but the laws had little effect on rising costs. Twenty-two of the states authorized pooling arrangements that allowed insurers to share the risk of providing malpractice coverage.

Medical Devices

Moving to expand the federal government's regulatory power in a long-neglected area, the Senate April 17 approved legislation (S 510) giving the Food and Drug Administration (FDA) authority to ensure the safety and effectiveness of medical devices ranging from heart pacemakers to intrauterine birth control devices (IUDs). The bill won final approval in 1976. *(p. 46-A)*

It drew widespread support because of the FDA's inability to assure patients that the life-sustaining devices of the 1970s were safe. Under existing law—unchanged since passage of the 1938 Food, Drug and Cosmetic Act—the FDA had clear-cut authority to regulate devices only if they were unsanitary or mislabeled. The administration supported expanding the FDA's powers in the device field.

Background

Congress passed the 1938 act to get clearly fraudulent devices off the market. Such devices included machines that would diagnose either "arthritis" or "meningitis" when patients stood on them.

But by the early 1960s, it was clear that the 1938 act did not give the FDA the powers it needed to cope with the more subtle dangers that might be posed by highly sophisticated new devices. The FDA found it had to develop extensive evidence that would hold up over long periods of court action to get the new dangerous devices off the market.

While court decisions in 1968 and 1969 broadened the FDA's authority to regulate some devices with drug-like qualities, the agency continued to indicate that it would need new legislative authority to expand regulation substantially. While waiting for such legislation, the FDA began the process of classifying devices according to their potential for harm on the recommendation of an ad hoc study group.

The study group, set up after President Nixon indicated his interest in new device legislation in 1969, surveyed medical literature from 1963 to 1969 to determine how much damage faulty or ineffective devices caused. It found

A 40-Year-Old Decision Lingers

The congressional decision to provide separate definitions of a "drug" and a "device" in the landmark 1938 Food, Drug and Cosmetic Act had been partially responsible for the FDA's limited authority to regulate medical devices. From an examination of how Congress arrived at that decision, however, it is clear that the legislators of the 1930s did not intend this result.

Sen. Royal S. Copeland (D N.Y., 1923-38), chief sponsor of legislation considered in 1935 that was similar to the bill enacted in 1938, adamantly supported inclusion of devices under the definition of drugs. But during floor debate on the bill, Sen. Joel Bennett (Champ) Clark (D Mo., 1933-45) objected to this provision, claiming it would make a bathroom scale a drug.

Support developed for Clark's position and those opposing Copeland's definition had a semantic field day. They finally settled on crutches as the most absurd example of what the bill would define as a drug.

Copeland then agreed to offer an amendment to the bill providing a separate definition of a medical device. He wanted to give the federal government the means to regulate quack devices, with the understanding that the drug definition would be read broadly enough to cover devices used to treat or cure disease. Later versions of the bill retained the dual definitions.

The impact of this decision was not apparent immediately, but it ultimately affected the FDA's authority under the 1938 act. The act authorized the FDA to require pre-market testing of "new drugs" to ensure safety, but gave the agency no such authority for new medical devices. Subsequent amendments to the drug provisions of the act also did not affect devices because they were defined separately.

accounts of 10,000 injuries resulting in 731 deaths; most of the deaths were attributed to heart valves.

Earlier Congressional Action

Device legislation was introduced in the early 1960s, but languished for a decade. Congressional interest heightened after a House Government Operations Subcommittee held hearings in 1973 on the dangers of IUDs.

The Senate had passed legislation similar to S 510 in 1974, but it died in a House subcommittee.

Senate Action

The Senate passed the bill April 17 after making one change in the bill as reported (S Rept 94-33) by the Labor and Public Welfare Committee. The amendment made all implanted devices, such as IUDs, heart valves and pacemakers, subject automatically to pre-market review by the FDA.

Basic provisions of S 510 required the FDA to classify devices into three categories: 1) those needing no regulation, 2) those that should meet standards set by outside groups or federal agencies, and 3) those subject to approval by panels of scientific experts before they could go on the market.

In general, the bill required pre-market approval for life-sustaining as well as implanted devices.

Other provisions expanded HEW's authority to regulate device advertising, to inspect device testing records and to ban devices if necessary.

Drug Abuse Prevention

The House and Senate passed different versions of legislation (HR 8150, S 2017) extending federal drug abuse prevention and treatment programs, but the legislation did not clear until 1976. *(p. 48-A)*

Debate over the legislation focused on whether to continue the life of a special White House office charged with coordinating all federal drug abuse programs. The Special Action Office for Drug Abuse Prevention was created by Congress in 1972 in response to a request by President Nixon.

Sponsors of the legislation decided that some sort of White House office should continue to coordinate federal drug abuse policy because drug addiction remained a serious problem. The administration wanted to transfer all of the special office's responsibilities to the National Institute on Drug Abuse within the Department of Health, Education and Welfare (HEW).

The House and Senate, in effect, only set future policy by extending the life of the White House office because Congress did not clear the bill before the 1972 legislation expired. The special White House office went out of existence on schedule on June 30.

While the final version of the bill created a permanent White House office, the legislation passed in 1975 provided only for temporary extensions. This approach was designed to give Congress time to evaluate the recommendations of a White House Domestic Council task force. In October, the task force recommended use of a Cabinet-level committee to coordinate drug abuse programs, aided by a small staff at the Office of Management and Budget.

Need

Those supporting an extension of the White House office argued that drug abuse problems still required high-level attention that the HEW institute could not provide.

Heroin addiction was moving into rural areas, "poly-drug" abuse (hazardous combined use of several drugs) was on the rise and drug-related deaths were mounting, the Senate Labor and Public Welfare Committee said when it reported (S Rept 94-218) its version of the bill June 20.

While the White House office did not seem to have made much of a dent in drug abuse problems, the committee argued that it had helped to assure that drug enforcement efforts did not completely overshadow prevention and treatment.

"The fact that in the short space of three years the accumulated problems of more than a century have not been definitely dealt with casts no discredit on anyone," the committee said. "It is merely a reflection of the serious difficulty of coming to grips with a major social ill."

The committee maintained that the HEW institute would be in a poor position to take over the White House office's functions. A 1974 reorganization left the institute at the "fourth echelon" of the HEW bureaucracy, the committee argued.

Senate Action

The bill reported by the Labor and Public Welfare Committee would have extended the White House office until the President proposed a reorganization plan, subject to congressional veto.

On the floor June 26, sponsors agreed to set aside this version and accepted a compromise (S 2017) that extended the office for only six months.

Charles H. Percy (Ill.), the ranking Republican on the Government Operations Committee, insisted on the modification.

Percy favored giving the White House office's responsibilities to the HEW institute, arguing that Congress could not continue to ask the President to run every program. But he agreed to the six-month extension so that the Domestic Council could finish its report.

As passed, the Senate bill authorized $205-million in each of fiscal 1976-78 to continue basic drug abuse prevention programs run by the HEW institute.

House Action

The House Interstate and Foreign Commerce Committee approved (H Rept 94-375) a one-year extension of the White House office on July 18. It provided specific funding of $10-million for the office.

An effort to kill the extension failed on the floor Sept. 11 when the House passed the bill.

Tim Lee Carter (R Ky.) pointed out that the White House office already had gone out of business, seeing no point in "resurrecting a corpse."

Paul G. Rogers (D Fla.), chief sponsor of the bill, argued that the HEW institute was too far down in the federal hierarchy to coordinate drug abuse policy. He doubted whether the institute's director "could even get his telephone calls returned."

Disease Control, Health Education

The Senate July 30 passed a bill (S 1466) providing a major expansion of public and private efforts to encourage consumers to adopt healthier life styles. Other provisions of the bill extended programs designed to control infectious diseases and venereal disease. Final action on the measure came in 1976. *(p. 50-A)*

The bill authorized $105-million in fiscal 1976-78 to control diseases such as tuberculosis, measles and polio and $145-million over the same period to control venereal disease. It made no major changes in the programs, which had expired June 30.

A second section of the bill established a high-level office in the Department of Health, Education and Welfare (HEW) to promote health education and a private center receiving some federal funds with the same mission.

The Labor and Public Welfare Committee, which reported (S Rept 94-330) the bill July 24, argued that it would take changes in personal habits to bring about notable improvement in illness, disability and premature death rates.

"We eat the wrong foods, drive too fast and drink too much," the committee said. "Ours is a generation of excess."

Noting that only 4 per cent of all health spending in the United States was devoted to preventive medicine and health education for consumers, the committee argued that the federal government should play a larger educational role.

Nursing Homes

A drive to provide better care for more than one million elderly persons living in nursing homes got under way in 1975, but no major legislation addressed to nursing home problems made it through the 94th Congress.

The drive to improve nursing home care was spearheaded by Frank E. Moss (D Utah), chairman of the Senate Special Committee on Aging's Subcommittee on Long-Term Care. Drawing on more than five years of hearings, the subcommittee began issuing a monthly series of reports in November 1974 detailing the problems found in nursing homes and recommending corrective steps.

The Committee on Aging, however, had no legislative authority. The key committees that would write nursing home legislation—Senate Finance and House Ways and Means—were tied up with other matters during the year.

Major Problems

Nursing home critics agreed that there had been major improvements in nursing homes since the federal government began regulating them under the Medicare and Medicaid programs enacted in 1965. They also stressed that there were many fine nursing homes in the United States, particularly church-affiliated homes run on a nonprofit basis.

But despite this progress, the Moss subcommittee concluded in a series of 1975 reports that serious and life-threatening violations of state or federal standards could be found in more than 50 per cent of U.S. nursing homes. The major abuses cited by the subcommittee included deliberate physical injury of patients, unsanitary or unsafe conditions, improper use of drugs, and profiteering and cheating by nursing home operators—caused in part by the for-profit nature of most of the nursing home industry. The subcommittee said that staff shortages and heavy reliance on untrained personnel, as well as negative attitudes toward the elderly infirm, were major factors contributing to these problems.

Proposals

Most of the proposals to reform nursing home operations addressed the three most glaring problems that had developed in federal long-term care programs:

● Extremely limited nursing home coverage under Medicare.

● Extremely limited coverage under both Medicare and Medicaid for alternatives to nursing home care.

● Limited federal authority to enforce nursing home standards under both Medicare and Medicaid even though public funds paid more than half of the nation's total nursing home bill.

The Moss subcommittee proposed expansion of the types of care covered under Medicare, federal financing of alternative types of care and supplementary federal enforcement of standards as basic steps needed to meet these problems.

School Lunch Extension

Congress Oct. 7 enacted into law, over a veto, an extension of the school lunch and other child nutrition programs (HR 4222—PL 94-105) that survived a formidable obstacle course. During the seven months of congressional consideration, the bill went through two rounds of debate on the House floor, two separate conferences and a veto by President Ford.

The bill extended all the non-school food programs, including a supplemental feeding program for mothers and their young children, and made the school breakfast program permanent. It also expanded the school lunch and breakfast programs to include children's residential institutions, increased the income eligibility level for reduced-price lunches and made children of unemployed parents eligible for free and reduced-price lunches. The bill required an estimated $2.7-billion in fiscal 1976 outlays.

Background

In the fiscal 1976 budget, the Ford administration proposed to replace categorical child nutrition programs with block grant assistance to the states. The categorical programs included the school lunch, school breakfast and summer feeding programs and a supplemental food program for women, infants and children. Funding authority for all but the school lunch program, a permanent activity, expired June 30, 1975.

The administration also proposed to end the general federal subsidy under the school lunch program to 15 million children not from needy families. The subsidy amounted to about 22 cents per meal, according to an Agriculture Department assistant secretary.

He argued before a House subcommittee March 4 that the change would target federal assistance on the most needy children, pointing out that states would be free to subsidize meals for middle-income children.

A third administration proposal would have narrowed eligibility for free and reduced-price lunches. The proposal would have limited free meals to children from families with annual income of $4,510 or less and reduced-price lunches to those from families with income up to $5,638.

The Agriculture Department had estimated that its proposals would reduce the number of children participating in the school lunch program to 19 million from 25.2 million if the states did not replace the subsidies for middle-income children. The drop was expected because regular prices for school lunches would have to increase by $1.10 a week to cover the loss of federal subsidies.

The administration put the fiscal 1976 cost of the block grant program at $1.9-billion, compared to estimated spending of $2.3-billion under the categorical programs.

House Action

The Education and Labor Committee reported HR 4222 (H Rept 94-68) March 17 after agreeing to add a provision requiring supplemental federal subsidies to cover the difference between a maximum 25-cent lunch price and the price in effect on Jan. 1, 1975. The full committee added the provision to a version of the bill approved March 5 by the Elementary, Secondary and Vocational Education Subcommittee recommending less controversial changes in child nutrition programs.

The committee estimated that the changes contained in its bill would add $1.4-billion to the projected $2.3-billion cost of continuing child nutrition programs without revisions in fiscal 1976. It estimated that the additional subsidies necessary to roll back school lunch prices to 25 cents for all children would amount to $655-million annually. It justified the decrease in price on economic grounds, arguing that the expected increase in participation would create 50,-000 new jobs and actually decrease the cost of preparing a meal because of the economies of scale.

The committee met again March 24 before floor debate began to consider criticisms that the bill would allow schools claiming exorbitantly high child lunch costs to collect unlimited new subsidies. In response, it prepared a floor amendment to allow schools to claim costs no higher than the escalation in the index measuring the cost of food eaten away from home.

To reward schools that had kept prices close to the 25-cent ceiling, the committee also approved an amendment to increase the minimum additional subsidy per meal to 15 cents from 10 cents. The change would provide a five-cent bonus, for instance, to schools that had held prices to 35 cents a meal, or 10 cents below the national average.

After approving a scaled-down proposal to provide new federal subsidies for the school lunch program, the House April 28 passed HR 4222 by a 335-59 vote.

Floor action on the bill had been suspended March 25 after the House easily defeated efforts by Democrats on the Education and Labor Committee to set a maximum price of 35 cents for a school lunch in lieu of the 25-cent maximum approved by the committee. The federal government would have had to subsidize the difference between the actual price of a school lunch on Jan. 1, 1975, and the 35-cent price.

Recognizing that the House would turn down any extensive subsidy program, a majority of Democrats on the committee decided after the March 25 vote to back a compromise proposal to provide a supplemental federal payment of five cents per lunch in fiscal 1976 only. The five-cent supplemental subsidy proposal was approved 213-176.

The compromise did not win the support of key Republicans on the committee, however, including Albert H. Quie (Minn.), ranking minority member. Republicans complained that the proposal would provide unnecessary subsidies for children from middle-income families who could afford the actual price of a school lunch.

The scaled-down subsidy program would cost an estimated $125-million, bringing the total cost of the legislation to slightly more than $3-billion in fiscal 1976.

Floor debate in both March and April focused on the need to provide any new subsidies for middle-income children participating in the school lunch program.

Senate Action

The Senate Agriculture and Forestry Committee June 26 reported by voice vote an amended version of HR 4222 (S Rept 94-259).

The Senate committee rejected two key provisions of the House-passed bill for budgetary reasons:

● A controversial five-cent subsidy for fiscal 1976 for school lunches served to children who did not qualify for free or reduced-price meals.

● Expansion of eligibility for reduced-price lunches, those costing a maximum of 20 cents, to include children from families with income up to 100 per cent above the income poverty guideline.

While the Senate committee sided with the House in rejecting an administration-backed plan to consolidate categorical child nutrition programs into a block grant system, the cost of the Senate program in fiscal 1976 would be lower, at $2.8-billion, than that of the House. The length of program extensions also differed from the House version.

After rejecting an amendment to expand eligibility for reduced-price lunches, the Senate July 10 passed HR 4222 by a vote of 81-8 in essentially the same form as reported. That version would have cost almost $2.8-billion in fiscal 1976. Floor amendments added an estimated $1.5-million, leaving the Senate bill still below the $3.1-billion version approved by the House.

The amendment offered by George McGovern (D S.D.) to expand eligibility for reduced-price lunches was defeated primarily on budgetary grounds. Budget Committee Chairman Edmund S. Muskie (D Maine) said it would add $150-million or more to a bill that already was $300-million over the fiscal 1976 budget targets adopted by Congress earlier in the year.

Two Conferences

The first conference report on HR 4222, filed July 30 (H Rept 94-427, S Rept 94-347), included modified versions of two expensive provisions voted by the House and knocked out of the bill by the Senate committee.

● Conferees reduced to three cents from five cents the House-approved additional subsidy to states for each lunch served in fiscal 1976 that was not a free or reduced-price meal. (In the only change between the first and second conference reports, this provision was deleted from the final version of the bill.)

● They cut the increased income eligibility level for reduced-price lunches to 95 per cent above the income poverty guideline, 5 per cent less than the House-approved figure.

The Senate, by a 76-0 vote, recommitted the bill to conference Sept. 5 with the understanding that Senate conferees would seek to eliminate both provisions to reduce the cost of the bill.

The Senate previously had delayed action on the conference report Aug. 1 when Muskie called for defeat of the conference version of HR 4222 because it would add $362-million in budget outlays over fiscal 1976 targets.

Muskie's success in defeating the conference report on a military procurement bill (HR 6674), also for budgetary reasons, was a factor in Senate conferees being willing to go back to conference to reduce the cost of the bill.

Conferees filed their second report on HR 4222 in the House Sept. 15 (H Rept 94-474) and in the Senate Sept. 17 (S Rept 94-379), after deleting the three-cent subsidy provision.

Conferees kept the increased eligibility level for reduced-price lunches of 95 per cent above the income poverty guidelines that had been provided in the first conference report.

Bill Cleared

The House Sept. 18 adopted the second conference report by a 380-7 vote with little debate.

The Senate approved the conference report Sept. 19 by voice vote, clearing the bill for the President.

Sen. Henry Bellmon (R Okla.), ranking minority member of the Senate Budget Committee, said that the second conference resulted in a cost reduction of $75-million. This left outlays in the bill $287-million above the budget target. The bill as originally passed by the Senate July 10 would have exceeded outlay targets by $291-million.

Veto, Override

Ford vetoed HR 4222 Oct. 3, charging it exceeded his budget request by $1.2-billion and extended federal subsidies to non-needy children through the increased eligibility level for reduced-price lunches.

"I cannot accept such fiscal irresponsibility," Ford wrote in his veto message, "when we face the real danger that the budget deficit could reach $70-billion instead of the already high limit of $60-billion I set earlier this year."

He gave Congress two alternatives: to extend current categorical programs, or enact the block grant program of assistance to states which he proposed in his fiscal 1976 budget.

Rejecting those alternatives, the House and Senate Oct. 7 overrode the veto. The House vote was 397-18, 120 more than the two-thirds majority required; the Senate overrode the veto by a 17-vote margin in a key vote of 79-13: R 20-13; D 59-0.

Supporters of the override, both Republicans and Democrats, said during floor debate that Ford's claim of a $1.2-billion increase was unfounded, since his budget request was based on the proposed block grant program that was never implemented. At the same time, they said that the bill, as cleared, was only $216-million over the cost of continuing the categorical programs at existing levels. That $216-million would be the only saving if the veto stood, they argued. Other members challenged the President's claim that the bill would increase subsidies to non-needy persons. In the House, only 14 Republicans and 4 Democrats voted to sustain the veto; 123 Republicans and 274 Democrats voted to override.

Major Provisions

As enacted into law over the President's veto, major provisions of HR 4222 (PL 94-105):

● Made the school breakfast program permanent and required that it be made available in all eligible schools where needed.

● Extended the summer food program through Sept. 30, 1977, required that meals be served without cost, and allowed all eligible summer feeding sponsors to enter the program upon request.

● Extended the special supplemental food program for women, infants and children (WIC) through Sept. 30, 1978, and authorized appropriations of $250-million per year for fiscal years 1976-78; required the Agriculture Secretary to use Section 32 funds, derived from U.S. customs receipts, to make up the difference in fiscal years 1976 and 1977 if the entire $250-million was not appropriated and also required that, during this time period, any unspent WIC funds from the prior fiscal year must be carried over until fiscal 1978.

● Revised the year-round phase of the special food service program to establish a child care food program for children in nonresidential child care institutions through Sept. 30, 1978.

● Increased eligibility levels for reduced-price lunches to 95 per cent above the income poverty guidelines, as revised annually by the Secretary of Agriculture, and required schools participating in the school lunch program to offer reduced-price lunches to eligible children. Under income poverty guidelines currently in effect, children from families of four with income up to $9,770 would be eligible for reduced-price lunches.

● Allowed any child whose parent or guardian was unemployed to receive either a free or reduced-price lunch during the period of unemployment if the family income during that period fell within the income eligibility criteria for those types of lunches.

● Expanded eligibility for the school lunch and breakfast programs to include any public or licensed nonprofit private residential child care institution, such as orphanages and homes for the mentally retarded or emotionally disturbed.

● Extended through Sept. 30, 1977, the Agriculture Secretary's authority to purchase agricultural commodities for child nutrition programs and programs for the elderly; required that cereal, shortening and oil products be included among these commodities. States which had phased out their commodity distribution facilities prior to July 1, 1974, could choose to receive cash instead of donated foods.

Summer Feeding Program

The extended controversy over HR 4222 made it necessary for Congress to pass a stop-gap extension of the summer feeding program for children operated by non-residential institutions and summer camps. The program, last extended in 1972, was scheduled to expire June 30, 1975. The extension to Sept. 30, 1975, was cleared April 18 (S 1310—PL 94-20).

The Senate passed S 1310 (S Rept 94-57) by voice vote March 26. The House passed it in different form April 9 by a 396-2 vote. Final action came April 18 when the Senate agreed by voice vote to the House changes.

As enacted, PL 94-20 provided for financing of the program through direct appropriations, for cost adjustments in summer meal reimbursement rates to reflect changes in operating costs since the period May-September 1974. The measure required the Agriculture Secretary to issue regulations for the program within 10 days of enactment. Funding for the program subsequently was provided in the second supplemental appropriations bill for fiscal 1975 when Congress cleared June 11 (HR 5899—PL 94-32).

Medicare Amendments

After throwing out a Senate proposal to allow individuals under age 65 to buy into the Medicare program for the aged, Congress Dec. 19 cleared legislation (HR 10284—PL 94-182) making a number of changes in the Medicare program.

Final action came when the Senate agreed to accept House changes in the heavily amended version of the bill passed by the Senate Dec. 17.

The House refused to accept the Senate provisions that would have allowed individuals aged 60 to 64 to buy into the Medicare program at cost. Most individuals did not qualify for subsidized Medicare coverage until they reached age 65.

But the House agreed to two other key Senate amendments modifying an existing law (PL 92-603) requiring local medical groups to set up professional standards review organizations (PSROs) to monitor the quality of in-patient care received by Medicare and Medicaid patients. These amendments would give physician groups that had not opposed the peer review program an extra two years to set up PSROs and enable doctors in a few states to place control of a PSRO program under a state medical society. *(PSROs, p. 34-A)*

The original House version of the bill would have made only minor changes in the Medicare program.

Legislative Action

House Action. By voice vote, the House Nov. 17 passed HR 10284. The House Ways and Means Committee was considering more fundamental revisions of Medicare and had held hearings on the program in 1975, but decided that Congress should act quickly on the issues covered by HR 10284.

The House passed the bill under the suspension of the rules procedure barring floor amendments, so no changes were made in the measure as reported by the Ways and Means Committee on Nov. 6 (H Rept 94-626).

The House version dealt only with a three-year extension for rural hospitals to comply with a requirement that they provide Medicare patients with registered nurse service, protection for doctors against a reduction in charges they could collect under Medicare as a result of new regulations, and a stipulation that a physician could not receive less for a service in fiscal 1976 than 1975.

Senate Action. The Senate Finance Committee reported HR 10284 (S Rept 94-549) on Dec. 12. The committee modified two of the provisions of the House-passed bill and added several amendments dealing with PSROs, physician charges and rural hospital nursing.

By voice vote, the Senate Dec. 17 passed a version of HR 10284 that would allow several million Americans age 60 to 64 to buy into the federal Medicare program for the aged at cost. This and other amendments added on the floor were adopted by voice vote, without debate, as were the Finance Committee amendments.

Final Action. The House voted 371-16 under suspension of the rules Dec. 19 to amend the broadened Senate version of the original House bill. The amendment retained some of the new Senate provisions, reworked others and killed several altogether.

The more important Senate amendments rejected by the House would have set up the Medicare "buy-in" program and restricted the medical malpractice liability of PSROs.

The Senate-passed amendments accepted by the House changed implementation of the PSRO program and clarified that medical peer review committees did not need to monitor the hospital admission of every Medicare patient. The House also insisted on its original version of provisions included in both the House- and Senate-passed measures.

The Senate cleared the bill by accepting the House amendment by voice vote later on Dec. 19.

Provisions

As signed into law, HR 10284: (PL 94-182):

● Stipulated that federal reimbursements to physicians for care of Medicare patients in fiscal 1976 could not be any lower than comparable reimbursements in fiscal 1975.

● Extended to Jan. 1, 1979, from Jan. 1, 1976, the authority of the Department of Health, Education and Welfare (HEW) to waive a requirement that rural hospitals provide Medicare patients with the services of a registered nurse around the clock.

● Directed HEW to poll doctors in states where the department had established more than one PSRO area as to whether they preferred to establish a PSRO serving the entire state instead of several PSROs within the state; limited the polling requirement to states where HEW had not designated a group to serve as a conditional PSRO in any PSRO area within the state.

● If a majority of doctors responding to the poll in each PSRO area within a state preferred the statewide approach, directed HEW to establish a statewide PSRO area.

● Authorized federal reimbursements for the cost of PSRO activities carried out directly by a PSRO as well as those carried out by established hospital committees selected by a PSRO to carry out the required review.

● Delayed the effective date of HEW's authority to designate a PSRO not controlled by a professional medical group to Jan. 1, 1978, from Jan. 1, 1976; reaffirmed HEW's authority to select a PSRO not controlled by physicians after Jan. 1, 1976, in areas where the largest professional medical group or the state medical society had voted to oppose the program or had rejected a PSRO.

● Clarified provisions of a 1972 law (PL 92-603) so that they would not require medical peer review of the need for the hospital admission of every Medicare and Medicaid patient.

● Corrected a technical error in existing law so that the monthly premium for physician services under Medicare could increase to $7.20 from $6.70 on July 1, 1976.

● Stipulated that states need not comply with an existing law requiring them to deduct, at the option of a welfare recipient, money needed to cover food stamp purchases from welfare checks until Oct. 1, 1976.

1976

Congress approved a batch of health bills in 1976, but with one or two exceptions, they just extended existing programs.

Legislators appeared more cautious about moving to any national health insurance program. To some extent, Congress did not bother considering health insurance proposals in 1976 because it wanted to see whether Jimmy Carter, a health insurance supporter, would be elected as President. But the cost of a national program, coupled with public disenchantment with federal regulatory efforts and criticism of existing federal health care programs, also discouraged congressional action.

Congress did finish work in 1976 on legislation that experts had called for before the country moved to a national health insurance system. The measure revised medical education programs in ways encouraging more young doctors to practice in rural and inner-city areas and in primary care fields. It was the most important health measure cleared during the year.

Other important legislation winning final approval dramatically upgraded the federal government's authority to assure the public that medical devices such as heart pacemakers were safe.

The administration concentrated its efforts during the year on a massive "swine flu" immunization program proposed by President Ford after this type of flu broke out at Ft. Dix, N.J. Scientists feared that the flu might be related to a strain that caused a deadly epidemic in 1918-19.

The Ford administration's two other major proposals in the health area—a health block grant program for the states and changes in Medicare coverage—got a frosty congressional reception.

Congress also was unwilling to live with the President's health budget in general. Twice in 1976, it overrode vetoes of appropriations bills boosting health spending.

Health Manpower

Congress Sept. 30 completed three years of work on a major health bill (HR 5546—PL 94-484) charting a new course for training programs for doctors and other health professionals.

HR 5546 made the first important changes in federal support for medical education since 1971, when worries about a national shortage of doctors prompted Congress to provide basic federal grants to medical schools.

Since then, health manpower experts worried less about the overall physician supply and more about getting enough doctors in the right places and the right medical fields. Data pointed to continuing shortages of doctors in rural areas and urban ghettoes and a need for more physicians providing basic kinds of care. Experts also were concerned by increasing U.S. reliance on often poorly trained graduates of foreign medical schools.

Congress began to grapple with these new problems in 1974 when most basic provisions of the 1971 act expired. Unable to come up with a final bill in 1974, it started work again in 1975 as an administration policy shift opened the way for development of a compromise. *(pp. 21-A, 33-A)*

Sponsors of the bill considered a number of ways to use federal control over medical school funding to correct the doctor distribution problems. Acting in 1975, the House agreed to require all medical students to repay the federal government "capitation" grants paid on their behalf to medical schools if they did not practice for a while after graduation in the doctor shortage areas.

The Senate version, passed in July 1976, built on some Republican recommendations. It cut off capitation support to medical schools that did not reserve an increasing number of student slots and advanced residency training positions for students accepting scholarships requiring service in an underserved area later and for young doctors entering primary care medical fields.

House-Senate conferees found the student "payback" and scholarship "quota" proposals too drastic. They simply agreed to increase funding for the scholarships requiring service later, believing that more students would seek scholarships voluntarily if the program were expanded.

This key decision was a victory for medical schools and organized medicine after a long lobbying campaign. The American Medical Association, for one, expressed its pleasure with the outcome by telling conferees that they "did a difficult job very well."

Conferees did retain a modified version of the residency training "quota" for primary care, but eliminated all vestiges of a stiffer Senate proposal for national allocation of residencies. Other key provisions imposed curbs on the flow of often poorly trained foreign doctors into the country.

While imposing some new requirements, the bill also guaranteed continuation of basic federal support for medical, dental and other health professions schools through fiscal 1980. For students, the bill offered a new federally guaranteed loan program as well as the big expansion in scholarships requiring practice in doctor shortage areas as a member of the National Health Service Corps. For fiscal 1978-80, the bill authorized a total of $2.3-billion.

President Ford decided to sign the bill, but expressed reservations about its cost and some of its provisions.

Senate Action

After rejecting a proposed allocation scheme for the advanced training of doctors in medical specialties, the Senate passed its version of the bill on July 1. It carried a total price tag of $2.8-billion in fiscal 1977-80.

As reported (S Rept 94-886) May 14 by the Labor and Public Welfare Committee, the bill had contained a controversial proposal that would have allowed the federal government to decide how many medical school graduates could enter advanced residency training programs in each medical specialty. The proposal was designed to get more doctors into primary care.

Faced with a threatened presidential veto over the issue, the Senate dropped the committee plan. Instead, it approved a substitute by J. Glenn Beall Jr. (R Md.) requiring a national council to set numerical goals for residency positions by specialty. The proposal allowed the health care profession to meet the goals on a voluntary basis without direct federal regulation. Edward M. Kennedy (D Mass.), chief backer of the strong allocation proposal, did not have the votes to fight the substitute on the floor.

The Senate bill also contained other provisions, not included in the House version, that were designed to make more young doctors enter primary care fields. They required the reservation of an increasing number of residency training positions for those going into primary care.

Conference Action

House-Senate conferees issued a report (H Rept 94-1612) on Sept. 17.

Controversy during the conference meetings quickly focused on the Senate provisions requiring medical schools to reserve increasing percentages of their student slots and residency training positions for students holding service scholarships and for doctors in primary care fields.

In return for dropping the scholarship quota requirement, House conferees accepted a modified version of the Senate quota requirement for primary care residencies. House conferees also went along with the Senate provisions limiting entry of foreign medical graduates into the United States and setting up the new guaranteed student loan program. The provision of the final bill requiring medical schools to accept U.S. students transferring from foreign schools was suggested by House conferees, but was not included formally in either version of the bill.

Conferees killed the substitute approved on the Senate floor that would have set up the national council to set goals for the number of new doctors entering each medical specialty.

Provisions

As signed into law, HR 5546:

Construction of Teaching Facilities

● Extended the Department of Health, Education and Welfare's (HEW) authority to make grants for the construction of teaching facilities for health professionals through fiscal 1980; authorized special grants for the construction of facilities to train students in the primary care of ambulatory patients.

● Extended HEW's authority to provide loan guarantees and interest subsidies for the construction of health training facilities through fiscal 1980.

Student Assistance

● Created a new program authorizing HEW to insure private loans to students in the health professions; limited the amount of insured loans to $500-million in fiscal 1978, $510-million in fiscal 1979 and $520-million in fiscal 1980.

● Limited the annual amount of an individual insured loan to $10,000 for most students and $7,500 for pharmacy students; required students to finish repaying the loan by 15 years after they completed their residency training; limited maximum interest on such loans to 10 per cent a year.

● Limited students eligible for insured loans to those attending schools in compliance with requirements for receipt of basic federal aid.

● Barred recipients of insured loans from using bankruptcy proceedings to escape repayment for five years after repayment was required to begin.

● Allowed HEW to assume insured loan repayment of $10,000 for each year a student agreed to practice in a medically underserved area as a member of the National Health Service Corps or in private practice; if a student defaulted on the service requirement, made him liable for three times the amount repaid by the government.

● Extended the direct federal loan program for students in health professions through fiscal 1980; increased the maximum annual amount of a federal loan to the cost of tuition plus $2,500 from an existing total limit of $3,500; increased the interest on such loans to 7 per cent from 3 per cent; barred direct federal loans to medical students graduating after June 30, 1979, unless they were exceptionally needy.

● Expanded the scholarship program for health professions students who agreed in return to practice in a medically underserved area after graduation; discontinued a general scholarship program.

● Gave priority, beginning in the 1978-79 school year, to scholarship applications from students who had already received scholarships and then to first-year students.

● Required students receiving these scholarships to serve in the National Health Service Corps in a health manpower shortage area after graduation for a period of two years or, if greater, one year for each year they received scholarship support; allowed medical, osteopathic and dental students to complete up to three years of advanced training before beginning service.

● Limited annual scholarship support to the cost of tuition and other reasonable education expenses plus a stipend of $4,800.

● As an alternative, allowed a student receiving a scholarship to fulfill his service requirement by private practice in a medically underserved area for the same required period of time; allowed HEW to release students showing promise in medical research fields from the service requirement.

● Required students defaulting on their service requirement to repay the federal government three times the amount of their scholarship support plus interest.

● Authorized HEW to make annual grants of $12,500 for two years to health professionals who completed their required service in the National Health Service Corps and agreed to continue in private practice in a medically underserved area.

● Stipulated that appropriations for National Health Service Corps scholarships must equal at least half of the appropriations for all health manpower programs if appropriations for basic per-student ("capitation") grants to medical and dental schools were at least 75 per cent of their authorized amounts; reserved 90 per cent of available scholarship funding for medical, osteopathic and dental students.

● Created a new scholarship program for exceptionally needy first-year students at health professions schools; gave priority for scholarships to medical, osteopathic and dental students; limited the amount of the scholarship to the cost of tuition and other necessary educational expenses plus an annual stipend of $4,800.

● Authorized at least 10 scholarships a year (known as Lister Hill scholarships) to medical students who agreed to enter family medicine practice in a medically underserved area after graduation.

National Health Service Corps

● Authorized HEW to pay monthly bonuses of up to $1,000 for a period of three years to doctors and dentists practicing in medically underserved areas as members of the National Health Service Corps.

● Stipulated that HEW could assign corps members to serve rural or inner-city areas, particular population groups or particular medical facilities experiencing health manpower shortages.

● Allowed HEW to waive requirements that communities contribute to the cost of paying salaries for corps personnel and other costs; authorized HEW to make a loan of up to $50,000 to a community to help it set up a practice for a corps member.

Aid to Schools

● Authorized annual "capitation" grants to health professions schools of 1) $2,000 in fiscal 1978 for each medical, osteopathic or dental student, $2,050 in fiscal 1979 and $2,100 in fiscal 1980; 2) $1,400 in each of fiscal 1978-80 for each student of public health; 3) $1,450 in each of fiscal 1978-80 for each student of veterinary medicine; 4) $765 in each of fiscal 1978-80 for each student of optometry; 5) $695 in each of fiscal 1978-80 for each student of pharmacy, and 6) $965 in each of fiscal 1978-80 for each student of podiatry.

● In general, barred grants to schools with decreased enrollments of first-year students.

● If, on July 15, 1977, all U.S. medical schools as a group did not fill 35 per cent of the first-year residency training positions in their affiliated hospitals with doctors entering the primary care fields of internal medicine, family medicine and pediatrics, then the bill barred grants to an individual school unless it met such required percentage by July 15, 1978; increased the required percentage, if "triggered" by group failure to comply, to 40 per cent on July 15, 1979, and 50 per cent on July 15, 1980, for an individual school.

● Barred grants to medical schools that did not agree to reserve places for qualified U.S. students who had finished two years of study at a foreign medical school and wanted to complete their training in the United States; allowed HEW to waive this requirement.

● Barred grants to schools of osteopathy that, beginning in fiscal 1978, did not devise a plan to provide at least six weeks of training for graduating students in areas remote from their main campus or in medically underserved areas.

● Barred grants to schools of dentistry that, beginning in the 1978-79 school year, did not reserve at least 70 per cent of any new residency training positions for students entering the fields of general dentistry or pedodontics (care of children); required dental schools to increase enrollment by 5 or 10 per cent depending on size or to train students in areas remote from their main campus or in areas that are medically underserved.

Health Manpower Program Authorizations

HR 5546 authorized funding for a variety of continuing programs in fiscal 1977 and the following specific amounts in fiscal 1978-80 *(in millions of dollars):**

	Fiscal 1978	Fiscal 1979	Fiscal 1980
Construction of Teaching Facilities			
Grants	$ 40.00	$ 40.00	$ 40.00
Loan guarantees, interest subsidies	2.00	3.00	3.00
Student Assistance			
Insured loan fund	1.50	—	—
Loans	26.00	27.00	28.00
National Health Service Corps scholarships	75.00	140.00	200.00
Scholarships for exceptionally needy students	16.00	17.00	18.00
Lister Hill scholarships	.16	.24	.32
National Health Service Corps	47.00	57.00	70.00
Aid to Health Professions Schools			
Capitation grants to medical schools	124.18	131.68	139.40
Capitation grants to schools of osteopathy	8.68	9.34	10.16
Capitation grants to dental schools	45.80	45.40	46.91
Capitation grants to schools of public health	9.74	10.46	11.06
Capitation grants to schools of veterinary medicine	10.22	10.55	10.71
Capitation grants to schools of optometry	3.20	3.27	3.37
Capitation grants to schools of pharmacy	16.99	17.11	17.37
Capitation grants to schools of podiatry	2.27	2.27	2.29
Public health traineeships	7.50	8.00	9.00
Health administration traineeships	2.50	2.50	2.50

	Fiscal 1978	Fiscal 1979	Fiscal 1980
Public and Allied Health			
Graduate programs in health administration	$ 3.25	$ 3.50	$ 3.75
Special projects in public health, health administration	5.00	5.50	6.00
Allied health personnel project grants	22.00	24.00	26.00
Allied health personnel advanced training	4.50	5.00	5.50
Aid to disadvantaged allied health students	1.00	1.00	1.00
Special Projects			
Departments of Family Medicine	10.00	15.00	20.00
Area health education centers	20.00	30.00	40.00
Education of U.S. students returning from foreign medical schools	2.00	3.00	4.00
Programs for physician and dental assistants	25.00	30.00	35.00
Training in pediatrics, internal medicine	15.00	20.00	25.00
Occupational health training	5.00	8.00	10.00
Family medicine, general dentistry	40.00	45.00	50.00
Aid to needy students	20.00	20.00	20.00
Aid to schools for start-up costs, financial distress, miscellaneous programs	25.00	25.00	25.00
Operational aid to new medical schools	1.50	—	—
Nurse Traineeships	25.00	—	—
Total	$662.99	$759.82	$883.34

* *Some figures have been rounded.*

● Required schools of public health, veterinary medicine, optometry and podiatry to make enrollment increases or satisfy other requirements.

● Authorized HEW to make grants to schools of public health and other graduate schools for student traineeships in the fields of public health, health care administration or health planning.

Foreign Medical Graduates

● Eliminated immigration preferences for alien graduates of foreign medical schools who had not passed qualifying examinations and demonstrated competency in written and oral English.

● Denied "exchange visitor" visas for foreign medical graduates unless they 1) proved that they had been accepted by a medical school or affiliated hospital for advanced training, 2) passed qualifying exams and demonstrated command of written and oral English, 3) agreed to return to their countries after completion of training and showed that skills acquired in the United States would be fully used in those countries and 4) agreed to leave the United States after two years of training in general, with provision for a one-year extension under some circumstances.

● Allowed waiver of the new requirements for exchange visitor visas through Dec. 31, 1980.

Other Provisions

● Authorized new grants for support of graduate programs in health care administration and health planning; extended support for training in allied health professions such as dental hygiene.

● Authorized grants for a long list of special projects including development of residency programs in family medicine and general dentistry, training of U.S. students returning from foreign medical schools, dental team training, occupational health, relief of financial distress and other specialized programs.

● Authorized special traineeships for nurse practitioners, who assume many responsibilities often performed by physicians, if they agree to practice in medically underserved areas or if they reside in such areas.

● Extended funding for existing health manpower programs through fiscal 1977; authorized advanced funding of any health manpower authorizations.

Swine Flu Program

Medical history books probably will record 1976 as the year of the swine flu immunization program, perhaps the most widely publicized—and trouble-ridden—federal health effort ever undertaken.

President Ford proposed the program in March after flu usually found in swine affected humans at Ft. Dix, N.J., and killed one soldier. Scientists suggested that the flu was related to a strain that caused a worldwide epidemic taking 20 million lives in 1918-19.

President Ford urged everyone to get a shot. Government health officials enthusiastically promoted the program as an important opportunity to take a preventive step that could avert a major health disaster. But after the flu failed to show up anywhere else in a few months, critics accused the administration of overreacting and using scare tactics to encourage participation in the program. (Two isolated cases of the flu were reported late in the year.)

The program was suddenly halted in mid-December so that the Department of Health, Education and Welfare (HEW) could investigate a possible connection between swine flu shots and a rare paralytic disease, Guillain-Barre syndrome, which was turning up around the country. The inoculation program was not resumed before President Ford left office in January 1977.

Congressional Role

While some members remained skeptical about the need for the program, Congress gave its approval twice in 1976 to the immunization program.

Appropriation. Anxious to avoid any blame if a swine flu outbreak should occur, Congress quickly passed a $135-million appropriations bill for the program (H J Res 890—PL 94-266). The House approved the measure April 5 (H Rept 94-1004) and the Senate passed it April 9 (S Rept 94-742). The House cleared the bill by accepting a Senate amendment on April 12.

The appropriations bill included $100-million to pay for production of vaccine used against the flu and $26-million to help state and local officials set up community immunization programs. The rest of the money was used by the federal government for research, testing and national organization.

Four private drug companies began production of the vaccine amid predictions that the immunizations could start in August. But the program hit a major snag in mid-June when the drug companies indicated that their insurance would not cover them against claims attributed to the swine flu vaccine. Without coverage, drug company officials told the Department of Health, Education and Welfare (HEW), they were not interested in manufacturing the vaccine.

Indemnity Bill. The administration promptly proposed legislation (HR 14409) requiring the federal government to indemnify the drug makers against swine flu claims not related to negligence on the manufacturers' part.

HEW officials argued that the legislation was reasonable because of the unique federal role in the swine flu program. The federal government, not the manufacturers, was responsible for the testing of the vaccine, development of warnings and supervision of inoculation programs, they pointed out.

But members of the House Interstate and Foreign Commerce Subcommittee on Health and the Environment were skeptical. Several said they would not be stampeded into approval of the proposal.

The subcommittee and administration officials were equally critical of the insurance industry for its refusal to write coverage for swine flu. Industry representatives argued that insurers were worried about a mass program using a new vaccine that would be given on an emergency basis. Even though government tests found the vaccine safe, they added, the size of the program posed incalculable risks. Some insurers indicated that their greatest fear was a large number of baseless suits that still would involve legal costs.

At an impasse, the subcommittee July 1 refused to approve the legislation. Paul G. Rogers (D Fla.), subcommittee chairman and a swine flu program supporter, asked HEW officials to try again to negotiate some solution with the vaccine makers that would not require legislation.

New Approach

These negotiations produced no agreement, but an outbreak of a mysterious killer disease in Pennsylvania in early August was the necessary spur to congressional action. The disease, called "Legionnaires' disease" because it affected persons who had some connection with a July American Legion convention, was not swine flu. Health officials in early 1977 identified a previously unknown bacterium as the cause of the disease.

HEW officials used the outbreak, which took 29 lives, to illustrate how quickly a disease could spread. The department drafted new legislation to deal with the swine flu insurance problem.

Under the bill, anyone claiming injury from the program could sue the federal government only. They would sue under the federal torts claims law protecting federal employees in agencies such as the Public Health Service. Drug manufacturers, and doctors and other health personnel who administered the vaccine without charge, were protected from suits under this arrangement. But if the government lost a case and had to pay a claim, it, in turn, was empowered to sue a drug company or a doctor to collect claims it attributed to nongovernmental negligence.

HEW officials argued that this approach was better than the earlier one because it would use federal procedures to weed out baseless suits, would limit lawyers' fees under the torts claims law and would simplify the claims process.

Legislative Action

On Aug. 5, Rogers and House Republicans urged the full Commerce Committee to act quickly to get the measure to the floor, but the panel balked. Several committee Democrats said they would not be rushed.

The bill's supporters then used short-cut procedures to try to clear the measure before Congress recessed for the Republican national convention. When the House Commerce Committee could not get a quorum together to report the bill, House sponsors worked with the Senate to get around the committee obstacle. The Senate passed a modified version (S 3735—PL 94-380) of the administration bill Aug. 10 after agreeing to discharge the Labor and Public Welfare Committee from further consideration of the measure.

The same day, House sponsors quickly got the House Rules Committee to clear the Senate bill for floor action in the House under a rule allowing no amendments. House passage Aug. 10 thus cleared the Senate version for the President.

Other Problems

While the insurance situation was the major roadblock, the immunization program ran into a host of other problems delaying its initial starting date until Oct. 1. They included additional testing needed to figure out how to make the vaccine effective for those under age 25 and delays in delivery of the vaccine to state and local immunization programs.

The program hit another bump in the road in mid-October when news reports highlighted the deaths of about 40 elderly or chronically ill persons after they received shots. HEW officials repeatedly stressed that the deaths had nothing to do with the swine flu vaccine. But evidence indicated that this initial adverse publicity made many afraid of the program. Health officials were particularly disturbed in late 1976 by the low rate of immunization among the urban poor.

About 35 million Americans—far short of the original goal—had received swine flu shots as of mid-December, when the program was suspended pending investigation of a possible link between the shots and Guillain-Barre syndrome. Government officials agreed that because of the scare, it was unlikely the public would take the shots even if the program were resumed later.

While no connection between the shots and the syndrome had been confirmed, HEW's swine flu surveillance system had found that the syndrome was turning up more frequently in persons who had received shots than in those who had not.

National Health Insurance

Congress took a "why bother" attitude toward national health insurance legislation in 1976.

President Ford remained opposed to a new insurance program, arguing in his Jan. 19 State of the Union message that "we cannot realistically afford federally dictated national health insurance providing full coverage for all 215 million Americans."

The only insurance proposal supported by Ford would have protected the elderly against the cost of a "catastrophic" illness while requiring them to pay more out of their own pockets for short-term care. Congress paid no attention to the proposal. *(See Medicare in 1976 chronology, p. 56-A)*

Waiting to see if the country would elect a new President more sympathetic to a health insurance program, the House Ways and Means and House Interstate and Foreign Commerce Committees continued sporadic hearings on the issue in 1976, but took no further action.

Continuing questions about the cost of a national program and the same disagreements about the right approach also stalled congressional action. But the congressional budget resolution for fiscal 1977 included $50-million for some initial planning of health insurance.

The two House committees did not resolve their jurisdictional dispute before adjournment. A September report by the House Democratic Study Group recommended creation of a special ad hoc committee to deal with health insurance. But, by the end of the year, the two committees were expected to work out a compromise informally with Speaker-elect Thomas P. O'Neill Jr. (D Mass.).

Carter Position

At the end of another four years of inaction on health insurance, prospects for creation of some sort of national health system brightened when Democrat Jimmy Carter was elected President.

Throughout his campaign, Carter expressed support for a comprehensive national health insurance program. While many specifics were missing, two features of Carter's proposal came directly from organized labor's plan. He supported a mandatory program that would be financed through a combination of general tax revenues and new payroll taxes. But, in contrast to labor's position, Carter also suggested that private insurers should play some role in the operation of the program.

To reduce the budget impact of the program, Carter said he would implement it in stages—although he did not say in 1976 which stage would come first.

Abortion

Abortion opponents won what was primarily a symbolic victory in 1976 when Congress voted to restrict federal funding for abortions, but their major goal—overturning the 1973 Supreme Court decision legalizing abortion—remained an elusive one.

Funding Ban

The House and Senate fought all summer over the abortion funding ban, holding up final action on a $56.6-billion fiscal 1977 appropriations bill (HR 14232—PL 94-439) for the Departments of Labor and Health, Education and Welfare (HEW).

Hyde Amendment. The dispute began June 24 when the House, by a key vote of 207-167 (R 94-34; D 113-133) adopted an amendment by Henry J. Hyde (R Ill.) to bar use of funds in the appropriations bill to pay for abortions. The amendment applied primarily to the Medicaid health program for the poor, which paid for 250,000 to 300,000 abortions a year at a federal cost of about $45 million.

Supporters of the funding ban argued that no tax dollars should support a procedure many considered the equivalent of murder.

Opponents argued just as vehemently that the amendment would discriminate illegally against the poor, who would be forced to seek unsafe abortions.

Senate Opposition. Opponents were in the majority in the Senate. On June 28, the Senate voted 57-28 to drop the House amendment from the bill. One factor affecting the Senate vote was the fact that the amendment allowed no exceptions to the abortion ban, outlawing abortions to save the life of the mother as well as those sought for convenience.

Deadlock. An initial attempt by House-Senate conferees to come up with a compromise failed. They reported (H Rept 94-1384) the abortion amendment in disagreement Aug. 3, and in a new series of votes, the House and Senate deadlocked again.

On Aug. 10, the House voted 150-223 against a move to drop the Hyde amendment and then, by voice vote, insisted that it wanted the funding ban in the bill.

The Senate insisted on its opposition to the amendment again by a 53-35 vote Aug. 25, sending the issue back to conferees once more.

Compromise Reached. As the scheduled adjournment date of Oct. 2 neared, pressure to find a compromise grew intense in order to clear the massive appropriations measure. After 10 weeks of off-and-on wrangling, conferees finally found some language most of them could live with (H

Rept 94-1555). It outlawed federal funding of abortions except when the life of the mother would be endangered if the pregnancy were carried to term.

The House endorsed the compromise Sept. 16 by a 256-114 vote. Acting as if it had little other choice in the matter if it wanted to clear the appropriations measure, the Senate gave the amendment its grudging approval Sept. 17 by a key vote of 47-21 (R 18-8; D 29-13).

Senators, in fact, had very little to say about the amendment, deciding to vote first and then open the floor to discussion. The *Congressional Record* then was rearranged to make it look as if all the discussion preceded the vote.

Opponents of the abortion language argued that it would not survive a legal challenge. "I hope and expect that it will be struck down by the courts as unconstitutional," said Rep. Bella S. Abzug (D N.Y.), a leading supporter of abortion rights.

Veto, Override. While he generally supported the funding ban, President Ford Sept. 29 vetoed the appropriations bill because it was nearly $4-billion over his budget. The following day both houses of Congress voted by wide margins to override the veto, more because of the popularity of programs funded under the bill than because of the abortion language. The House overrode the veto by a 312-93 vote; the Senate followed suit hours later by a key vote of 67-15 (R 19-11; D 48-4).

The courts, however, immediately acted to prevent the language from taking effect. The Supreme Court was expected to rule in 1977 in a test case related to the amendment.

All of the abortion votes during 1976 revealed that sentiment on the issue did not respect party lines. But, in general, Republicans were more likely to favor restrictions on abortion while Democrats sometimes split almost evenly over the issue.

Constitutional Amendments

Proposed constitutional amendments to overturn the 1973 Supreme Court decision remained lodged in committee in 1976.

On April 28, the Senate voted 47-40 against a move to start debate on a proposed constitutional amendment to guarantee unborn children the right to life. It was the first time either house of Congress had given even procedural consideration on the floor to proposed anti-abortion amendments to the Constitution since the 1973 decision.

Basically, Jesse A. Helms (R N.C.), sponsor of the amendment, was seeking a vote to put senators on the record on the abortion issue in the election year. He used a procedural maneuver to place his proposal on the Senate calendar without committee action. A Senate Judiciary subcommittee rejected a number of anti-abortion proposals in 1975. *(p. 31-A)*

Three hours of low-key debate preceded the vote. Those supporting restrictions on abortion stressed that unborn children had as much right to live as anyone else. "What we are talking about is what value our society is going to place on human life," said James L. Buckley (Cons-R N.Y.).

"The American Congress is the last hope for the millions whose lives will be terminated unless we act now," added Helms.

Opponents of the proposal argued that the Senate had no business getting involved in such a touchy moral issue or interfering with women's rights. "Are we going to relapse to the Dark Ages or are we going...to let one-half of our pop-ulation...have the same rights that we have?" Jacob K. Javits (R N.Y.) asked the all-male Senate.

In the House, a Judiciary subcommittee held hearings on abortion, but took no further action. Subcommittee Chairman Don Edwards (D Calif.) said a majority of the panel opposed anti-abortion proposals.

Court Ruling

In another setback for abortion opponents, the Supreme Court July 1 struck down state laws requiring a husband's or parent's consent before a woman could get an abortion during the early stages of pregnancy. The decision invalidated a Missouri law.

Campaign Issue

The abortion issue made several appearances in the political spotlight during the presidential campaign—as abortion opponents hoped it would.

But the outcome of the election was a disappointment to them. Jimmy Carter, while personally opposed to abortion, said he was unlikely to support proposed constitutional amendments outlawing the procedure. President Ford's position was slightly more to the right-to-life movement's liking. He said he could support a constitutional amendment that would leave regulation of abortion up to the states, but he never proposed such an amendment during his administration.

Medical Devices

Congress May 13 gave final approval to landmark legislation (S 510—PL 94-295) establishing the federal government's clear-cut power to oversee the safety and effectiveness of medical devices ranging from crutches to life-supporting kidney dialysis machines. The legislation, pending for more than a decade, updated laws written 38 years earlier.

Under the bill, most life-supporting devices and devices implanted in the body could not be sold without prior approval by the Food and Drug Administration (FDA). The FDA also could ban very risky devices.

The pre-market review requirement applied only to the most dangerous devices. The FDA was authorized to set performance standards for less risky devices and to exert general controls over all devices. These controls allowed the FDA to require manufacturers to repair or replace faulty devices.

The administration supported the bill, and industry groups had played a major role in drafting the legislation. It had strong bipartisan support.

Legislative Action

The Senate had passed S 510 in 1975. *(p. 35-A)*

The House-passed version, approved March 9, was similar to the Senate version, but more detailed about the regulatory process.

As written (H Rept 94-853) by the Interstate and Foreign Commerce Committee, the House version, for instance, made a distinction between "new" devices, which generally would need pre-market clearance, and devices on the market before enactment of the legislation.

The final bill, drafted by House-Senate conferees (H Rept 94-1090), generally followed the lines of the House version. One change loosened a House provision that would have required automatic pre-market review of new devices that were implanted in the body.

Provisions

As signed into law, S 510:

Classification

● Required the Secretary of Health, Education and Welfare (HEW) to establish panels of experts to recommend classification of medical devices into three categories; required the panels to recommend classification of devices on the market before enactment of the legislation within one year of receiving funding for their work.

● Based classification on the type of regulation needed to assure the safety and effectiveness of a device.

● Established three classification categories: 1) Class I devices subject to general controls, 2) Class II devices subject to general controls and performance standards and 3) Class III devices subject to general controls and pre-market approval.

● In general, required the panels to recommend Class III classification for life-sustaining or life-supporting devices and devices implanted in the body that were 1) on the market before enactment or 2) substantially similar to devices on the market before enactment; if a panel recommended placing these devices in some other class, required it to state its reason for doing so.

● Upon receipt of a panel's recommendation for classification of devices on the market before enactment, required the HEW Secretary to propose regulations classifying these devices; allowed the Secretary to change a panel's recommendation for Class III classification if he stated his reasons for doing so and identified any possible health risks; allowed the Secretary to reclassify devices based on new information.

● Required the Secretary to classify into Class III all devices that were not 1) on the market before enactment or 2) substantially similar to devices on the market before enactment; allowed the manufacturer of such a "new" device to petition for a change in Class III classification; required the Secretary to deny a petition for reclassification of a new implantable or life-supporting device unless he determined that pre-market approval was not needed to assure its safety and effectiveness.

Performance Standards

● Allowed the Secretary to select an outside organization or a federal agency to set performance standards for Class II devices.

● Stipulated that the standards could govern the construction and components of a device, testing requirements and actual performance of a device.

● Allowed the Secretary to accept existing standards instead of seeking the development of new standards.

● In general, stipulated that performance standards could not take effect until one year after they were proposed as regulations by the Secretary; allowed the Secretary to set an earlier effective date to protect public health.

Pre-Market Approval

● Required the Secretary, by regulation, to require devices on the market before enactment that had been classified as Class III to receive pre-market approval before they could continue to be sold; required manufacturers of these "existing" devices to file applications for pre-market

approval within 90 days after these regulations were issued or within 30 months after a device was classified Class III.

● Required manufacturers of both new and existing devices seeking pre-market approval to submit applications describing manufacturing processes, testing results and other information about the devices; required manufacturers to submit samples of these devices under most circumstances.

● Required the Secretary to approve or disapprove an application within six months of its receipt; allowed the Secretary to withdraw approval of an application at a later date.

● Allowed a manufacturer to gain pre-market approval of a device by setting forth standards for its development and then meeting them; allowed the Secretary to deny his approval if final testing results differed substantially from those initially set forth by the manufacturer.

● Allowed manufacturers to petition for review when denied pre-market approval of devices.

General Controls

● Subjected devices in all three classes to the following general controls and existing prohibitions against adulteration and mislabeling.

● Allowed the Secretary to ban a deceptive device or one posing an "unreasonable and substantial" risk of illness or injury.

● Allowed the Secretary to require notification of device users, health professionals, manufacturers and others if a device posed an unreasonable risk to public health; allowed the Secretary to let health professionals provide notice of risks to device users if this posed less danger to patients.

● Allowed the Secretary to order manufacturers to repair, replace or provide refunds for devices posing risks because of poor manufacturing.

● Allowed the Secretary to require manufacturers to keep certain records and make reports as required to HEW; allowed the Secretary to exempt certain manufacturers, such as those making devices generally regarded as safe, or small businesses, from these requirements.

● Allowed the Secretary to require a prescription for the sale of certain devices; allowed the Secretary to restrict the use of certain devices to persons with special training if needed to assure the safety and effectiveness of the devices.

● Required device manufacturers to register with HEW.

● Allowed the Secretary to set standards for the manufacture, packing, storage and installation of devices in conformance with good manufacturing practices.

Other Provisions

● Allowed the Secretary to exempt from certain regulations custom devices ordered by doctors for individual patients or devices used in scientific investigations.

● Required the Secretary to make public information about the safety and effectiveness when he approved, disapproved or withdrew approval of an application for pre-market approval.

● Required HEW to establish a special unit to provide technical assistance to small manufacturers of devices.

● Allowed the Secretary to approve the export of devices that cannot be sold in the United States if he determined that export was not contrary to public health and if the country importing the devices approved.

● Defined a "device" as an instrument, apparatus, implant or other related article 1) intended for use in the diagnosis, treatment or prevention of disease or intended to affect structure or functions of the body and 2) which did not achieve any of its principal intended purposes through chemical action or the process of metabolism.

Drug Abuse Prevention

Despite administration objections, Congress insisted that a high-level White House office should coordinate federal drug abuse programs. Legislation (S 2017—PL 94-237) cleared March 4 created the new office for a three-year period and authorized $689-million in fiscal 1976-78 to prevent drug abuse and treat addicts.

Although he signed the legislation, President Ford refused to use appropriations provided for the office or name a director during the remainder of his term. So the unit remained a "paper" organization in 1976. Sponsors of the bill planned to push for creation of the office in the new Carter administration.

Although its responsibilities would be more limited, the new office would replace the White House Special Action Office for Drug Abuse Prevention created in 1972 as a visible focus for the Nixon administration's drug abuse prevention efforts. President Ford dismantled the special office on June 30, 1975, shifting its duties to the National Institute on Drug Abuse within the Department of Health, Education and Welfare (HEW).

Congressional sponsors of S 2017 questioned how a fourth-level agency in HEW could coordinate the federal government's far-flung drug abuse programs run by agencies ranging from the Veterans Administration to the Agriculture Department. In June 1975, the Senate voted to extend the life of the special White House office through the end of 1975. The House-passed version of the bill, approved in September 1975, extended the office through June 30, 1976. *(p. 36-A)*

The temporary extensions were designed to give Congress time to evaluate White House Domestic Council recommendations that a Cabinet-level committee coordinate federal drug abuse programs. Key sponsors of the bill decided they still wanted to have a White House office so that one person would be accountable to Congress for the smooth operation of drug abuse programs.

The administration opposed creation of a new office, arguing that it would restrict the President's flexibility and duplicate policy-coordination mechanisms preferred by the White House. However, the administration supported continued funding for basic drug abuse prevention and treatment programs run by the HEW institute.

Conference Action

Conferees filed a report (H Rept 94-839) Feb. 24 that technically stated they had been unable to reach agreement since the three-year extension of the White House office went beyond the scope of either version of the bill. But conferees actually drafted a compromise version then acccepted by the House and Senate.

Conferees agreed the new office should be an advisory unit that would recommend priorities and goals for drug abuse programs to the President and seek to coordinate programs within this framework. Basic operational authority to run drug abuse prevention and treatment programs should be shifted to the HEW institute, conferees decided.

In light of this decision, conferees dropped provisions of both the House and Senate versions that would have given the White House office a special fund to support innovative programs run by other agencies.

Provisions

As signed into law, S 2017:
- Established an Office of Drug Abuse Policy within the Executive Office of the President; authorized the President to appoint the director of the office subject to Senate confirmation; barred the director from holding any other office in the federal government.
- Required the director to make recommendations to the President regarding priorities, goals and policies for federal drug abuse programs and to coordinate all federal drug abuse activities; required the director to review all federal regulations related to drug abuse programs and to evaluate the effectiveness of the programs.
- Required the Attorney General to notify the director when he made changes in legal restrictions on the distribution of drugs that potentially could be abused.
- Authorized $1.2-million for the activities of the White House office through Sept. 30, 1976; authorized $20-million for the office in each of fiscal 1977-78.
- Barred private and public hospitals receiving any federal support from using admission or treatment policies to discriminate against any patient solely because of his drug abuse or drug dependence problems.
- Authorized $45-million in each of fiscal 1976-78 and $11.25-million for the three-month transition period between fiscal 1976 and 1977 for formula grants to the states for drug abuse prevention and treatment activities.
- Authorized $160-million in each of fiscal 1976-78 and $40-million for the three-month transition period between fiscal 1976 and 1977 for project grants awarded by the Department of HEW for drug abuse prevention and treatment activities; required HEW to give "a high priority" to grant applications for primary prevention programs designed to discourage initial use of drugs.
- Transferred basic operational responsibility for federal drug abuse prevention, treatment and research programs to the National Institute on Drug Abuse within HEW; authorized $7-million in each of fiscal 1976-78 and $1.75-million for the transition period between fiscal 1976 and 1977 for the testing and development of drug detoxification agents and substitute maintenance drugs that were less addictive than heroin.

Health Maintenance Organizations

Redoing its earlier handiwork, Congress Sept. 23 gave final approval to legislation (HR 9019—PL 94-460) easing requirements for health maintenance organizations (HMOs) seeking federal aid under a 1973 law. HMOs provided a range of health services for a periodic set fee.

In exchange for federal aid provided under the 1973 act, Congress required federally supported or approved HMOs to offer a long list of benefits, to open enrollment to even the sickest of patients and to charge the same fees for healthy families and those with health problems. After passage of the 1973 act, HMO groups decided that some of the requirements—while theoretically desirable—made their plans so expensive that they could not compete with traditional health insurers. *(p. 4-A)*

The House agreed in late 1975 to repeal or delay many of the requirements. The Senate, acting in 1976, was more anxious to hold on to them at least in some form. *(House action, p. 32-A)*

Key provisions of the compromise allowed HMOs to trim the list of services they must offer and required only large and well-established HMOs to open enrollment to patients with health problems. The bill also gave new HMOs three years to adopt a fee system that did not distinguish between healthy and less healthy families.

Another key section of the measure revised provisions of the 1973 act requiring some employers to offer the HMO option and clarified the bargaining power of unions in these situations.

The administration generally supported the bill.

Legislative Action

Senate. The Senate passed its version of the legislation on June 14.

Edward M. Kennedy (D Mass.), chairman of the Health Subcommittee of the Labor and Public Welfare Committee, voted against the bill to protest the committee's decision to weaken the open enrollment requirement. He argued that the change would hurt the very sick who could not obtain regular health insurance.

Required HMO Services

As revised in 1976, the law required a federally funded or federally qualified HMO to offer the following basic services to its members. An HMO could offer the following supplemental services at its own option at an additional cost to members.

Basic Services

Physician health care, including consultation and referral
Inpatient and outpatient hospital services
Emergency health services, if medically necessary
Short-term (limited to 20 visits) outpatient services for mental health crises and evaluation
Diagnostic laboratory and diagnostic and therapeutic X-ray services
Home health services
Preventive health services, including voluntary family planning and infertility services, immunizations, well-baby care, periodic checkups for adults, and preventive vision care and ear exams for children
Medical treatment, including referral, for alcohol and drug abuse

Supplemental Services

Services of facilities for intermediate or long-term care (such as nursing homes)
Vision care (excluding preventive care for children)
Dental care (including preventive care for children)
Mental health care not covered by basic services
Physical medicine and rehabilitation (including physical therapy) on a long-term basis
Prescription drugs required as part of care by an HMO

As reported (S Rept 94-884) by the committee and then passed, the bill applied a limited open enrollment requirement only to large and well-established HMOs. This proposal, however, went beyond the House bill, which repealed the provision entirely.

The Senate also decided not to delay some other requirements of the 1973 act as long as the House did.

Conference Action. In general, House-Senate conferees found some middle ground between the House and Senate positions. Their report (H Rept 94-1513) spelled out the compromises, which, in general, made the law more complicated.

Provisions

As signed into law, HR 9019:

● Revised the basic benefits that an HMO must offer to qualify for federal aid or federal approval; eliminated preventive dental care for children from the list of required basic benefits; added to required benefits immunizations, well-baby care, periodic checkups for adults and ear examinations for children to determine need for hearing correction.

● Repealed a provision of the 1973 act that required federally approved or funded HMOs to offer other benefits, known as supplemental benefits, to enrollees who wanted to pay extra fees for them.

● Revised provisions of the 1973 law barring HMOs from contracting with individual health professionals to provide infrequently used services for HMO enrollees; allowed such contracting if the amount of care contracted for did not exceed 30 per cent of the value of a rural HMO's total doctor services and 15 per cent of a non-rural HMO's services.

● Revised provisions of the 1973 law requiring HMOs to use health professionals who devote at least half of their time to HMO patients; stipulated instead that such professionals individually must devote over half their time to group practice (although not necessarily HMO practice) and that the group as a whole must devote a substantial portion of its time (defined by conference language as over 35 per cent) to HMO practice; allowed HEW to waive this new requirement for three years.

● Modified a provision of the 1973 act requiring HMOs to open their enrollment to anyone during a 30-day period each year; stipulated instead that an HMO that 1) had been in existence for at least five years or 2) had at least 50,000 enrollees, must open enrollment for 30 days annually following a year in which it did not incur a financial deficit; limited the number of persons an HMO was required to enroll during this period to 3 per cent of its total increase in enrollment the previous year; allowed an HMO to deny enrollment to persons institutionalized with chronic illness or permanent injury and to delay coverage of any benefits for these enrollees for 90 days after enrollment.

● Revised a provision of the 1973 act requiring HMOs to base enrollment fees on the health experience of their communities ("community rating") instead of the individual experience of a family group; instead delayed the requirement for four years for existing HMOs while continuing to apply it to new HMOs.

● Increased limits on federal assistance to an individual HMO for feasibility surveys, planning, initial development and initial operation.

● Allowed the Department of Health, Education and Welfare (HEW) to provide loan guarantees for private, non-profit HMOs.

• Required employers to offer their employees the option of joining a federally approved HMO plan if they offered traditional health insurance coverage only when at least 25 of their employees resided in an area served by an HMO seeking inclusion in a company's health benefits plan.

• Clarified that an employer need not offer the HMO option to individual employees if the union that bargained for them rejected the HMO option; once the option had been approved by the bargaining agent, required the employer to offer it individually to employees to accept or reject.

• Set civil penalties of up to $10,000 for employers who did not comply with the HMO "dual choice" requirements.

• Revised authorizations for federal aid to HMOs to extend funding through fiscal 1979; changed an authorization of $85-million in each of fiscal 1976-77 to authorizations of $40-million in fiscal 1976, $45-million in each of fiscal 1977-78 and $50-million in fiscal 1979.

• Required HEW to administer the HMO assistance program, except for its regulatory aspects, through a single agency.

• Authorized $15-million through fiscal 1977 for federally supported home health services.

Disease Control, Health Education

After rewriting the legislation to ward off a presidential veto, Congress June 7 cleared a two-part bill (S 1466—PL 94-317) providing a new focus for federal support for disease control and immunization programs.

Faced with strong administration objections, the House and Senate retreated from a more extensive plan to provide federal support for public and private programs promoting healthy habits and appropriate use of health services. The administration argued that the plan would require duplication of existing programs.

Senate Action

The Senate had passed the bill in 1975. Supporters argued that it was time to expand government efforts to stamp out health risks that consumers imposed on themselves. *(p. 36-A)*

House Action

The House passed its version of the bill April 7, 1976, after rejecting, 185-207, a move to kill the section of the bill expanding consumer health education programs.

Republicans opposing this section questioned the effectiveness of the legislation, suggesting that everyone knew that habits like smoking or excessive eating were unhealthy. "All of us in Congress know this. All this information has been available to us...," noted Del Clawson (R Calif.). "But how many of us practice all of these things, even after we know about them?"

Sponsors of the bill countered that new efforts were needed to find out exactly what would motivate people to adopt healthier habits.

The House-passed version was similar to the Senate bill. It continued various disease control programs. The second part of the bill established a high-level office in the Department of Health, Education and Welfare (HEW) to promote health education and proposed creation of a private health promotion center receiving some federal startup aid.

The Interstate and Foreign Commerce Committee, which reported (H Rept 94-1007) the measure April 2, made one addition to the Senate version. It extended funding for a lead-based paint prevention program, previously extended in 1973. The Senate had passed separate legislation (S 1664) Feb. 19 to continue the lead poisoning prevention program, but later agreed to consider it as part of S 1466. *(1973 action, p. 9-A)*

Final Compromise

House and Senate sponsors of the bill worked with the administration to draft a final version acceptable to the White House. There was no formal House-Senate conference.

The final compromise essentially provided a higher-level focus for health education and information programs within HEW, required improved coordination of such programs and provided congressional goals for the kind of programs that should receive HEW's support. The compromise reduced the three-year authorization for the programs, eliminated the new private health education center and dropped a provision requiring HEW review of the health impact of other departments' policies.

Another feature of the final bill provided for a special program to immunize children against communicable and other diseases. Several members of Congress argued that the government should be doing more to promote these immunization programs before it put so much effort into an administration-backed "swine flu" immunization program. *(p. 44-A)*

Provisions

As signed into law, S 1466:

Health Promotion

• Directed the Secretary of Health, Education and Welfare (HEW) to develop a strategy for the promotion of good health care and appropriate use of health services and to support programs aimed at achieving these goals.

Authorizations

As signed into law, S 1466 authorized the following amounts *(in millions of dollars)*:

	Fiscal 1976	Fiscal 1977	Fiscal 1978
Health information and promotion*	—	$ 7	$ 10
Immunization of children	$ 9	17.5	23
Control of diseases borne by rodents	13.5	14	14.5
Other disease control programs	4	4.5	5
Venereal disease research	5	6.6	7.6
Venereal disease control	32	41.5	43.5
Lead-based paint poisoning prevention	10	12	14
Total	**$73.5**	**$103.1**	**$117.6**

* The bill authorized an additional $14-million in fiscal 1979 for health information and promotion.

• Stipulated that such programs could include research programs, community-based programs, information programs and training programs; authorized the Secretary to make grants to private nonprofit organizations working in health promotion and information areas.

• Required the Secretary to make a periodic survey of the needs, attitudes and knowledge of U.S. citizens regarding health care.

• Required the Secretary to conduct a study to determine the extent of coverage under health insurance plans for preventive health services and health education services.

• Required HEW to establish an Office of Health Information and Health Promotion within the Office of the Assistant Secretary for Health to coordinate health promotion and information programs.

Disease Control

• Authorized grants to the states and other public agencies for disease control programs through fiscal 1978.

• Required HEW to give special consideration to grant applications for programs that 1) will increase to 80 per cent the immunization rate for any group that has not received immunizations against general diseases, and 2) will cooperate with private groups and volunteers.

• Required HEW to give priority to grant applications for disease control programs aimed at communicable diseases.

• Stipulated that programs eligible for support should be aimed at the prevention or reduction of tuberculosis, rubella, measles, polio, diphtheria, tetanus, pertussis, mumps and other communicable diseases, and arthritis, diabetes, diseases borne by rodents, hypertension, heart and lung diseases, and Rh disease.

• Authorized separate funding for programs to immunize children against communicable diseases and to control diseases borne by rodents.

• Extended through fiscal 1978 special programs to prevent and control venereal disease.

• Extended through fiscal 1978 special programs to prevent and treat lead-based paint poisoning.

• Required agencies receiving grants for the detection and treatment of lead-based paint poisoning to develop programs to remove the paint hazard from the homes of children treated for the disease.

• Barred the use of lead-based paint on cooking, eating and drinking utensils, toys, furniture, and residential buildings supported with any form of federal assistance.

• Within one year of enactment, limited the allowable lead content in interior residential paints to .06 per cent by weight unless the full Consumer Product Safety Commission set another allowable content limit (up to a maximum of .5 per cent) within six months of enactment.

Biomedical Research

Congress cleared legislation (HR 7988—PL 94-278) April 12 extending funding for a number of popular health programs that had expired on June 30, 1975. The House and Senate had passed different versions of the bill in 1975. *(p. 33-A)*

As cleared, the bill authorized a total of $752-million in fiscal 1976-77 for federal programs to combat heart, lung and blood diseases. It provided an additional $90-million in fiscal 1976-78 for efforts to help parents who suspected they might carry genetic diseases. Other sections of the measure continued funding for medical student loans and

Authorizations

As signed into law, HR 7988 authorized the following amounts *(in millions of dollars):*

	Fiscal 1976	Fiscal 1977	Fiscal 1978
Heart, lung and blood diseases			
Prevention and control	$ 10	$ 30	—
Research	339	373	—
National Research Service Awards	165	185	—
Genetic disease testing, counseling and information	30	30	$30
Arthritis centers*	8	20	—
Physician shortage area scholarships	2	—	—
Health manpower student loans	60	—	—
Total	**$614**	**$638**	**$30**

* Revised existing authorizations of $13-million in fiscal 1976 and $15-million in fiscal 1977.

scholarships and for special awards to students in biomedical research training programs.

House-Senate conferees drafted (H Rept 94-1005) a final version April 2. They dropped Senate provisions authorizing a separate program to combat sickle cell anemia, which caused genetic disorders in blacks. They accepted the Senate provisions adding an authorization for the student loan program.

These programs were noncontroversial, but an important rider to the bill dealing with vitamin regulation ended a four-year debate. *(See separate story on vitamin regulation, p. 52-A)*

Provisions

As signed into law, HR 7988:

• Extended specific authority to conduct prevention, control and research programs related to heart, lung and blood diseases through fiscal 1977; renamed the National Heart and Lung Institute the National Heart, Lung and Blood Institute to underline the institute's responsibility for programs related to blood diseases and the management of blood resources.

• Authorized the establishment of 10 special research and training centers focusing on heart diseases, 10 centers focusing on lung diseases and 10 on blood diseases.

• Extended a national award program for doctors and scientists in biomedical research training fields through fiscal 1977.

• Authorized HEW to conduct voluntary testing and counseling programs for parents who may carry genetic diseases; required HEW to give special consideration to funding for existing programs to detect sickle cell anemia.

• Authorized HEW to use its general research program authority to support research related to genetic diseases; gave priority to basic research related to sickle cell anemia or Cooley's anemia.

• Authorized HEW to pay stipends to "visiting scientists" who agreed to help universities with large numbers of minority students develop programs in biomedical sciences.

● Extended through fiscal 1976 HEW's authority to make loans to students in the health professions and to award scholarships to medical students headed for practice in physician shortage areas.

Vitamin Regulation

Ending a dispute that started in 1973, Congress moved to narrow the federal government's authority to regulate vitamins and minerals. A biomedical research bill (HR 7988—PL 94-278), cleared April 12, contained the vitamin regulation rider. *(See separate story on other provisions of the biomedical research bill, p. 51-A)*

As enacted, the rider barred the Food and Drug Administration (FDA) from regulating the composition or maximum potency of vitamins, minerals or combinations of these substances unless they were toxic, habit-forming or needed to be administered by a doctor. But the FDA could continue to impose such restrictions on vitamins or minerals used in dietary treatment of certain diseases, those intended for children under age 12 and those taken by pregnant or lactating women.

In return, the bill also gave the FDA the authority in certain circumstances to seize or take other enforcement actions against vitamin and mineral products if they were falsely advertised. The Federal Trade Commission (FTC), however, had a 90-day option to act on FDA-proposed enforcement actions first. The FTC had authority to regulate vitamin advertising under existing law.

The FDA strongly opposed the legislation.

Background

A battle over control of vitamins began in 1973 when the FDA issued regulations designed to protect consumers from what the agency considered the harmful effects of taking large doses of certain vitamins over extended periods of time.

The FDA had been concerned about the $350-million-a-year vitamin industry since 1962, when it first proposed rules to regulate the content and labeling of vitamin and mineral preparations. The agency argued that many of these products were sold in unnecessarily high dosages and that some contained substances not needed for nutrition. It also believed that false medical claims were made for some vitamin and mineral products.

Vitamin manufacturers and health food organizations argued that regulation would destroy consumer freedom of choice and the health food industry.

The regulations proposed in 1973 would have required a prescription for high doses of Vitamins A and D, limited the dietary and medical claims that could be made for certain products, and prohibited certain combinations of vitamin and mineral supplements.

The regulations never took effect, but they set off a massive mail campaign to convince Congress to rein in the FDA's regulatory powers. Congressional offices received an estimated one million letters and cards protesting the FDA regulations.

Legislative Action

The Senate had approved an amendment to a health manpower bill in 1974 that would have restricted vitamin regulation, but that measure died in conference at the end of the year.

In 1975, by a 7-4 vote, the Senate Labor and Public Welfare Committee added the rider to the biomedical research bill (S Rept 94-509) and the Senate approved the bill Dec. 11. The House version contained no comparable provision.

Sens. William Proxmire (D Wis.) and Richard S. Schweiker (R Pa.), chief backers of the amendment, argued that the dosage guidelines issued by the FDA in 1973 were arbitrary and unscientific.

An FDA spokesman complained that the bill would require the FDA to prove that vitamins and minerals in certain dosages or combinations were toxic rather than requiring industry to prove the safety of a product before it was marketed. "It just takes us out of regulating vitamins and minerals," he maintained.

House-Senate conferees generally accepted the Senate proposal (H Rept 94-1005). But they broadened the list of vitamin and mineral products the FDA could continue to regulate. They also stressed that the FDA would retain its authority to regulate the potency of vitamins in conventional foods such as milk or bread and products that simulated conventional foods or were promoted as the sole item of a meal.

Indian Health Care

Congress Sept. 16 ended a three-year, bipartisan campaign to improve federal health programs for Indians, clearing legislation (S 522—PL 94-437) authorizing a $480-million increase in spending for Indian health activities through fiscal 1980.

The bill created new scholarship programs for Indians seeking training in health care professions, upgraded health services available to Indians and provided support for construction of health facilities and water and sewer systems serving Indians. The measure, which also was directed at Alaskan natives, set up special health programs for Indians in urban areas.

The Department of Health, Education and Welfare (HEW) maintained that it could fulfill the bill's goals without new legislation. But Republicans as well as Democrats gave the proposal their warm support. Chief Republican supporters included House Minority Leader John J. Rhodes (Ariz.).

As passed originally by the Senate in 1974 and 1975, the bill laid out a seven-year program. The 1975 Senate version (S Rept 94-133), passed May 16, authorized a total of $1.6-billion in fiscal 1977-83.

While still envisioning a seven-year program, the House July 30 reduced funding to $475-million in fiscal 1978-80 (H Rept 94-1026). The Senate accepted the House version.

Major Provisions

As signed into law, S 522:

● Authorized the Department of Health, Education and Welfare (HEW) to support programs to recruit Indians interested in attending health professional schools and to provide two-year scholarships for the pre-professional college training of such students.

● Created a scholarship program for Indian students attending health professional schools to be run in conjunction with other health scholarship programs; required Indians receiving scholarships to repay their support with service in the Indian Health Service or in a private practice serving Indians.

● Provided stipends for the summer employment of Indian scholarship students in the Indian Health Service.

● Provided continuing education allowances for professionals employed by the Indian Health Service.

● Increased funding available to the Indian Health Service for the provision of patient care, field health care, dental care, mental health, alcoholism treatment and general maintenance of the service.

● Increased funding available for the construction and renovation of Indian Health Service hospitals, clinics and staff housing; provided separate funding for the construction of safe water supply and waste disposal systems for Indians.

● Allowed HEW to give preference to Indian-controlled businesses for construction projects.

● Allowed Indians to get federal reimbursement under the Medicare and Medicaid programs for care provided at Indian Health Service facilities; required substandard facilities to use their reimbursements to improve conditions.

● Required HEW to enter into contracts with Indian organizations to meet the health care needs of urban Indians.

● Required HEW to study the feasibility of establishing a medical school solely for Indians.

Authorizations

As signed into law, S 522 authorized the following amounts in fiscal 1978-80 plus open-ended sums in fiscal 1981-84:

	Fiscal 1978	Fiscal 1979	Fiscal 1980
	(figures in thousands of dollars)		
Indian Health Manpower			
Recruitment	$ 900	$ 1,500	$ 1,800
College scholarships	800	1,000	1,300
Professional school scholarships	5,450	6,300	7,200
Summer intern stipends	600	800	1,000
Continuing education allowances	100	200	250
Health Services			
Patient care	10,025*	8,500	16,200
Field health	*	3,350	5,550
Dental care	*	1,500	1,500
Mental health	*	3,400	5,075
Maintenance and repair	*	3,000	4,000
Alcoholism	4,000	9,000	9,200
Health Facilities Construction and Renovation			
Hospitals	67,180	73,256	49,742
Health centers	6,960	6,226	3,720
Staff housing	1,242	21,725	4,116
Water and waste disposal facilities	43,000	30,000	30,000
Services for Urban Indians	5,000	10,000	15,000
TOTAL	$145,257	$179,757	$155,653

The $10-million is authorized as a total amount for the first five categories of service in fiscal 1978; alcoholism funding is separate.

● Required HEW, by Dec. 31, 1979, to recommend to Congress additional authorizations for the Indian health programs in fiscal 1981-84.

Alcoholism Programs

Congress voted June 29 to continue special federal programs for the prevention and treatment of alcoholism. Regular funding authority for the programs was set to expire the following day.

Legislation (S 3184—PL 94-371) sent to the President after routine final approval authorized a total of $600.5-million in fiscal 1977-79 to help the estimated 10 million alcoholics and problem drinkers in the United States. The bill also continued special grants for states whose laws treated alcoholism as a medical problem, not criminal behavior. Twenty-seven states had adopted such laws as of early 1976.

Congress also asked the administration to pay special attention to the growing numbers of female and teenage alcoholics.

The final funding figure—decided by House-Senate conferees (H Rept 94-1285)—was a compromise between the $755-million approved by the Senate March 29 (S Rept 94-705) and the $481.5-million authorization passed by the House May 21 (H Rept 94-1092).

The administration had proposed to make the programs covered by the bill part of a new health block grant system.

Provisions

As signed into law, S 3184:

● Authorized $70-million in fiscal 1977, $77-million in fiscal 1978 and $85-million in fiscal 1979 for formula grants to the states for the prevention and treatment of alcoholism.

● Authorized $85-million in fiscal 1977, $91-million in fiscal 1978 and $102.5-million in fiscal 1979 for project grants for the prevention and treatment of alcoholism and for special grants to states that had adopted a model statute designed to treat alcoholism as a disease, not a criminal offense.

● Increased the maximum annual grant to a state that had adopted the model statute to $150,000 plus 20 per cent of its basic formula allotment from a previous maximum of $100,000 plus 10 per cent of the formula allotment.

● Required states to survey the need for the prevention and treatment of alcoholism in women and teenagers; required states to assess their progress under the program every three years.

● Required the Department of Health, Education and Welfare (HEW) to give special consideration to project grant applications for programs designed to prevent and treat alcoholism in women and teenagers.

● Specifically authorized the National Institute on Alcohol Abuse and Alcoholism to conduct research related to alcoholism and alcohol abuse; authorized $20-million in fiscal 1977, $24-million in fiscal 1978 and $28-million in fiscal 1979 for such research.

● Authorized $6-million in each of fiscal 1977-79 to support outside centers coordinating research and training programs related to alcoholism; limited the maximum annual grant to any center to $1-million.

● Barred discrimination against patients with alcohol problems in outpatient clinics, as well as hospitals; ordered HEW to issue regulations implementing the ban on discrimination by Dec. 31, 1976.

Emergency Medical Services

Congress Oct. 1 granted a three-year extension of federal support for 300 local systems providing emergency treatment for accident victims and other patients.

As cleared, the popular legislation (S 2548—PL 94-573) authorized $215-million in fiscal 1977-79 to continue emergency medical services programs begun in 1973. These programs had expired June 30. The bill also authorized $22.5-million over the same period to fund a new burn injury treatment program. *(1973 action, p. 7-A)*

The bill made changes in the existing programs that were designed to ensure that emergency medical systems would continue to exist once federal funding ran out. It also took steps to improve coordination between various emergency medical programs and to heighten emphasis on the training of doctors in emergency medicine.

Because differences between the House and Senate versions of the bill were not too substantial, sponsors drew up a final version without a formal conference.

Compromise Agreement

The compromise agreement generally accepted Senate provisions attempting to assure the continued existence of a local emergency medical treatment program once it had reached the end of its five-year federal funding cycle. The Senate version (S Rept 94-889), approved June 10, required the emergency systems to get detailed promises of continued support from local governments in order to qualify for federal grants in the third through fifth years of assistance. The House bill (H Rept 94-1089), passed Aug. 24, contained no comparable provisions.

The other major difference between the two versions centered on training programs in emergency medicine. The Senate included this funding in the emergency medical services bill while the House added it to a health manpower measure (HR 5546). The Senate version also reserved specific funding for the training of doctors in emergency medicine.

Under the compromise agreement, the training money was included in the emergency medical bill. The agreement reserved 30 per cent of available funds for physician training.

Provisions

As signed into law, S 2548:

• Continued support for emergency medical services, training and research programs through fiscal 1979.

• Authorized the Department of Health, Education and Welfare (HEW) to make a second annual grant for planning in order to study use of advanced life-support techniques or to improve services in rural or inner-city areas.

• Required an emergency medical system seeking a first annual grant for establishment and initial operation to assure HEW that it has the support of volunteer groups and local governments; required a system seeking a second such grant or grants for expansion and improvement to provide detailed assurances that local governments would continue to support the system.

• Clarified the list of required components of an emergency medical system.

• Required greater coordination of emergency medical treatment programs.

• Earmarked 30 per cent of training funds for the training of doctors in emergency care fields.

Authorizations

As signed into law, S 2548 authorized the following amounts in fiscal 1977-79 *(in millions of dollars):*

	Fiscal 1977	Fiscal 1978	Fiscal 1979
Development of emergency medical systems	$45	$55	$70
Research in emergency medicine	5	5	5
Training in emergency medicine	10	10	10
Burn injury program	5	7.5	10
Total	**$65**	**$77.5**	**$95**

• Authorized HEW to support research, training and treatment programs dealing with burn injuries; gave priority for grants to proposed burn injury programs in areas without such services.

• Extended the life of the National Commission for the Protection of Human Subjects of Biomedical and Behavioral Research for one year, through Dec. 31, 1977.

Arthritis, Diabetes Research

Acting on one last health bill before adjournment, Congress Oct. 1 quickly cleared legislation (S 2910—PL 94-562) extending research and training programs dealing with arthritis and diabetes through fiscal 1979. The programs were created in 1974. *(p. 26-A)*

The bill authorized a total of $128.5-million in fiscal 1977-79 to run the arthritis and diabetes programs, to set up national advisory boards on these two diseases and to establish a national commission to draw up a plan for a coordinated attack on digestive diseases such as gallstones and liver diseases.

The Senate passed the bill Oct. 1 by voice vote without waiting for formal committee approval.

The House cleared the measure by accepting the Senate version without change later the same day by voice vote.

Drug Regulation

The Food and Drug Administration (FDA) continued to draw criticism from Congress and consumer activists dissatisfied with its drug approval procedures.

Sen. Edward M. Kennedy (D Mass.) held follow-up hearings on charges first publicized by two subcommittees in 1974 that the FDA often was swayed by industry pressures to approve new drugs for marketing and had punished employees who resisted those pressures.

Kennedy and other critics were unconvinced that the charges had been adequately investigated. A second report on the charges, issued by a Department of Health, Education and Welfare panel, called for further investigation—so yet another report was expected in 1977.

The agency also was criticized during the year for relying too heavily on advisory panels in an effort to escape responsibility for hard decisions, and for laxity in supervising testing of new drugs.

Hearings and preliminary discussions got underway in the House and Senate on proposed legislation to require more detailed labeling of prescription drugs and increase the FDA's power to halt sales of potentially dangerous drugs and food additives.

Clinical Laboratories

Congress ran out of time at the end of the session to finish action on legislation giving the federal government authority to set stiffer standards for medical laboratories. Sponsors were expected to revive the bill in 1977.

The legislation was a response to growing congressional concern about lab test errors, sloppy procedures, rising costs and evidence of fraud.

Nationally, federal officials estimated that perhaps 15 per cent of the five billion lab tests performed each year yielded inaccurate results. Increasing reliance on such tests boosted the national bill for lab work to $12-billion in 1975.

The Department of Health, Education and Welfare (HEW) had authority to regulate some labs under two existing laws. Under Medicare and Medicaid, the government technically set standards for about 10,000 hospital and independent labs. But critics contended that enforcement of these standards by the states or accreditation organizations had been lax.

Under a 1967 law, HEW's Center for Disease Control licensed about 1,000 other labs—those engaged in interstate commerce. Sponsors of the legislation rated this program as competent, but charged HEW with poor coordination of its two regulatory programs.

In addition, some states set standards for nearly 5,000 other labs not covered by the two programs and an estimated 50,000 to 80,000 labs in doctors' offices. But sponsors of the legislation argued that only five states had adequate regulatory programs, while 26 states set no requirements for lab performance.

Senate Action

The Senate passed its version of the bill (S 1737—S Rept 94-764) April 29. The legislation had bipartisan support.

Basic provisions of the bill allowed the federal government to use licensing procedures to set standards for lab performance, quality control procedures and competence of lab personnel. HEW was empowered to revoke or suspend the license of labs that violated the standards or those found guilty of fraud. A Senate committee report had suggested that fraud and abuse cost the taxpayers an extra $1 for every $4 paid under Medicare and Medicaid for lab services.

The bill allowed the states to take over licensing procedures if they set requirements as strict as those required by HEW. The measure also exempted rural labs and labs in doctors' offices from regulation under some circumstances.

House Action

The House Interstate and Foreign Commerce Committee reported its labs bill (HR 14319—H Rept 94-1484) on Sept. 8. The committee version followed the outlines of the Senate bill, although it contained some differences of detail.

The committee also beefed up the anti-fraud provisions of the Senate version.

But the House rejected the bill, 193-188, on Sept. 20 under the suspension of the rules procedure requiring a two-thirds vote for passage. Dissatisfaction with the suspension procedure (which allowed no amendments), conservative opposition to more regulation by the federal bureaucracy, and fears about the impact of the measure in rural areas contributed to the bill's defeat.

The bill had been scheduled to come up for action again under regular procedures requiring only majority approval, but it never made it to the floor before Congress adjourned Oct. 2.

Health Block Grants

Congress greeted a Ford administration proposal to combine funding for many health programs with legislative disinterest and partisan opposition. The proposal did not even get a committee hearing in either house.

The Ford plan would have combined 15 categorical health programs and the Medicaid program for the poor into a single system giving the states health "block grants." The categorical programs included most health services programs, disease control programs and the health planning program created by Congress in 1974.

President Ford argued that the plan would give the states more flexibility in their use of federal health dollars and streamline the federal bureaucracy. Administration officials also maintained that the plan would eliminate a lot of federal red tape.

Congressional opponents of the plan argued that the plan would reduce funding available for health services for the sick and poor because the uncontrollable Medicaid program would eat up most of the money the administration proposed to make available for the block grants. While in favor of gaining more control over health funds, state and local groups also expressed concern because the proposal would force them to absorb Medicaid costs beyond what the administration proposed to pay.

Administration officials used the proposal during the campaign as an example of how President Ford wanted to trim the federal bureaucracy. But the White House did not seriously push for the measure on Capitol Hill in the face of widespread support for the categorical health programs. Congress routinely extended many of the programs that would have been covered by the proposal.

Veterans' Medical Care

Congress approved legislation (HR 2735 — PL 94-581), the Veterans' Omnibus Health Care Act of 1976, giving veterans with service-connected medical problems priority consideration in outpatient care over veterans with non-service-connected medical problems.

Related legislation (S 2908) initially was reported by the Senate Veterans' Affairs Committee (S Rept 94-1206). A minor House-passed bill (HR 2735) then was considered and amended to contain the language of S 2908, and HR 2735, as amended by the committee was passed by the Senate Sept. 16 and returned to the House.

On Sept. 29 the House passed the bill a second time after deleting from the Senate version programs for treatment of alcohol and drug abuse, preventive health care and readjustment counseling. The Senate Oct. 1 concurred in the House amendments, completing action on the bill.

Provisions. As signed into law, HR 2735 (PL 94-581):

● Established by statute priority in outpatient care for service-connected medical problems over non-service-connected problems.

● Authorized comprehensive VA health care benefits for any veteran with a service-connected disability rated at 50 per cent or more (lowered from 80 per cent under existing law).

● Provided certain counseling, training and mental health services to the families of veterans being treated for service-connected conditions when such services were essential for a veteran's treatment.

● Authorized the VA as part of a national immunization program to provide immunization to veterans receiving treatment in VA hospitals.

Medicare-Medicaid

Despite sweeping proposals by President Ford and influential members of the Senate Finance Committee, and reports of widespread abuses in the Medicaid program, Congress made only minor changes in Medicare and Medicaid in 1976.

Medicare

Congress July 1 cleared a bill (HR 13501—PL 94-368) that permanently barred any reduction in federal reimbursement rates to physicians below fiscal 1975 levels, delayed changes in reimbursements for doctors in teaching hospitals until Oct. 1, 1977, and required the government to continue to update allowable reimbursement rates on July 1 of each year rather than the start of the fiscal year which was changed to Oct. 1. A 1975 law (PL 94-182) had prevented a rollback in fiscal 1975 rates during 1976 for physicians caring for the aged in the Medicare program.

The House passed HR 13501 May 13 by voice vote (H Rept 94-1114). The Senate passed an amended version by voice vote June 30 (S Rept 94-993). The Senate dropped its changes July 1, clearing the measure.

Inspector General

In the wake of persistent reports of abuses in the Medicaid health program for the poor, Congress completed action Sept. 29 on a bill (HR 11347—PL 94-505) aimed at controlling fraud and abuse in programs run by the Department of Health, Education and Welfare (HEW). It established an Office of Inspector General in the department to carry out investigation and audit activities dealing with all departmental programs. The inspector general was to set up a special staff to handle investigations of Medicaid, Medicare and other health programs. The final provisions, added to a minor tax bill, were derived from separate measures passed by the House and Senate.

Congressional action came several weeks after Sen. Frank E. Moss (D Utah), chairman of the Long-Term Care Subcommittee of the Special Committee on Aging, estimated after a dramatic investigation that fraud and abuse ate up $1.8-billion of the $15-billion-a-year Medicare program.

1977

The Carter administration showed no lack of initiative in proposing health programs in 1977 and promised there would be more to come. Within weeks of assuming office, the new secretary of Health, Education and Welfare (HEW), Joseph A. Califano Jr., mobilized his massive agency to deal with one of the nation's major social problems — the skyrocketing cost of hospital care.

However, Congress moved slowly on the Carter hospital cost cap proposal and by the end of the session, only one of the four committees with jurisdiction over the legislation had reported it.

On Sept. 26, HEW proposed a set of guidelines for local health planning agencies that were patterned after some of the provisions in the cost control bill. The guidelines would limit the number of acute care hospital beds and restrict certain types of medical procedures and care. In early November, HEW moved on another front to control costs by announcing that Medicare would start paying for second opinions before surgery was done, and urging that all Americans obtain a second opinion before surgery. Critics had charged that much of the surgery performed in the United States was unnecessary as well as costly.

Although the lack of congressional action on cost control had a delaying effect on national health insurance proposals, the two federal health programs, Medicare and Medicaid, figured prominently in health news in 1977. Congress easily passed HR 3, a bill it had been working on for several years, aimed at curbing fraud and abuse in the two programs.

In other action, Congress passed legislation that delayed a proposed ban on the controversial artificial sweetener, saccharin. Also cleared was a bill easing the requirement that U.S. medical schools must admit a certain number of American citizens studying medicine abroad to their third-year classes in order to qualify for federal aid. Responding to the apparent shortage of doctors in rural areas, Congress cleared a bill intended to increase the supply of medical practitioners in areas that lacked adequate health care facilities.

Unresolved at the end of the session were several issues, including proposed controls on research using recombinant DNA (deoxyribonucleic acid). Also in abeyance was the extension of major federal health programs; Congress passed a temporary, one-year authorization, with a view to examining and revising the programs at a later date.

Hospital Cost Control

President Carter's hospital cost control legislation, proposed in an April 25, 1977, message to Congress, was viewed by the administration as a first major step in controlling soaring health care costs. However, by the end of the first year, only one of four committees with jurisdiction over the measure had acted on it. The hospital industry had strongly opposed mandatory controls, and many members of Congress were unenthusiastic about the legislation.

Continued opposition to his plan led even President Carter to declare it unpassable in mid-1978. Toward the end of the session, however, the Senate unexpectedly approved a compromise version. But the measure never reached the House floor, and died with adjournment.

In 1979, the House effectively killed the Carter plan when it approved a bill that eliminated cost controls altogether and merely established a study commission on the problem. *(Details, see Hospital Cost Control chapter)*

Health Programs Extension

President Carter Aug. 1, 1977, signed into law (PL 95-83) a one-year extension of major federal health programs, authorizing $3.4 billion for health planning, biomedical research and a variety of health services programs in fiscal 1978.

The routine extension was sought in order to meet the reporting requirements of the congressional budget act. During 1978, the appropriate congressional committees examined the programs closely with an eye to revising them before granting a longer extension. *(1978 action on health planning systems, p. 66-A; 1978 action on biomedical research and mental health programs, p. 64-A; 1978 action on health services, p. 64-A; 1978 action on family planning and sudden infant death syndrome programs, p. 65-A. See also Health Planning chapter)*

The largest single amount authorized by the bill (HR 4975) was $1 billion for cancer control and research programs. *(Authorizations box, this page)*

The House had passed three separate extension measures by wide margins March 21; the Senate combined them before approving the bill by a 92-1 vote May 4.

The three House bills (HR 4974 — H Rept 95-116, HR 4975 — H Rept 95-117, HR 4976 — H Rept 95-118) were reported from the House Interstate and Foreign Commerce Committee March 26. As recommended by the committee and passed by the House, authorization levels for the biomedical research and most of the health services programs were simply raised 15 per cent above the actual fiscal 1977 appropriations for the programs. Because they were new, the health planning programs were authorized at a higher level — the same as the fiscal 1977 authorization level.

The bill (HR 4975 — S Rept 95-102) reported by the Senate Human Resources Committee April 26 set most of the authorizations at 20 per cent above the fiscal 1977 appropriations.

Conferees filed their report July 14 (H Rept 95-500, S Rept 95-349), after resolving all major disagreements over authorization levels by approving figures halfway between the higher and lower amounts. The Senate adopted the report by voice vote July 15, and the House cleared the measure July 20.

Medicare, Medicaid Fraud

Congress moved to clean up fraud and abuse in the Medicare and Medicaid programs in 1977 when it cleared HR 3 Oct. 13.

The bill (PL 95-142) was a result of three years of congressional consideration, following discovery by federal and state investigators that kickbacks, fraudulent billings, unnecessary medical treatment and other problems were occurring in the federal health programs. The

Health Programs Authorization

As signed into law Aug. 1, 1977, HR 4975 authorized the following amounts for fiscal 1978 *(in millions of dollars):*

Health Planning	$176.00
Resources Development	322.50
Health Services Research	28.60
Health Statistics	33.60
Total, Health Planning	560.70
Medical Libraries	14.60
Cancer Programs	1,008.15
Heart, Blood Vessel, Lung and Blood Disease Programs	456.32
National Research Service Awards	161.39
Total, Biomedical Research	1,640.46
Grants to states for comprehensive health services	106.75
Hypertension programs	12.68
Migrant health centers	39.26
Community health centers	262.72
Family planning	208.50
Sudden infant death syndrome programs	3.65
Hemophilia programs	4.55
Blood separation centers	3.45
Community mental health centers	102.70
Maternal and child health programs	399.90
Home health services	12.00
Total, Health Services	1,156.10
Grand Total, all programs	**$3,357.28**

Department of Health, Education and Welfare (HEW) estimated that these abuses cost the government close to $900 million a year.

The bill increased penalties for fraud and abuse, strengthened the oversight responsibilities of professional standards review organizations (PSROs), required more ownership information from program providers and made other administrative changes.

Herman E. Talmadge (D Ga.), chairman of the Senate Finance Subcommittee on Health, described the bill as "a clear and loud signal to the thieves and the crooks and the abusers that we mean to call a halt to their exploitation of the public and the public purse."

The bill was seen by many members as a necessary forerunner of national health insurance. As Al Ullman (D Ore.), chairman of the House Ways and Means Committee, said, "This legislation represents an important step toward getting our health financing programs under control. We should take this first step now, before we are called upon to consider major changes in the nation's health care financing policy." *(See National Health Insurance chapter)*

Background and Legislative Action

With the cost of Medicare and Medicaid continually rising — they were estimated to cost $47 billion in fiscal 1977 — Congress set out in 1975 to cut back on some of the illegal practices. However, only minor changes were made in the Medicare program during 1976 and major revisions were postponed until the 95th Congress.

In its July 12 report on HR 3 (H Rept 95-393, Part

II), the House Commerce Committee detailed the numerous instances of fraud in shared health facilities, clinical laboratories, nursing homes and activities by independent practitioners. (The Ways and Means Committee, which shared jurisdiction over the legislation, filed Part I of H Rept 95-393 on June 7.)

The shared health facilities, some of which were known as "Medicaid mills," had been involved in some of the "more flagrant" activities, the Commerce Committee said. Many were set up in storefronts in poor areas and staffed by foreign-educated physicians, who were forced to split much of their income with the owners of the mills under complicated lease and fee arrangements. The facilities relied on heavy volume, and violations included unnecessary referral of patients to other physicians in the facility, filing of claims for family members who accompanied a patient or for services not rendered, and kickbacks.

"Factoring" was also still a problem in these facilities, although it was banned in 1972. Under factoring, physicians and institutions providing services reimbursable under Medicare and Medicaid sold their receivables to organizations called factoring agencies. The receivables (money owed to the doctor or institution) were sold for a percentage of their face value and the factoring agency collected from the government.

Although factoring was outlawed by the Social Security Amendments of 1972 (PL 92-603), the committee said the law was circumvented through use of powers of attorney.

The committee said kickbacks were one of the main problems with clinical laboratories, which entered into such arrangements to receive Medicaid business. The kickbacks took the form of cash, gifts, long-term credit and other arrangements. Some labs also "rented" small offices in medical clinics for exorbitant fees.

Such activities occurred in nursing homes as well. In addition, some homes misrepresented costs, juggled their accounting procedures to make auditing impossible and were involved in collusion with their suppliers, the report said. The committee said there was much less fraud and abuse among individual practitioners than in institutions.

Differences between the House version, passed by a 362-5 vote Sept. 23, and the Senate version (S 143 — S Rept 95-453), passed by voice vote Sept. 30, were generally over details. A provision concerning the confidentiality of medical records was controversial during House committee consideration, but never came up on the House floor and was not in the Senate bill. Both the House and Senate adopted the conference report (H Rept 95-673) on HR 3 Oct. 13.

Provisions

As signed into law, HR 3 included the following major provisions:

● Upgraded most existing misdemeanors for fraud against the Medicare and Medicaid programs to felonies; increased penalties to $25,000 in fines, five years in prison or both, from $10,000 and one year in prison.

● Allowed states to suspend Medicaid recipients convicted of defrauding the program.

● Required the HEW secretary to suspend from the two programs any doctor or other practitioner convicted of a criminal offense related to the program and to notify the appropriate state licensing agency about the suspension.

Abortion Riders Added To Several Bills

The continuing controversy over the questions whether and when to provide federal funds for abortion — issues that had surfaced in the early 1970s — continued to rage in the latter part of the decade.

For half of 1977, Congress hotly debated whether to permit the use of Medicaid funds for abortions for low-income women. Passage of a $60 billion appropriations bill for the Departments of Labor and Health, Education and Welfare (HEW) was held up until December while Congress haggled over the conditions under which federally funded abortions would be allowed. After months of negotiations and roll-call votes, Congress finally agreed on a provision that would permit Medicaid abortions when the mother's life was endangered or when two doctors certified that severe and long-lasting physical health damage would result from continued pregnancy. The compromise also permitted "medical procedures" for victims of rape or incest, if the offense were reported promptly to police or to a public health agency.

Though the final 1977 abortion provision was less restrictive than one passed in 1976, "pro-choice" supporters complained that their side had done all the compromising during the long stalemate.

The following year, anti-abortion forces in the House broadened their efforts to put tighter restrictions on the use of federal funds to pay for abortions — with several notable successes.

Their biggest victory in 1978 was attaching abortion restrictions to the fiscal 1979 appropriations bill for the Department of Defense, which in 1977 funded about 26,500 abortions for military personnel and dependents. Congress also prohibited the use of Peace Corps funds to pay for abortions for Peace Corps volunteers. Similar restrictions on abortions for low-income women were finally attached to the appropriations bill for the Departments of Labor and HEW. In addition, House anti-abortion activists successfully delayed action on family planning, health planning and pregnancy disability bills during the year.

In 1979, Congress wrestled with the issue of federally funded abortions as never before when the House added strong anti-abortion language to six fiscal 1980 appropriations bills and two continuing appropriations resolutions. After a protracted battle over one of these, the Senate finally accepted language that was essentially the tough House position on the emotional issue. As in 1977, the language permitted Medicaid funding of abortions only when required to save the mother's life or in cases of rape or incest that were promptly reported to a law enforcement or public health agency. Dropped was a provision contained in 1977 legislation that would permit an abortion if the mother's health were endangered. The House also added anti-abortion provisions to two authorization bills — the Department of Education and the Child Health Assurance Program, but conferees dropped the provision from the education bill. *(See Child Health Programs chapter)*

• Required providers of services under the programs to name any person owning five per cent or greater interest; required owners to provide similar information for any subcontractor of which a provider owned more than five per cent.

• Extended the conditional designation period for local PSROs to 48 months from the existing 24 months; allowed an additional 24 months in unusual circumstances; provided that the HEW secretary give priority to PSRO requests to review care provided in shared health facilities; increased the authority of the states in establishing and evaluating PSROs.

• Provided federal funding to states for fiscal 1977 through fiscal 1980 to finance up to 90 per cent of the cost of establishing and operating a separate office to prosecute cases of suspected Medicaid fraud, up to a $500,000 limit.

• Required states to ensure that 90 per cent of Medicaid claims submitted by practitioners in individual or group practice or shared health facilities be reimbursed within 30 days and 99 per cent within 90 days, effective July 1, 1978.

• Prohibited use of powers of attorney by providers to pool Medicare and Medicaid claims in illegal "factoring" arrangements.

Clinical Lab Standards

A bill (S 705) strengthening federal regulations for clinical laboratories passed the Senate in July 1977, but the House took no action on the legislation that year. Although two House committees reported a bill in 1978 similar to the Senate-passed version, it never came to the floor and the measure died at the end of the session. *(1978 action, p. 71-A)*

The Senate had passed a clinical lab regulation bill in April 1976. A House bill was reported but was not acted on in the 94th Congress. *(1976 chronology, p. 55-A)* Congressional action to set federal standards for the quality of laboratory work resulted from reports of startlingly high error rates in laboratory work on even the simplest of blood tests, and from a number of malpractice suits stemming from deaths or serious injury incurred as a result of faulty laboratory work. The error rate for results from some laboratories ranged as high as 25 per cent, one of every four tests performed, according to the Department of Health, Education and Welfare (HEW).

Under the laws authorizing the Medicare program, HEW was responsible for accrediting and regulating the approximately 10,000 clinical laboratories that received funds under that program. The Clinical Laboratories Improvement Act (PL 90-174) placed another 950 laboratories under federal supervision, specifically under the authority of the Center for Disease Control (CDC).

The lack of uniformity in the standards set out by the two accrediting and regulatory agencies was in part responsible for the ineffectiveness of the federal regulatory scheme, in the view of the Senate Human Resources Committee. Furthermore, as many as 55,000 to 85,000 laboratories — in hospitals, independently run, and in doctor's offices — were not subject to any federal control.

Many of these, according to the committee, had never been inspected or performance-tested. Some used broken and dirty equipment; others employed inexperienced personnel.

Immunization Program

A crash program to immunize American children against major childhood diseases was announced by Health, Education and Welfare Secretary Joseph A. Califano Jr. April 6, 1977.

Califano termed "shocking" the lack of a coherent national immunization policy. He said almost 40 per cent of the 52 million American children under 15 had not been vaccinated against such diseases as polio, measles, German measles, mumps, whooping cough, diphtheria and tetanus.

Of the estimated 20 million unvaccinated children, 13 million came from lower-income families, 7 million from upper-income homes, Califano said. The goal of the new program was to immunize more than 90 per cent of U.S. children by 1979.

As outlined by Califano, the program would be local, rather than federal, in emphasis. It would use the $19 million included in the fiscal 1978 federal budget for immunization programs as "leverage" to train immunization personnel, provide technical assistance to local health agencies, buy vaccines, set up a permanent immunization system and reacquaint parents and community groups with the critical necessity for preventive immunization.

Some health experts said the absence of epidemics in recent years had caused parents and health professionals to be apathetic about vaccinations.

Attention had been focused on the immunization problem earlier in the year, when the Center for Disease Control (CDC) reported a 62 per cent increase in measles cases in the first three months of 1977 as compared to the same period in 1976.

Senate Action

The Senate Human Resources Committee reported S 705 (S Rept 95-360) July 22, and the Senate passed the bill July 28 by voice vote and without change.

S 705 authorized $16 million a year for carrying out the provisions of the act. It authorized the HEW secretary to establish national standards to ensure accurate and reliable testing by clinical laboratories and required that those standards include adequate quality control procedures in each laboratory, proper maintenance of records, equipment and facilities, and adequate proficiency of employees. The bill further created a new office within HEW, called the Office of Clinical Laboratories, to license all labs in the United States except those under the jurisdiction of the Department of Defense and Veterans Administration.

Although he supported the concept of uniform clinical lab standards, HEW Secretary Joseph A. Califano Jr. said he opposed establishment of a new agency to enforce them.

Rural Health Clinics

A bill designed to improve health care services in medically underserved rural areas was cleared by Congress Nov. 29 and signed into law Dec. 13, 1977 (HR 8422 — PL 95-210).

The bill extended Medicare and Medicaid reimbursement to services provided by nurse practitioners and physician assistants in rural health clinics, which often were the only source of medical care in doctor-shortage areas. It also provided for demonstration projects in which selected clinics in medically underserved urban areas would be reimbursed for services provided by the specially trained paraprofessionals. *(Related action on health planning guidelines, p. 61-A)*

Under existing law, only medical services provided by physicians could, in most cases, be reimbursed by the federal health programs for the elderly and the poor. *(Further details, Rural Health Care chapter)*

Proponents of the bill said it was needed to encourage the development and utilization of rural health clincs and to keep some existing clinics from going broke. Without Medicare or Medicaid coverage of clinic services, many rural residents either did not get adequate care, had to pay for it themselves despite financial hardship or had to be treated as bad debts by the clinics, the bill's sponsors said. Financial problems had forced some clinics to close and threatened the existence of others, they noted.

About half of the 3,000 U.S. counties and numerous subcounty areas were officially classified as medically underserved, Robert Dole (R Kan.) told the Senate Nov. 29. William D. Hathaway (D Maine) said HR 8422 "has the potential of assisting 31.6 million Americans who live in small towns and rural areas which are medically underserved."

The Congressional Budget Office estimated the cost of the bill at about $118 million in fiscal 1978, rising to $164 million in fiscal 1982.

Background

Clinics operated by trained paraprofessionals had grown up in areas that could not attract or keep a doctor. They were generally under the supervision of a physician, although in many cases the supervision was long-distance, such as in the case of "satellite" clinics in rural areas set up by doctors in a nearby urban area.

In other, more populated communities that could support a full-time physician, doctors often used paraprofessionals to provide many medical services, easing the burden of a heavy patient load.

Because Medicare reimbursed for medical services only if they were provided by a physician, and two-thirds of state Medicaid plans had similar restrictions, many elderly and low-income persons could not pay for clinic services, creating serious financial problems for the clinics.

In Appalachia, some clinics had received special grants from the Appalachian Regional Commission to help meet their costs, but the grants were due to expire shortly.

Legislative History

Because jurisdiction over Medicare and Medicaid was split, the bill was reported (H Rept 95-548) by both the House Ways and Means Committee (Part I, July 29) and the House Interstate and Foreign Commerce Committee (Part II, Sept. 19).

The bill passed by the House Oct. 17 by voice vote included all of the Medicare reimbursement provisions reported by the Ways and Means Committee and the Medicaid reimbursement provisions added by the Commerce Committee.

The Senate passed a similar version of HR 8422 Oct. 19 by voice vote. Both chambers adopted the conference report (H Rept 95-790) by voice votes Nov. 29.

Major Provisions

As cleared by Congress, HR 8422:

● Authorized Medicare reimbursement for direct medical care provided in rural health clinics by nurse practitioners and physician's assistants.

● Defined direct medical care as services provided by nurse practitioners (including nurse midwives) and physician's assistants that would be reimbursable if provided by a physician.

● Also covered part-time or intermittent nursing care and related medical supplies furnished to a homebound individual by a rural health clinic located in an area with a shortage of home health agencies.

● Required rural health clinics, to be eligible, to be directed by a physician or to have an arrangement with one or more physicians to review periodically the services furnished by the paraprofessionals, supervise and guide them, prepare necessary medical orders for patient treatment and be available for referral, consultation or emergency aid or advice.

● Required clinics to maintain clinical records on all patients, have an arrangement with one or more referral hospitals, provide routine diagnostic services and have prompt access to certified facilities for more complicated diagnostic services, provide drugs and biologicals that the secretary of Health, Education and Welfare (HEW) determined were necessary to treat emergencies, have appropriate procedures to review utilization of services, and meet any other requirements determined by the secretary to be in the interest of the health and safety of clinic patients.

● Required that, to be eligible, a clinic must be located in an area that is not urbanized and is designated by HEW as having a medically underserved population or a shortage of primary medical care personnel. Rural clinics not in those designated areas could be eligible if the secretary determined the supply of physicians in the area was insufficient.

● Required nurse practitioners and physician's assistants to meet the legal requirements of the state in which they practice and whatever training, education and experience requirements HEW established.

● Required all states that authorized medical practice by nurse practitioners and physician's assistants to reimburse Medicaid services performed in rural health clinics.

● Authorized the National Institute of Occupational Safety and Health (NIOSH) to continue its program of obtaining from the Internal Revenue Service the addresses of persons who were previously employed in occupations in which they were exposed to known or suspected occupational hazards.

Foreign Medical Students

Congress Dec. 7, 1977, cleared a bill (HR 9418 — PL 95-215) easing the requirement that U.S. medical schools must admit certain American citizens studying medicine abroad to their third-year classes in order to qualify for federal aid.

A number of top medical schools had said they would give up the aid, known as capitation grants, rather than obey the 1976 law (PL 94-484) that imposed the requirement. They said the law violated their academic freedom to choose their own students.

The bill also removed the 1976 restrictions on the academic standards the schools applied in admitting transfer students. Proponents of the bill said it represented a compromise between the medical schools, which did not want to be forced to accept any students who did not meet their criteria, and those American students attending foreign medical schools who wanted to return to the United States to finish their medical educations.

Background

The provision permitting U.S. students studying medicine abroad to transfer to a U.S. school in their third year had been slipped into the 1976 bill during conference. It was not in either the original House or Senate version.

The new provision became known as the "Guadalajara clause" because of the large number of American students enrolled in it and other foreign medical schools as competition for scarce openings in U.S. medical schools became more intense. The families of those students formed an effective lobby to pressure Congress to allow their children to "come home" and finish their training at generally superior U.S. schools.

The 1976 provision required all U.S. medical schools, in order to qualify for capitation grants, to reserve positions in their third-year classes in school years 1978-79, 1979-80 and 1980-81 for a pool of students that met certain criteria.

Some estimates placed the potential pool of students as high as 1,500, and a number of schools announced in the fall of 1977 that they would rather refuse federal aid than follow the regulations.

Legislative Action

The House Oct. 17 passed a bill (HR 9418 — H Rept 95-707) to loosen the requirement substantially. The Senate version (S 2159 — S Rept 95-545), passed Nov. 4, repealed the transfer provision altogether.

Conferees generally went along with the House version but reduced the percentage by which schools were required to expand their third-year classes and limited the requirement to one school year, 1978-79. The Senate adopted the conference report (H Rept 95-828, S Rept 95-608) Dec. 1; the House adopted it Dec. 7, completing action.

Major Provisions

As cleared by Congress, HR 9418:

● Replaced the medical school third-year enrollment increase requirement of PL 94-484 with a provision requiring medical schools, as a condition of receiving federal capitation grants in fiscal 1978, to increase their third-year class enrollments in the 1978-79 school year by 5 per cent of their 1977-78 first-year or third-year enrollment, whichever was less. Schools could not count in the 5 per cent increase any transfer students who were not U.S. citizens; who came from U.S. medical schools that had third-year places for them, from schools of dentistry or osteopathy, or from unaccredited U.S. medical schools, or who first enrolled in a foreign medical school after Oct. 12, 1976.

Schools could count as transfer students U.S. citizens who enrolled in foreign medical schools before Oct. 12, 1976; students who had successfully completed two years of training in certain two-year medical or other special programs in U.S. schools, and students enrolled in a foreign school before Oct. 1, 1976, but accepted in the second-year class of a U.S. school.

● Allowed the secretary of Health, Education and Welfare to waive the requirement if it threatened a school's accreditation, if the school's clinical facilities were inadequate for a larger class, or if there were insufficient eligible students available.

● Exempted from the requirement schools whose first-year enrollment in 1977-78 exceeded their third-year enrollment by at least 25 per cent.

● Provided that a school that did not receive capitation aid in fiscal 1978 because of failure to comply with the act would also be ineligible for such aid in fiscal 1979 and 1980.

● Provided that students in ineligible schools would still be eligible to receive student loans.

● Exempted certain schools of dentistry from requirements that 70 per cent of their residency programs be in general or children's dentistry.

● Expanded eligibility for public health traineeships to students enrolled in other schools besides schools of public health; increased authorizations for traineeships by $1 million in fiscal 1979 and 1980.

● Made changes in the federally insured loan program for students in health professions schools, including deferral of interest payments, an increase in the maximum interest rate to 12 per cent, from 10 per cent, and the overriding of state usury laws.

Health Planning Guidelines

Upset by proposed national health planning guidelines aimed at eliminating excess hospital beds and services, the House Dec. 6, 1977, unanimously approved a resolution urging that the special needs and problems of rural areas be taken into account in the final version. The resolution (H Con Res 432) was adopted 357-0.

The day before, 42 senators signed a letter to Health, Education and Welfare (HEW) Secretary Joseph A. Califano Jr. endorsing the House position, but the Senate never acted on the resolution.

The sponsor of H Con Res 432, Berkley Bedell (D-Iowa) said he drafted it because of "grave grass-roots concern" that HEW's proposed guidelines would force small rural and community hospitals to close down. Other speakers said the same flexibility called for in H Con Res 432 for rural hospitals should be extended to urban hospitals.

The guidelines published by HEW Sept. 23 were meant to reduce the cost of the U.S. health care system by eliminating excess beds and underused hospital units and limiting specialized procedures to facilities that perform them regularly. The guidelines set a standard of four general hospital beds for each 1,000 persons and required an average annual hospital occupancy rate of 80 percent, two provisions that were part of the Carter hospital cost control package.

If the standards were fully implemented by the 205 local health planning agencies, HEW estimated, 100,000 unnecessary hospital beds could be eliminated. Each one was estimated to cost $80,000 in initial construction expense and $20,000 to $50,000 a year in operating costs, depending on location and type of hospital.

In addition, the guidelines proposed occupancy and patient volume standards for maternity and pediatric services, as well as for open heart surgery, other types of heart procedures and certain radiologic procedures, including the controversial body scans.

HEW admitted that the local health planning agencies would have up to six years to implement the objectives and that under existing law neither HEW nor the health planning agencies had any authority to close down or otherwise enforce the guidelines on existing hospitals. The planning agencies were directed to take them into account in approving any new hospital construction, however.

The guidelines were mandated by the 1974 Health Planning and Resources Development Act (PL 93-641). That act was extended through fiscal 1978 by PL 95-83; a more extensive revision died in 1978. *(See Health Planning chapter)*

Saccharin Ban Delay

Congress Nov. 4, 1977, cleared legislation (S 1750 — PL 95-203) delaying a proposed Food and Drug Administration (FDA) ban on the artificial sweetener saccharin.

The FDA had proposed the ban March 9 because of scientific evidence linking saccharin with an increase risk of bladder cancer. Congress was forced into the issue because of an avalanche of complaints from angry constituents who said they needed saccharin because of illness or obesity. Some members reported receiving more mail and phone calls on this than on any other issue in years.

Congress voted to delay the ban 18 months, pending new studies of saccharin and the whole question of carcinogenicity in food products.

In 1979, the House voted to extend the ban for two more years. Although the Senate took no action on the moratorium, it continued in effect. In June 1980, the Senate concurred in the House moratorium, clearing the bill by voice vote. *(See chapter on Food Law Revision)*

DNA Regulation

Congress appeared ready in early 1977 to place federal controls on research using recombinant DNA (deoxyribonucleic acid). But lobbying by scientists worried about government interference in scientific research derailed the efforts. By late autumn Congress was taking a new look at whether such controls actually were needed, and in 1978 legislation to regulate DNA research was shelved.

DNA research involves taking segments of the genetic material DNA from different organisms and species and putting them back together again in different combinations, thereby creating new forms of life. Such research could result in beneficial new drugs, agricultural products and industrial chemicals.

The call for federal regulation came after several scientists and others expressed fears that there was great potential danger to the public if DNA research proceeded unchecked. *(Details, 1977-78 legislative action, p. 68-A)*

Kidney Dialysis Program

The House passed legislation (HR 8423 — H Rept 95-549) Sept. 12, 1977, aimed at putting a lid on the soaring costs of the federal government's program to aid persons suffering from kidney failure.

Although the Senate Finance Committee did not act on the measure in 1977, it did report a bill in 1978, and Congress cleared a compromise version of the legislation that year. *(Details, 1977-78 action, p. 71-A)*

Child Nutrition Programs

Congress cleared for the President Oct. 28 a bill (HR 1139 — PL 95-166) making changes in the school lunch and some child nutrition programs.

The bill included provisions to curb fraud and abuse in the summer food service program for children, and extended that program through fiscal 1980. It also extended authority for commodity and equipment purchases under the National School Lunch and Child Nutrition Act of 1966, established a new nutrition education program and gave the secretary of Agriculture greater authority to control "junk" foods sold in schools participating in the school lunch and breakfast programs. *(1978 action on related programs, p. 73-A)*

Legislative Action

The House Education and Labor Committee reported HR 1139 (H Rept 95-281) May 10, and it passed the House eight days later by a vote of 393-19.

A companion bill reported by the Senate Agriculture, Nutrition and Forestry Committee June 16 (S 1420 — S Rept 95-277) added several new provisions to the House-passed version, notably a new nutrition education program and authority for the Agriculture secretary to ban sales of "junk" foods — non-nutritious food such as candy, gum and soft drinks.

In considering the bill June 20, the Senate accepted a major amendment to the nutrition education program that changed it from an annual appropriation to a five-year entitlement program before passing and sending the bill to conference.

Major compromises agreed to by the conferees were adoption of the three-year extension of the summer food program as passed by the Senate and the three-year extension of the equipment assistance special fund as passed by the House. Most of the separate provisions passed by both chambers were consolidated in the final version.

Conferees cut the nutrition education program to three years instead of the five passed by the Senate, and required that it be subject to the regular congressional appropriations process in the third year.

They modified the Senate's language on banning junk foods, providing instead that the secretary must approve the competitive foods that would be allowed in schools.

The House agreed to the conference report (H Rept 95-708, S Rept 95-504) Oct. 27. The Senate approved it Oct. 28, completing congressional action.

Provisions

As cleared by Congress, HR 1139 contained the following major provisions:
- Extended the summer food program for three years,

through fiscal 1980, established stricter criteria for sponsoring organizations, such as adequate administrative and financial ability, and added more stringent reporting and administrative requirements.

● Extended for three years the special fund that reserved one-third of equipment assistance to needy schools; required, with some exceptions, that all equipment assistance funds be used for on-site preparation of hot meals.

● Extended for five years the secretary of Agriculture's standby authority under Section 14 of the National School Lunch Act to purchase commodities in case of insufficient supplies from other sources; and required each state to set up an advisory council to coordinate the distribution of federal commodities with local districts.

● Eliminated the extra milk given to certain children participating in the school lunch and breakfast programs.

● Created an entitlement program, lasting three years, to make grants to state educational agencies to train teachers and cafeteria personnel in nutrition principles and to establish pilot nutrition education programs in schools; established a formula for funding based on 50 cents for each schoolchild; provided that in fiscal 1980 the program would be subject to the regular appropriations process.

● Required the secretary of Agriculture to approve the competitive foods that may be offered for sale in schools during the time the school lunch and breakfast programs are in operation.

1978

The rising costs of health care clearly dominated debate on federal health programs in 1978. U.S. medical costs were growing about twice as fast as the overall rate of inflation, and spending for health services in 1978 averaged out to more than $800 per man, woman and child. In six years the nation's aggregate medical bill had nearly doubled, in 15 years it had quadrupled, and since 1950 it had increased more than eleven-fold, according to the Congressional Research Service.

Despite these dramatic rises and a congressional mood of budget austerity, Congress had a mixed record in saving health dollars in 1978. While economizing on existing health programs, members balked at regulating hospital costs, the one step the Carter administration said would significantly slow the ominous acceleration of health care spending.

A bill to limit increases in hospital rates, seen as a necessary prelude to national health insurance, fell victim to lobbying by the health industry. And Carter's blueprint for national health insurance legislation not only met the expected opposition but also an attack by Sen. Edward M. Kennedy (D Mass.), the principal congressional advocate of national health insurance.

One of the most significant factors in 1978 health policy debates appeared to be members' heightened sensitivity to the highly emotional issue of access to health care — much of it due to a 1977 fracas over proposed federal health planning guidelines intended to eliminate underused hospital beds and facilities. In 1978, Congress called on the Department of Health, Education and Welfare (HEW) to accommodate rural needs, and the final version of the 1978 health planning bill clarified that the guidelines were advisory, not mandatory.

In other action, Congress cleared legislation authorizing federal aid to prepaid group medical practices, called Health Maintenance Organizations (HMOs); extended a variety of public health programs; reauthorized health care and cancer research programs; and revised Medicare coverage for kidney dialysis programs. However, Congress failed to clear measures that would have strengthened regulation of clinical laboratories, broadened health care coverage for poor children and extended local health systems agencies.

Hospital Cost Control

Hospital cost control legislation, which had been pronounced dead for the year repeatedly during 1978, was resurrected and passed by the Senate Oct. 12. But it never made it to the House floor, and the measure was buried three days later at the end of the 95th Congress.

The bill passed unexpectedly by the Senate was a watered-down version of the legislation the administration had first proposed in 1977 as a crucial element of its fight on inflation. President Carter also had said such legislation was a necessary prerequisite for any system of national health insurance.

The president's proposal had been gutted by the House Interstate and Foreign Commerce Committee in July and rejected by the Senate Finance Committee in August, so the fact that it re-emerged in any form came as a surprise to almost everyone.

Carter himself said in a speech Sept. 20 that he had given up any hope for passage of the legislation, blaming the "selfish concerns" of the hospital and medical lobby for its failure. But administration officials pushed the fight anyway, apparently to get what political mileage they could from the issue, and the surprise Senate victory was the result. *(Details, see Hospital Cost Control chapter)*

National Health Insurance

President Carter in 1978 found himself between a rock and a very hard place on the issue of national health insurance.

Prodded by labor and Sen. Edward M. Kennedy (D Mass.) to make good on his 1976 campaign promise of a "comprehensive national health insurance system with universal and mandatory coverage," Carter issued a statement of general principles on July 29 and directed Health, Education and Welfare (HEW) Secretary Joseph A. Califano Jr. to draft a health plan to be submitted to Congress in 1979. But he said that to hold down federal spending, the program would have to be phased in gradually.

Labor leaders criticized the president's plan as too little, too slow, and in October Kennedy launched a series of nationwide hearings on his own comprehensive, labor-backed Health Care for All Americans Act. Labor had hoped to make health insurance a campaign issue in the 1978 congressional elections, but that issue was overshadowed by concerns about inflation and federal budget-cutting.

While the administration still insisted the federal government could not afford a major new health program in the immediate future, at year's end it was exploring the possibility of linking its hospital cost containment proposal to a limited federal program of coverage for catastrophic health costs. Carter had insisted hospital cost control was a necessary prerequisite to national health insurance, but Congress failed to enact his plan in 1978. *(Story, p. 63-A)*

Carter formally submitted the health insurance plan to Congress June 12, 1979, after Kennedy offered his plan in May. During that year, the Senate Finance Committee started marking up its own bill, but no national health legislation cleared in the 96th Congress. *(Details, National Health Insurance chapter)*

Health Services, Centers

The 95th Congress in its last hours cleared omnibus health legislation (S 2474 — PL 95-626) extending support for health facilities serving doctor-short areas and for programs targeted on specific health problems such as hypertension.

The $2.9 billion authorization also included new initiatives to head off unwanted teen-age pregnancies through increased counseling and other services and to promote better health through preventive programs like water fluoridation. The various programs were authorized for one, two or three years.

The only objection to the final version came when Robert E. Bauman (R Md.) urged members to recommit (kill) the bill because conferees had removed a requirement that parents of young adolescents be notified if their children used the family planning or pregnancy prevention services. That issue, plus efforts by abortion foes to bar funding for abortion counseling or referrals, had helped defeat a major component of the bill in the House when it was first brought up under suspension of the rules. *(Abortion issue, box, p. 58-A)*

A second major objection to the reauthorizations — money — had surfaced and been dealt with earlier. House and Senate sponsors Paul G. Rogers (D Fla.) and Edward M. Kennedy (D Mass.) both cut funds on the floor from committee-recommended totals. Conferees did some additional fiscal trimming, cutting back on proposed spending levels for the teen-age pregnancy prevention program and new hospital-based primary care services.

Legislative History

The Health Services and Centers Act cleared for the president had a complicated legislative history. The Senate stitched together a health services reauthorization (S 2474 — S Rept 95-860), a disease prevention-health promotion package (S 3116 — S Rept 95-1196) plus a teen-age pregnancy bill (S 2910 — S Rept 95-1206) in floor action and passed them as S 2474 Sept. 29 by a vote of 82-4. Kennedy led off floor debate with a money-cutting substitute for the main bill (S 2474) under consideration. The Senate agreed to the funding cuts without objection. The only extended debate was on the abortion/teen-age pregnancy issue.

Meanwhile, the House passed its health centers bill (HR 12460 — H Rept 95-1186) on Sept. 19 by a 302-102 vote. It first rejected its health services bill (HR 12370 — H Rept 95-1191) by a 193-193 tie vote under suspension Sept. 25, then passed a cheaper version Oct. 13 by a 343-27 vote. The House then substituted HR

12370 and the health services portion of HR 12460 for the text of S 2474 and requested a conference with the Senate.

Conferees retained Senate-passed programs on water fluoridation, smoking and physical fitness; the House version did not contain anything comparable. Conferees also retained the primary care provisions of S 2474; the House had no similar provisions. Another difference was that the House bill provided a one-year authorization for a program to inoculate high-risk individuals against influenza. The Senate bill explicitly banned use of any funds in the bill for flu immunization. Conferees agreed to the House provisions with conditions. Both the House and Senate adopted the conference report (H Rept 95-1799) Oct. 15.

Absent from the final omnibus bill were a community mental health centers reauthorization that had passed the House as part of HR 12460, and reauthorizations for family planning and sudden infant death syndrome programs that had been part of HR 12370. The mental health centers were reauthorized along with biomedical research programs in S 2450, and the other two programs were transferred to S 2522 and cleared separately. *(S 2450, p. 69-A; S 2522, p. 65-A)*

Provisions

As signed into law Nov. 10, S 2474 authorized a total of $2.9 billion for one-, two- and three-year extensions and new authorizations for a variety of public health programs. Most of the funds were for comprehensive health services; community health centers for the needy in rural or inner-city areas; and migrant health centers. *(Authorizations box, p. 71-A)*

The bill also:

Primary Care

●Established new authority for grants to public and private non-profit community hospitals for planning, developing and operating primary care centers in medically underserved areas.

●Required the new primary care centers to be administered separately from the hospital sponsoring them, to deliver primary health care services and appropriate supplemental services, and to be staffed by at least three primary care physicians (except that one nurse practitioner or one physician assistant could substitute for one doctor in physician-short areas).

●Required primary care grants to be awarded so as to assure equitable urban-rural distribution.

●Limited planning and development grants to $150,000 per project.

●Required the General Accounting Office to submit by March 1, 1981, a comparative study of the hospital-based primary care centers and community health centers.

●Established new authority for grants and contracts to public and private entities to either demonstrate new methods of delivering primary health and dental services or to conduct research on delivery of services; required the projects to serve medically underserved areas, and barred funds for projects eligible for other types of federal support; provided separate authorizations for urban and rural projects, with rural projects receiving more than four times the amount of urban projects. This provision provided statutory authority for continuing research and demonstration projects, funded with appropriations since

1975, known as Health in Underserved Rural Areas (HURA) Programs.

Health Services

● Continued formula grants to states for comprehensive public health services through fiscal 1979; converted this support to health incentive grants of at least $1 per capita, depending on state contributions, for fiscal 1980.

● Continued formula grants to states for hypertension programs (screening, detection, diagnosis, prevention, referral for treatment) through fiscal 1979; converted this support to project grants for fiscal 1980 and 1981.

● Authorized grants to state and local governments for community and school-based fluoridation projects, for fiscal 1980 and 1981.

● Authorized, for fiscal 1979 only, funds for immunizing high-risk individuals against influenza; prohibited spending any appropriated funds for this purpose unless the Health, Education and Welfare (HEW) secretary submitted by June 30, 1979, a complete report on health and legal liability problems of immunization programs, including the 1976 swine flu program.

● Required the secretary to provide cost-sharing grants for fiscal 1980-82 for state preventive health services; required states to provide detailed plans for dealing with at least one of the five leading causes of death within the state.

● Required the secretary to conduct five demonstration programs to test, in rural and urban areas, methods for delivering comprehensive disease prevention services to specific populations; authorized funds for fiscal 1979-81.

● Required the secretary to establish research and community- and school-based programs to identify causes of childhood smoking and alcohol consumption and to discourage these behaviors; authorized the programs for fiscal 1980-81.

● Assigned to an existing HEW health information office new authority to make grants for state physical fitness councils, for model projects to improve physical fitness, for research on sports injuries, and for a national conference in 1979 on teaching and fitness.

● Created a new national panel for promotion of child health; directed the panel to set child health goals, develop a national child health plan and report legislative and other recommendations within 18 months of enactment.

● Authorized for fiscal 1979-81 support for community-based health and other services targeted on unwanted adolescent pregnancies, and called for a study of the problem.

● Continued for fiscal 1979-81 federal support for the following categorical health programs: childhood immunization, rodent and other disease control, venereal disease control, genetic disease screening and counseling, and hemophilia programs (including blood separation centers).

Migrant and Community Health Centers

● Authorized centers to fund improvements to private property, with the permission of the owner, to eliminate the source of an environmental health hazard, if no other funds were available; authorized the HEW secretary to earmark appropriated funds for this purpose.

● Made pharmaceutical services a required rather than a supplemental service.

● Authorized the secretary to make grants for conversion to a prepaid basis for providing services for some or all of the population a center served.

● **For Migrant Health Centers Only:** Redefined a "high impact area" as one with 4,000 migratory and seasonal agricultural workers in residence (instead of 6,000), and required the secretary to rank programs by need and distribute funds according to that ranking.

● Made aged or disabled former migrant workers and members of their families eligible for services.

● Required applicants for migrant health center funding to set priorities on certain environmental and supplemental health services and required the secretary to fund those priorities, if the center as a whole were funded, or explain why he did not.

● Repealed authority for grants to pay for converting existing facilities into migrant health centers.

● **For Community Health Centers Only:** Required the centers to develop referral relationships with one or more hospitals.

● Barred the secretary from requiring a center to provide a full range of services in rural areas where such services "are not practical."

● Required the secretary to provide grant recipients with lists of federal and non-federal resources to improve the environment and nutritional status of individuals in the center's service area.

● Required the secretary to equalize urban-rural distribution of the centers when approving grants for the centers.

Family Planning, SIDS

Withstanding a final assault by anti-abortion House members, Congress Oct. 15, 1978, cleared legislation authorizing funds for three years for family planning and sudden infant death syndrome programs.

The bill (S 2522 — PL 95-613) authorized $1.07 billion for family planning services and $12.5 million for sudden infant death syndrome (SIDS) programs in fiscal 1979-81.

Family Planning

Until the 1960s, family planning services generally were available only through private physicians and clinics. In 1967, however, Congress passed the Child Health Act as part of the Social Security Amendments of 1967 (PL 90-248). It required states to make family planning services available to Aid to Families with Dependent Children (AFDC) recipients and provided special project grants for the services.

In 1970 Congress passed the Family Planning Services and Population Research Act (PL 91-572), which established an office of Population Affairs in the Department of Health, Education and Welfare (HEW), and added a Title X to the Public Health Service Act, which authorized funds for family planning services, training, information and education programs, and population research. The act stipulated that all family planning services must be provided only on a voluntary basis, and it contained a prohibition against using Title X funds for abortions; however, funds were provided to clinics that provide abortion counseling and referrals.

Nearly 4,300 of the nation's 5,000 family planning clinics received some Title X funds in 1978.

Teen-age Pregnancy. Of special concern was the high number of pregnancies among teen-age women. According to the Senate Human Resources Committee, approximately one million teen-agers became pregnant annually, and almost 600,000 gave birth.

These pregnancies were frequently unwanted. A higher incidence of low birthweight infants, a higher percentage of pregnancy and childbirth complications and higher rates of school dropout, unemployment and welfare dependency were some of the problems that plagued teen-age mothers.

The rate of elective abortions among teen-agers was also high. In 1976, one-third of the estimated 1,100,000 abortions performed in the United States involved teen-agers.

Sudden Infant Death Syndrome

An estimated 6,000-7,000 infants succumbed each year to sudden infant death syndrome. These children died suddenly, unexpectedly and quietly in their cribs, during what had been considered normal sleep. SIDS, or "crib death," was the leading cause of death of infants one to 12 months old, according to the Human Resources Committee.

In 1974, Congress passed the Sudden Infant Death Syndrome Act (PL 93-270), which provided funds for research on the causes and prevention of SIDS. *(See p. 26-A)*

Legislative History

As originally passed by the Senate June 7, S 2522 (S Rept 95-822) authorized $2.6 billion for fiscal 1979-83 for family planning programs and $49 million for SIDS programs.

Lower authorizations were brought to the House floor as part of an omnibus health services bill (HR 12370 — H Rept 95-1191). That bill first came to the floor Sept. 25 under suspension of the rules and was defeated on a 193-193 tie vote. The defeat was aided by anti-abortion members angered that the suspension procedure prohibited them from offering any amendments. When the bill was brought back to the floor Oct. 13 under regular procedures, the House rejected a series of abortion amendments and then easily passed the bill. It then agreed by voice vote to substitute the family planning and SIDS provisions for the text of the similar Senate bill.

The Senate approved the lower House authorizations by voice vote Oct. 15, clearing the bill for the president.

Provisions

As signed into law Nov. 8, S 2522:

● Authorized $200 million in fiscal 1979, $230 million in fiscal 1980 and $264.5 million in fiscal 1981 for family planning services, including natural family planning services, services for infertile couples and family planning services for teen-agers.

● Authorized $3.1 million in fiscal 1979, $3.6 million in fiscal 1980 and $4.1 million in fiscal 1981 for programs to train family planning personnel.

● Authorized $105 million in fiscal 1979, $120.8 million in fiscal 1980 and $138.9 million in fiscal 1981 for family planning and population research programs, including biomedical research projects and programs to develop new contraceptive devices.

● Authorized $700,000 in fiscal 1979, $805,000 in fiscal 1980 and $926,000 in fiscal 1981 for programs to develop and make available family planning information, including

educational materials, to all persons desiring such materials.

● Required that family planning pamphlets and other information materials be suitable for the group or community to which they are to be made available, taking into account educational and cultural background and community standards; required review and approval of such materials by an advisory committee broadly representative of the community or group.

● Authorized $3.5 million in fiscal 1979, $4 million in fiscal 1980 and $5 million in fiscal 1981 for programs to provide information on the causes of sudden infant death syndrome (SIDS) and to provide counseling to families affected by SIDS.

Doctor Recruitment Aid

Congress cleared legislation Oct. 13, 1978, designed to help government agencies recruit and retain physicians by providing bonus payments of up to $10,000 a year.

The measure (S 990 — PL 95-603) was intended to alleviate the difficulties experienced by many agencies in hiring physicians at normal government pay scales or for assignment in geographically unpopular locations.

The bill passed the Senate by voice vote May 25 after being reported May 15 by the Governmental Affairs Committee (S Rept 95-864). The House passed the bill by voice vote under suspension of the rules Oct. 3, and the Senate Oct. 13 accepted the bill as amended by the House, clearing the measure for the president.

The legislation did not apply to physicians in the Defense Department or Veterans Administration, who were eligible for bonus payments of up to $13,500 under legislation cleared in 1974 and 1975. In 1980, President Carter vetoed legislation increasing bonus payments to doctors in the armed services. *(See Veterans Programs chapter)*

Health Planning Bill Dies

A three-year extension of the controversial system for allocating health resources such as hospital beds and expensive diagnostic machines went down to a surprise defeat under suspension of the rules in the House Sept. 18, 1978.

The health planning measure (HR 11488) later was granted a rule, but never made it back to the floor in the crush of last-minute legislation. Instead, the programs in the bill received a simple one-year extension under an omnibus continuing resolution (H J Res 1139 — PL 95-482) passed at the end of the session. *(Details, Health Planning chapter)*

The Senate July 27 had approved a three-year extension of the health planning system (S 2410) that included a stiff limit on doctors buying very expensive diagnostic and treatment equipment.

The House vote on the bill was 261-141. Under suspension, which required a two-thirds vote, 268 votes were needed to pass the bill. The House defeat was blamed on a volatile mix of rumor, irritation with the planning system and annoyance over the short-cut procedure used to bring the $1.49 billion reauthorization bill to the floor. The controversial health planning system, enacted in 1974, charged a new national network of local planning panels

— called health systems agencies — with preventing unnecessary development, establishing priorities for development of services and facilities that were needed and monitoring uses of federal health funds. The 1974 act was given a one-year extension in 1977 to give the Carter administration time to review the program and recommend changes. In 1979 Congress enacted a three-year extension.

Federal Aid to HMOs

Legislation that would convert federal aid for health maintenance organizations (HMOs) from an experimental, demonstration project basis to more substantial, continuing support cleared Congress Oct. 14, 1978.

S 2534 was a three-year, $164 million reauthorization for federal grants and loans for the prepaid group medical practices. The final bill was a scaled-down version of the administration's proposal and the version reported by the Senate Human Resources Committee. *(Details, see HMO chapter)*

As reported May 15 by the Senate Human Resources Committee (S 2534 — S Rept 95-837), the bill reflected many of the president's proposals, authorizing $415 million for the federal HMO program for five years through fiscal 1983.

But renewed charges of fraud in certain HMOs and the widespread anti-spending mood in Congress took its toll during Senate floor debate. Before passing the bill July 21, by a 71-1 vote, the Senate sliced two years and $230 million from the committee version and beefed up anti-fraud provisions by adding criminal penalties. The bill authorized $185 million for fiscal years 1979-81.

As cleared by the House Sept. 25 by a 327-60 vote, the bill (HR 13655 — H Rept 95-1479) authorized $151 million for HMOs for fiscal 1979-81. Like the Senate bill, HR 13655 raised loan ceilings and loosened certain service requirements for the prepaid plans, relaxations intended to make the HMOs more competitive in price with conventional health insurance plans.

The biggest difference between House and Senate bills was in overall authorization levels. Conferees in their Oct. 13 report (H Rept 95-1784) leaned toward the less generous House bill. In most of the major policy changes, the differences were relatively minor, and conferees traded off the differences without making major changes. Both chambers adopted the conference report easily.

Major Provisions

As signed into law Nov. 1, S 2534 (PL 95-559):

● Authorized a three-year total of $164 million for grants, contracts and loans for health maintenance organizations — $31 million for fiscal 1979, $65 million for fiscal 1980 and $68 million for fiscal 1981.

● Increased to $2 million, from $1 million, the maximum amount an entity could receive for initial HMO development grants, contracts or loan guarantees, beginning Sept. 30, 1979; made grants available for up to three years.

● Permitted established HMOs to receive initial development funds for significant expansions of services or membership.

● Increased to $4 million, from $2.5 million, the total amount an HMO could receive in initial operating loans and loan guarantees; raised to $2 million, from $1 million,

the maximum amount an HMO could receive under this section in any given year.

● Authorized the HEW secretary to take possession of property or take any other steps needed to keep an HMO from defaulting on a federal operating loan or guaranteed loan.

● Authorized the secretary to provide loans and loan guarantees up to $2.5 million for constructing and equipping HMO ambulatory care (outpatient) facilities.

● Established a new HMO management internship program, providing stipends for individuals and support funds for HMOs or other training entities.

● Required the secretary to provide HMO technical assistance grants, for both start-up and operating phases.

● Required certain employers, with the consent of an employee, to provide payroll deductions for HMO payments.

● Required HMOs periodically to submit financial reports to HEW, identifying owners and describing transactions with "parties-in-interest" (persons with an interest in both the HMO and an entity providing goods or services to the HMO); required the reports to include evidence that the HMO was "fiscally sound," and to cover any organizations related to an HMO by common ownership or control.

● Required HMOs to disclose the financial reports to members upon request.

● Provided criminal penalties of up to $25,000 in fines and up to five years' imprisonment for intentional falsification of the financial reports.

● Limited HMO enrollment practices for Medicaid beneficiaries to methods approved by the secretary.

● Exempted public HMOs from a requirement that the HMO policy-making body must be one-third HMO members, with representation from medically underserved populations in its service area; required instead that they establish advisory boards with comparable membership; authorized the advisory boards to make policy decisions if the public HMO delegated that power to them.

● Removed an existing limit on HMO contracts for services with non-physician providers (hospitals, home health agencies, clinical laboratories, optometrists, dentists and others); retained an existing limit on HMO contracting with doctors not working full-time for the HMO; allowed HMOs to use medical groups not meeting statutory requirements for amount of total practice devoted to HMO patients, for up to 48 months after qualification.

● Authorized HMOs to collect workmen's compensation or private health insurance payments for services to HMO members eligible for these benefits.

● Required HMOs to reimburse members for health services that were provided by another entity only when the care was provided on an emergency basis.

● Limited to "good faith" efforts HMO responsibility for health care during natural disasters, wars or other uncontrollable events. Labor disputes were not included in this exemption.

● Permitted HMOs to refuse to cover unusual or infrequently provided services such as sex-change surgery.

● Exempted new HMO outpatient facilities and services from federal health planning system reviews, but only for purposes of Medicare-Medicaid reimbursement. (Existing law required certificate-of-need approval for such facilities before including an appropriate proportion of their cost in overall payments for Medicare and Medicaid services.)

Nurse Training Aid Veto

President Carter Nov. 11 pocket-vetoed legislation (S 2416) extending support for nurse training programs for two more years at existing spending levels. Congress had cleared the bill Oct. 15, the final day of the 1978 session.

Because a continuing resolution carried the nursing education programs at existing funding levels through fiscal 1979, the veto did not abruptly terminate nursing education programs. Furthermore, Congress in 1979 passed a one-year compromise extension of the program that President Carter signed into law. *(1979 action, p. 77-A; see also Rural Health chapter)*

Carter said he would not sign the 1978 nurse training bill because its spending levels were "excessive," particularly since two decades of federal aid to nursing schools had all but ended nursing shortages. Other forms of federal aid were available to nursing students, Carter pointed out, adding that "future federal assistance should be limited to geographic and specialty areas that need nurses most."

Carter had asked Congress to end most nurse training aid, except for $20 million worth of special projects and nurse practitioner training funds. But Congress had continued a broad range of grants — at more than $200 million a year — through 1980.

Both the Senate Human Resources and House Commerce committees had reported versions of the bill May 15 (S Rept 95-859, HR 12303 — H Rept 94-1180), which passed both chambers easily. Conferees retained most features of the similar House and Senate bills, and the report (H Rept 95-1785) was adopted by the House by voice vote Oct. 13, the Senate Oct. 15.

DNA Regulation

After two years of consideration, Congress in 1978 shelved efforts to enact legislation to regulate a controversial form of genetic research — recombinant DNA or "gene-splicing."

Two House committees reported a weakened version of legislation considered in 1977, but no floor action was taken. And for the second time in a year, Sen. Edward M. Kennedy (D Mass.), once a strong advocate of stiff regulation, withdrew his legislation to extend federal regulation to academic and commercial research involving the substance, deoxyribonucleic acid.

Instead, Kennedy suggested the Carter administration use existing authority under the Public Health Service Act to extend federal safety standards for DNA research to all laboratories. The administration had contended it needed specific authority from Congress to do so and never issued such sweeping regulations. Instead, in December 1978 it announced it was loosening existing restrictions on federally funded DNA research.

Background

The controversy over recombinant DNA research first erupted in 1974 when a group of concerned scientists called for a voluntary halt in the research until guidelines could be developed to protect the public from potential risks.

The scientists said they feared that unscrupulous or careless researchers could combine genes in such a way that new bacteria would be created against which humans would have no immunity, possibly resulting in terrible epidemics. Others warned of possible alteration of the normal evolutionary process, and other health and genetic dangers.

Although some scientists and environmental groups wanted to ban all recombinant DNA research, others felt that it should be allowed to continue under proper controls. The research could result in more powerful drugs, better strains of agricultural crops, possibly even cures for diseases such as cancer, proponents argued.

In June 1976, the National Institutes of Health (NIH) issued a set of guidelines establishing safety precautions for all DNA experiments funded by NIH and other federal agencies and banning some experiments altogether. The guidelines did not apply to private laboratories, which were quickly entering the DNA research field.

In 1977 a presidentially appointed Interagency Task Force on Recombinant DNA Research recommended that federal control be extended to all laboratories, both private and public, doing DNA research. The labs would be subject to registration, licensing and inspection by the federal government, but private firms would be allowed to protect trade secrets pending the granting of patents. The task force also recommended that federal requirements supercede local requirements.

The Carter administration proposal, presented in April 1977, generally followed the recommendations of the task force but requested that states and local areas be allowed to set more stringent standards than the federal government.

1977 Legislative Action

The Senate Human Resources Committee reported a bill (S 1217 — S Rept 95-359) in July 1977 establishing an independent federal commission to regulate DNA experimentation. A House bill (HR 7897) placing control of DNA research within the Department of Health, Education and Welfare (HEW) was approved by the House Commerce Subcommittee on Health and the Environment.

However, in September Kennedy, the chief Senate sponsor, withdrew his support from his own bill. Bowing to scientists' fears that the bill would set a precedent for future government control of scientific research, Kennedy proposed that existing federal guidelines be extended for one year while a new commission, to be formed, studied how dangerous DNA research actually was and how it should be regulated.

At the same time, House Commerce Committee Chairman Harley O. Staggers (D W.Va.) blocked a committee vote on the House subcommittee's bill, also citing scientists' fears that federal control might slow research and prevent new advances in science.

1978 Legislative Action

Continuing debate on federal regulation of DNA research resulted in the introduction of modified bills in 1978. The measure reported by the House Interstate and Foreign Commerce and the House Science and Technology committees (HR 11192 — H Rept 95-1005, Parts I and II) and Kennedy's amended version of the 1977 Senate bill would have extended the NIH safety standards for recombinant DNA research to all public and private laboratories for two years only. The 1977 version had set no time limit on the regulation.

The 1978 measures also would have directed the HEW secretary to regulate the research, but provided no blueprint. Local biohazard or biosafety review committees, mandatory in the 1977 bills, were made optional, and there was no explicit requirement for public-interest representation on a national advisory board.

But by 1978 a strong lobby of academic and commercial DNA researchers, professional organizations and university officials argued that fears of potential hazards from DNA research were groundless and that federal regulation would be an unwarranted interference in continued research. Their views were apparently persuasive; Congress took no further action on either measure.

New DNA Regulations

HEW Secretary Joseph A. Califano Jr. Dec. 15 announced new regulations that would relax federal safety rules for federally funded DNA research and provide for more input by non-scientists into decisions on what experiments should be done.

He also said he was asking the Food and Drug Administration and the Environmental Protection Agency to use existing authority to regulate commercial DNA experiments.

The new regulations exempted about one-third of the experiments from federal "containment" requirements and authorized the secretary to permit, on a case-by-case basis, hazardous experiments that had been banned. The regulations, effective Jan. 1, 1979, also increased the number of non-scientists serving on local review committees and a national advisory board.

Cancer Research, Ethics

President Carter Nov. 9, 1978, signed into law a bill mandating an intensive study of the ethics of genetic counseling and other difficult health issues, and adding a major new direction to federal cancer research.

The multi-part, $4 billion reauthorization (S 2450 — PL 95-622) re-established a national commission to study medical ethics problems and provided two-year extensions for disease research and control programs of the National Cancer Institute and the National Heart, Lung and Blood Institute. Half of the reauthorization, $2.1 billion, was for cancer programs. *(1977 action, p. 57-A)*

The bill also continued for two years various types of federal aid to community mental health centers and assistance programs for medical libraries.

The ethics of genetic counseling was one of several topics the ethics commission was directed to study. Its predecessor had focused on protection of human participants in medical research but the new commission had a broader charge, reflecting current concerns with such issues as a uniform definition of death ("brain death," for example, as compared with the traditional standard based on cessation of heartbeat and other "vital signs").

The reauthorization of the cancer programs reflected a judgment that what started out as President Nixon's "blitzkrieg" war on cancer had lengthened into a classic war of attrition, with no victory in sight. The 1971 National Cancer Act had conferred special status on the cancer institute and accepted the theory that massive infusions of money into targeted research could produce an early cure, in much the same way that stepped-up federal spending had put men on the moon.

1978 Changes

By 1978, however, there was strong statistical evidence that personal habits such as smoking and environmental factors such as pollution played a major role in the incidence of cancer. And many scientists viewed cancer as a highly complex group of diseases, with multiple causes, rather than as a single entity.

The 1978 reauthorization cleared by Congress included new statutory authority for the secretary of Health, Education and Welfare (HEW) to test substances for carcinogenicity (cancer-causing properties) and other harmful effects, and ordered research on low-level ionizing radiation, implicated in cancer.

The bill also mandated annual publication of a list of substances known or suspected to be carcinogenic. The list would have no legal force — that is, presence of a substance on it would not be grounds for another agency with regulatory responsibility to move against that substance. Still, the proposal had attracted considerable opposition from conservative members and chemical industry representatives, who argued that data on carcinogenicity was still too imprecise to justify the damage that would be done to a product by inclusion on the list.

The reauthorization also added new stress on disease-prevention measures, including new information programs for medical practitioners and for the public, to be conducted by the cancer and heart-lung-blood institutes. Funding authorization levels were not dramatically raised for either institute.

There were few changes for the mental health centers, other than a relaxation of service requirements for the start-up period of a center. Some centers had found that providing the mandated range of services from the first day of operation was too costly.

Legislative Action

Most of the policy changes, except for the ethics commission, originated in the House Commerce Committee. The Senate Human Resources Committee had decided on a simple one-year extension for the mental health centers and the health institutes, anticipating a full-scale review of the centers and all the National Institutes of Health in 1979. *(See National Health Research chapter)*

The final version of the legislation, approved by both chambers Oct. 15, was a compromise worked out by committee staff and members without a formal conference when it appeared that time was about to run out for the 95th Congress. It combined elements of several earlier bills.

The only piece of the final bill that the House initially passed was a three-year mental health centers reauthorization, approved Sept. 19 as part of a health centers bill (HR 12460 — H Rept 95-1186). The House had not acted on a bill (HR 12347) — H Rept 95-1192) reported in May by the Commerce Committee that extended the health institutes for three years and made policy changes stressing disease prevention and environmental and behavioral factors in the diseases. There had been no House legislation reported comparable to the ethics commission bill (S 2579 — S Rept 95-852) that passed the Senate

June 26. The Senate had added the provisions of S 2579 to a simple one-year extension (S 2450 — S Rept 95-838) for the two institutes and the mental health centers, which also was approved June 26.

Major Provisions

As cleared by Congress, S 2450:

● Authorized through fiscal 1980 grants to community mental health centers for costs of planning, initial operations, consultation and education programs and conversion of facilities; extended financial distress grants through fiscal 1979 only; authorized state mental health program support through fiscal 1981, and rape prevention programs through fiscal 1980.

● Raised to five, from three, the number of financial distress grants a center could receive, and broadened eligibility standards for the grants.

● Relaxed existing minimum service requirements for initial operations grants, to permit centers to begin operations with only six basic services, if the HEW secretary approved a plan for adding other mandated services within three years. The six services that had to be provided initially for all age groups were inpatient, outpatient, emergency, screening and referral, follow-up and consultation and education.

● Permitted centers to share certain services (inpatient, emergency, transitional or "halfway house" services), if the services were accessible to patients in both centers' service areas and if the secretary approved the arrangement.

● Extended federal assistance programs for medical libraries through fiscal 1981.

● Extended National Heart, Lung and Blood Institute and National Cancer Institute programs through fiscal 1980.

● Required both institutes to step up their efforts to provide information both to doctors and other health professionals and to the general public; directed the Heart-Lung and Blood Institute to include disease-related information on nutrition and environmental pollutants.

● Required the cancer institute to expand and intensify its research on preventing cancer caused by occupational or environmental exposure to carcinogens.

● Extended the National Research Service Award program through 1981; extended to five years, from three, the maximum period an individual could receive the awards; authorized cost-of-living adjustments in the stipends; relaxed some service pay-back requirements.

● Directed the secretary to conduct research and testing of substances for their capacity to cause cancer (carcinogenicity), severe birth defects (teratogenicity), significant and basic changes in genetic material (mutagenicity) or other harmful biological effects.

● Required the secretary to establish a research program on the biological effects of low-level ionizing radiation, and to review federal research programs on the topic.

● Directed the secretary to support research and information programs on human nutrition.

● Required the secretary to publish an annual report on carcinogens, including a list of all substances known or thought likely to be carcinogenic, evaluations of existing regulatory efforts to control specific substances, surveys of federal agency testing and research results.

● Established an 11-member President's Commission for the Study of Ethical Problems in Medicine and Biomedical and Behavioral Research, with representatives

Authorizations

As cleared by Congress, S 2450 authorized the following amounts for fiscal 1979-81 *(in millions of dollars)*:

	1979	1980	1981
Mental health centers			
Planning	$ 1.5	$ 1	—
Initial operations	34.5	35	—
Consultation, education	20	3	—
Conversion	30	25	—
Financial distress	25	—	—
Rape prevention	8	9	—
State mental health programs			
	5	20	$ 25
Medical libraries	15	16.5	18.5
Cancer Institute			
Control programs	90.5	103	—
Research, other programs	924.5	927	—
Heart, Lung and Blood Institute			
Prevention, control programs	40	45	—
Research, other programs	470	515	—
National Research Service Awards	197.5	210	222.5
Ethics Commission [1]	5	5	5
Totals	**$1,866.5**	**$1,914.5**	**$271**

[1] S 2450 also authorized $5 million for this program in fiscal 1982.

from biomedical and behavioral research, medicine, humanities, social sciences and other natural sciences. Full-time federal employees were barred from membership.

● Directed the commmission to report every two years on human research policies and their implementation in all federal agencies.

● Directed the commission to conduct special studies on the impact of income and place of residence on the availability of health services, and on the ethical and legal implications of these subjects:

Informed consent in medical contracts.

The desirability of a uniform legal definition of death.

Genetic counseling and information programs.

Confidentiality of patient records in research and access of patients to such records.

● Required publication of commission recommendations on programs or policies of a federal agency, with opportunity for public comment; required the agency to either adopt the recommendation within six months or publish its reasons for deciding not to do so.

● Barred the commission from disclosing trade secret information or medical records that were protected by the Freedom of Information Act.

Health Care Research

Congress Oct. 15, 1978, cleared a three-year, $378 million reauthorization (S 2466 — PL 95-623) for federal health statistics and health care research programs.

The bill provided statutory authority for a newly created health technology evaluation center in the Department of Health, Education and Welfare (HEW). It also authorized both the center and a related new national advisory body to advise the HEW secretary on whether and to what extent Medicare and Medicaid should pay for new health technologies applied to their beneficiaries.

Health economists had partially blamed spiraling health care costs on wasteful duplication and inappropriate use of such expensive equipment as the half-million-dollar computerized X-ray machine known as the CAT scanner. The medical and economic worth of certain specialized treatment units, such as hospital coronary care units, and certain surgical procedures had also been questioned. Paradoxically, there had also been some complaints that information about new medical developments was difficult for many practitioners to come by. The new center was authorized to address both of these problems through direct research and projects carried out under federal grants and contracts.

The increasing prominence of cost issues in health care also showed up in new authority for studies on environmental-related diseases and health conditions. The bill required the secretary to report periodically to Congress on a broad, ongoing study of the present and future costs of environment-related diseases and disabilities. A second new study was to evaluate the desirability of setting up a new federal program to study health effects of exposure to hazardous substances, locate victims of exposure and assist with medical follow-up.

Legislative Action. The bill had been substantially reduced from earlier proposals after opponents objected to higher spending levels and increased bureaucracy. The Senate June 26 rejected a committee bill (S 2466 — S Rept 95-839) authorizing a three-year total of $440 million and elevating the three health research, technology and statistics centers to the status of National Institutes of Health. A $318 million version was approved by the Senate Aug. 9; it kept the existing status of the centers. House approval of similar but more expensive legislation (HR 12584 — H Rept 95-1190), with a three-year total of $429 million, came Sept. 25.

The House approved the conference report on the bill (H Rept 95-1783) by voice vote Oct. 13, the Senate Oct. 15.

Provisions

As cleared for the president, S 2466:

● Authorized a three-year (fiscal 1979-81) total of $378 million, as follows: for the National Center for Health Services Research, $120 million; for the National Center for Health Statistics, $185 million; for the National Center for Health Care Technology, $73 million.

● Directed the HEW secretary to add certain priorities to health statistics and health services research, including health care costs and cost increases, and effectiveness and impact of health care technology.

● Required the secretary to support manpower training programs in health care research, statistics and technology evaluation.

● Established a National Center for Health Care Technology.

● Authorized the center to support evaluations of health care technology for safety, effectiveness and cost effectiveness; for social, ethical and economic impact, and for factors affecting use of technologies and methods of disseminating information about them.

● Authorized the center to make recommendations on health care technology with respect to all HEW statutory responsibilities, including reimbursement policy (such as Medicare and Medicaid payments for health services).

● Authorized the secretary to support existing or new facilities to conduct health care technology studies, with a goal of at least three such centers in operation by Sept. 1, 1981; stipulated that the centers were to be within established academic or research institutions and specified staff and other requirements.

● Established a National Council on Health Care Technology to advise the secretary and the center director on health care technologies, to develop "exemplary standards, norms, and criteria" for the use of particular technologies and to review certain research projects and grants.

● Directed the secretary to conduct an ongoing study of existing and future health costs of pollution and other environmental conditions (including those of the workplace). The study was to be conducted by the National Academy of Sciences, with a first report to congressional health committees within 18 months of enactment and subsequent reports every two years thereafter.

● Directed the secretary to submit to Congress by Jan. 1, 1981, a plan to standardize collection of statistical and epidemiological data on effects of environment on health.

● Directed the secretary to establish, within two years of enactment, guidelines for collection and processing of information relating to workplace and other environmental conditions and public health; required protection from disclosure for medical records and trade secrets; required review of the guidelines every three years and, if needed, revision.

● Directed the secretary to study the desirability of a federal system to locate individuals exposed to hazardous substances, study the health outcomes of such exposures and assist exposed individuals in securing medical care, if needed.

Clinical Lab Standards

For the third time in three years, Congress in 1978 failed to complete action on legislation to strengthen and broaden regulation of laboratories that do medical tests.

Two House committees reported a clinical laboratories bill (HR 10909 — H Rept 95-1004) similar to one (S 705) that the Senate had passed in 1977. The House briefly debated the bill Oct. 2, but when the end-of-session crunch came, there were six health reauthorizations to clear in three days and a cluster of amendments to the labs bill. House leaders refused to shove the labs bill onto their overcrowded schedule and Congress adjourned without a House vote. *(1977 Senate action, p. 59-A)*

Although the lab bill's chronic problems suggested blocking efforts by organized opposition, proponents said that was not the case, citing numerous exceptions and delays that had been written into successive versions of the bill to soften its immediate impact. Instead, health observers credited the House failure to vote to the legislative overload of other health bills, late-surfacing amendments from a few conservative opponents of regulation, and absence of an active sponsor in the House.

Kidney Dialysis Program

President Carter June 13, 1978, signed into law legislation (HR 8423 — PL 95-292) to encourage persons with end stage renal disease (kidney failure) to conduct their own dialysis treatments at home or in special self-care facilities with professional assistance, or to choose kidney transplants. Both were said by proponents to be less expensive and more healthful alternatives to costly hospital-based dialysis.

Under existing law, home dialysis patients had to bear a substantially greater portion of the treatment costs than those entering hospitals for the life-sustaining treatments.

The measure, a compromise between House- and Senate-passed measures, emphasized priorities of a network of regional planning groups and individual physicians and patients in selecting appropriate treatment. Provisions endorsed by the House in 1977 for a strong federal role involving national goals and sanctions for enforcing those goals were watered down. Health committee sources credited these changes partly to fallout from a controversy that erupted in the fall of 1977 over national health planning goals.

Soaring Medicare spending for hospital-based dialysis, coupled with a dramatic decline in less costly home care, prompted congressional action. Since 1972, when Congress created the Medicare renal disease program, the number of patients dialyzing at home had dropped to 10 per cent from 40 per cent, largely because of the financial incentives introduced for hospital treatment, according to proponents. The annual bill for the program was $1 billion and had been projected to reach $6 billion by 1992 — for a relatively small patient population (estimated to reach 75,000).

Legislative History

The House passed HR 8423 Sept. 12, 1977. The bill stated a national goal, that a majority of new renal disease patients use self-dialysis or receive a kidney transplant. It also established a network of regional peer review units and directed those units to set goals for identifying patients for self-care or transplants, and to review regional facilities' success in meeting those goals. Under the House bill a regional agency could report facilities that consistently failed to meet these goals to the secretary of Health, Education and Welfare (HEW), who could withhold a facility's certification. Areas with low self-dialysis rates could lose federal certification for additional facilities or beds. *(1977 action, p. 62-A)*

With no discussion and without objection the Senate April 10, 1978, passed HR 8423 by voice vote.

The Senate-passed bill, which was reported by the Finance Committee March 22 (S Rept 95-714), was in most respects identical to the version the House approved in 1977. But several changes made by the Finance Committee were disturbing to members of the House Ways and Means Committee, who requested a conference.

The House members were concerned with Senate deletion of provisions for a national dialysis policy and related language that spelled out responsibilities of the national network of peer review agencies. The Senate bill retained the review network but limited its functions to advice and review.

The final compromise followed Senate action in deleting the numerical national goal. Instead, each entity in the national network would establish goals for its own region. National goals could be articulated by federal guidelines, but these would only be advisory. However, HEW could end or suspend Medicare reimbursement of facilities that did not cooperate with regional goals established by the peer review organizations.

The House approved the compromise language May 1 without objection, and the Senate followed suit May 24 by voice vote, clearing the bill.

Provisions

As signed into law, HR 8423 contained the following major provisions:

● Waived the three-month waiting period for Medicare coverage of dialysis costs for patients who enroll in a self-dialysis training program.

● Authorized Medicare reimbursement for all supplies used in home care and for periodic monitoring and maintenance visits at home by trained dialysis personnel.

● Also authorized reimbursement to facilities that set up and maintained self-dialysis units for patients interested in self-care but unable to perform it at home.

● Authorized Medicare to reimburse dialysis facilities for the "reasonable cost" of buying and installing and maintaining dialysis machines in patients' homes.

● Broadened Medicare coverage for patients undergoing kidney transplant operations.

● Stipulated that Medicare covered kidney donors as well as recipients.

● Directed the HEW secretary to establish a network of renal disease peer review organizations that would set goals for identifying patients for self-care or transplants and oversee dialysis facilities; required patient membership in the organizations.

● Authorized the secretary to promulgate national guidelines, for advisory purposes only, for renal disease treatment.

● Directed the regional peer review organizations to identify facilities and providers "not cooperating" with the established goals and assist them in developing plans to facilitate cooperation.

● Authorized the secretary to suspend or end reimbursement to uncooperative facilities until the department found "reasonable efforts" toward cooperation with the goals.

Medicare-Medicaid Benefits

The House Sept. 18, 1978, passed legislation (HR 13097, HR 13817) to make home health care — nursing, physical therapy and similar services — more available to the elderly beneficiaries of Medicare.

However, the Senate's Medicare-Medicaid revisions were in legislation (HR 5285) that included hospital cost control provisions which died at the end of the session, so the benefit changes were not enacted. *(See Hospital Cost Control chapter)*

The Carter administration opposed new health benefits for budgetary reasons.

With only two dissenting votes the House agreed to unlimited home health visits for beneficiaries, dropping an existing curb on the number of visits that would be reimbursed. It also dropped a prior-hospitalization eligibility requirement, eliminated a $60 deductible and adopted other changes designed to make more home care available to more of the aged ill.

Benefits revisions for Medicare were included in HR 13097 (H Rept 95-1533) which passed by a 398-2 vote.

Changes affecting peer review, nursing care beds in acute-care hospitals and auditing procedures for both federal programs were included in a second bill (HR 13817 — H Rept 95-1534) which passed 359-40.

Child Health Program

Concern that legislation broadening health care coverage for poor children would mark the first step toward liberalization of cash welfare programs helped kill the measure in the last hectic days of the 95th Congress.

The legislation, called the Child Health Assurance Program (CHAP), would have replaced Medicaid's widely criticized Early and Periodic Screening, Diagnosis and Treatment Program. The program would have raised the average federal payment to the state to carry out the screening program and would have made more poor children eligible for Medicaid by expanding coverage in all states to children living in needy two-parent households. CHAP would have added another 1.7 million to 2.5 million children to the Medicaid rolls.

The legislation (HR 6076), proposed by President Carter in 1977, drew strong bipartisan and interest group support. However, neither the House nor the Senate version ever came to a vote on the floor. The Senate Finance Committee filed its report on the bill (S 1392 — S Rept 95-1310) late Oct. 12. The House briefly debated its CHAP bill (HR 13611 — H Rept 95-1481) Oct. 11, but the measure died with Congress' Oct. 15 adjournment.

"It was everyone's second priority," said a spokeswoman for the Children's Defense Fund, who along with the American Medical Association and a host of other health groups lobbied vigorously in support of CHAP.

But concerns about the program's cost and about the provision that liberalized Medicaid eligibility by allowing poor children from intact families to receive aid helped scuttle the legislation.

The House approved similar legislation in 1979. *(See Child Health Programs chapter)*

Child Nutrition Programs

Although he cited reservations about the final bill, President Carter Nov. 10, 1978, signed into law legislation (S 3085 — PL 95-627) extending certain child nutrition programs for four years, through fiscal 1982.

Carter said he signed the measure because he had received assurances from key committee members that the 96th Congress would make the changes necessary to satisfy his concerns, including a reduction in the spending entitlement for fiscal 1980 for the supplemental feeding program for women, infants and children (WIC). Although the Senate in 1979 did pass legislation reducing the authorizations, the House failed to act on the bill that year.

A spending level of $800 million for fiscal 1980, plus the conversion of the WIC program from an authorization to an entitlement for fiscal 1979 and 1980, had drawn a veto recommendation from the Office of Management and Budget (OMB), reportedly on grounds that the provisions were highly inflationary. However, other agencies, WIC backers and various anti-poverty activist groups, successfully lobbied the White House on behalf of the measure.

As originally reported by House and Senate committees (S 3085 — S Rept 95-884, HR 12511 — H Rept 95, 1153), the legislation would have made WIC an entitlement program for all four years of the authorization. The program had been plagued since its establishment by uncertain funding. However, the Senate Appropriations Committee objected to creating another entitlement program, and the Senate agreed to cut the entitlement provision to two years; the House went along with that compromise.

Although the spending levels and entitlement provision were "significant problems," Carter said, the bill contained other changes in the nutrition programs advocated or backed by the administration. Those changes included provisions to reduce administrative expenditures for the school feeding programs and to expand the child care food program.

Congress had refused to go along with several other administration proposals, including making the school breakfast program mandatory in schools with large numbers of poor children, eliminating children aged 3 to 5 from the WIC program, and ending the special milk program.

In extending both WIC and the child care food program, S 3085 made few major changes in existing law; principally it aimed to better target the food aid and to provide incentives for program expansion.

Like dozens of other bills passed by the 95th Congress, the fate of the bill remained uncertain until the final days of the session. Fearing that the bill would die, key legislators in the House and Senate began private negotiations. Early on Oct. 15, they reached agreement and quickly steered the final compromise bill through both chambers.

Major Provisions

As signed into law, S 3085 amended the National School Lunch Act and the Child Nutrition Act of 1966 as follows:

● Made the child care food program permanent and authorized such funds as necessary to carry out the program.

● Established eligibility requirements for participation in the program.

● Simplified payment rates for participating institutions, except family and group day care homes, for which a separate rate schedule was established.

● Increased to $6 million from $3 million the amount available for food service equipment assistance for child care institutions participating in the program.

● Extended the special supplemental food program for women, infants and children (WIC) for four years, through fiscal 1982.

● Established an entitlement for the program of $550 million for fiscal 1979 and $800 million for fiscal 1980; authorized $900 million for fiscal 1981 and $950 million for fiscal 1982.

● Limited program participation to pregnant, postpartum and breastfeeding women, infants and children up to age 5 who are determined to be at nutritional risk and whose incomes are below the standard for reduced-price lunches under the National School Lunch Act (195 per cent of the poverty level).

● Reduced in general the federal reimbursement rate to states for reduced-price school lunches by 10 cents, making the reimbursement rate 20 cents below the free lunch rate.

● Allowed schools to provide free milk to children who are eligible for free lunches.

● Increased the authorization for equipment funds for the school breakfast program to $75 million from $40 million.

● Provided increased assistance of 10 cents more per free breakfast for schools if they have high percentages of poor youngsters.

● Prohibited the secretary of agriculture from limiting or prohibiting the use during the 1978-79 school year of formulated grain-fruit products ("super donuts") currently used in the school breakfast program; allowed the secretary to issue final regulations banning the use of the products 60 days after notifying appropriate congressional committees.

1979

Three years after his campaign promise for an all-inclusive health insurance plan, President Carter finally came up with a proposal in 1979, but it turned out to be a very limited scheme instead. His plan effectively set the agenda for congressional debate on the issue, undermining his chief political rival, Sen. Edward M. Kennedy (D Mass.), who for years had identified himself with the issue.

By focusing on "catastrophic" coverage that would protect the middle class against ruinously expensive illnesses, Carter allied himself with the powerful head of the Senate Finance Committee, Russell B. Long (D-La.) He also pinpointed a major constituency, heretofore ignored by public programs.

By the end of the year, the Finance Committee had tentatively approved major elements of a mandatory national catastrophic health insurance program for workers, along with improvements in Medicare that would cap the amount elderly beneficiaries would have to pay each year for health care. Legislation to upgrade and expand Medicaid coverage for poor children and pregnant women was passed by the House and reported by the Finance Committee.

But there were major stumbling blocks to enactment of other health care bills. The child health bill had picked up several controversial anti-abortion amendments in the House. No agreement was in sight on additional improvements in Medicaid. And another critical element of the president's plan, annual revenue limits on hospitals, had been soundly defeated in the House.

On the other hand, Congress cleared measures extending the controversial health planning system, providing nurse training aid, subsidizing emergency medical services programs and extending alcohol and drug abuse programs.

Hospital Cost Control

After a three-year contest, controversial legislation to control soaring hospital costs was effectively killed when the House Nov. 15, 1979, rejected the administration's bill (HR 2626) and adopted instead a substitute that simply created a national study commission on hos-

pital costs and authorized some funds for state cost control programs. Four months earlier, the Senate Finance Committee had also rejected the administration's hospital cost control cap. *(Details, Hospital Cost Control chapter)*

The vote was a major legislative defeat for the president, who had called the bill his top-priority anti-inflation measure of the year and had personally lobbied for it. Under his proposal, the federal government would regulate hospital revenues if the industry failed through voluntary efforts to keep spending at a set annual rate of increase.

After voting to create only a study commission and rejecting a move to kill even that, the House voted 321-75 to pass the bill.

Committee Action

Committee action on the legislation was somewhat of a replay of previous years.

Human Resources. Of the four congressional committees with jurisdiction over the bill, only the Senate Labor and Human Resources Committee reported it relatively intact in 1979. As approved by that committee June 13 (no report was filed), the bill stuck closely to the president's plan, differing in these respects: it eliminated a national advisory commission; it specified certain exemptions which the Carter bill left up to the discretion of the secretary of HEW; it included a "sunset" provision ending the program after five years; it contained an "anti-dumping" provision to prevent hospitals from refusing to accept poor, uninsured patients or those with problems costly to treat, and it stipulated that the voluntary limit on hospital spending could not go below a fixed number. (The administration formula was based on the rate of inflation.)

The committee bill did not include a national cap on hospital capital investments, as Carter had proposed in 1977 but omitted in 1979.

Finance. As it had in 1978, the Senate Finance Committee July 12 rejected the administration's plan and agreed instead to report a bill (HR 934 — S Rept 96-471) that would only limit Medicare and Medicaid payments to hospitals — something HEW had already moved to do administratively.

Ways and Means. On the House side, the Ways and Means Committee July 17 approved a much amended version of the president's plan (HR 2626 — H Rept 96-404, Pt I). During four days of markup, the committee riddled the bill with exceptions and exemptions, cut its savings by a third and added a one-house veto provision. Altogether, the Health Subcommittee and the full committee added more than 30 amendments to the bill, most of them ensuring special treatment for certain hospitals in members' districts.

The administration itself offered 21 compromise amendments, fine-tuning various exemptions and adjustments, substituting the hospital industry's own 1979 goal for spending restraint as the minimum in the bill, and retracting much of the discretionary authority given to the HEW secretary in the original bill.

As reported by Ways and Means, HR 2626 authorized standby mandatory controls on hospital inpatient revenues if hospitals failed to keep 1979 spending from rising more than 11.6 percent above 1978 spending. Because of the exemptions added to the administration bill, HEW officials said mandatory controls would cover only 35 to 40 percent of the nation's hospitals under the bill.

Commerce. In a surprising reversal of its 1978 action, the House Commerce Committee voted 23-19 Sept. 26 to report HR 2626 (H Rept 96-404, Part 2), after rejecting a motion to gut it by a 21-21 tie vote.

Although HR 2626 could have gone to the floor no matter what the panel did, winning the approval of the second House committee was seen as an important psychological boost.

The Commerce bill was a modified version of the president's proposal, containing some but not all of the amendments added by Ways and Means. HEW officials said it would save more money than the Ways and Means bill but not as much as the administration's. It exempted fewer hospitals from cost-control requirements, and had a five-year sunset provision instead of four.

House Floor Action

The precarious position of the cost control bill was nowhere more evident than in the House Rules Committee. The panel did not give HR 2626 a rule until more than a month after the Commerce Committee reported the bill, and it did so then only because the administration insisted on a House floor vote Nov. 15.

The rule the committee approved and the House adopted (H Res 486) showed the administration's weak position. The panel refused the virtually closed rule that bill sponsors wanted in order to protect it from damaging floor amendments, and permitted a vote on a substitute sponsored by Richard A. Gephardt (D Mo.).

The House debated the legislation for five hours Nov. 15 before decisively rejecting Carter's cost control plan. The adopted Gephardt substitute created a 15-member, presidentially appointed commission to monitor voluntary industry efforts to cut costs, reporting back to Congress within a year, and to consider long-term solutions to hospital cost inflation. The proposal also authorized $10 million for fiscal 1980 and sums "as needed" through fiscal 1982 for grants to state cost control programs.

The substitute established as a national goal the industry's voluntary goal of keeping 1979 hospital cost increases no more than 11.6 per cent above 1977 increases, with adjustments in future years to reflect inflation.

Members who spoke for Carter's plan during debate — mostly younger, liberal Democrats — stressed the weakness of Gephardt's plan, the seriousness of hospital cost increases and the original bill's potential impact on inflation.

But opponents insisted that Carter wanted the bill for political reasons and that any potential savings would be far outweighed by the bill's two major defects: it was new government regulation, and it would freeze medical technology at its present status, closing off future growth and development.

National Health Insurance

While political skirmishing continued throughout 1979 over the rival national health insurance plans of President Carter and Sen. Edward M. Kennedy (D Mass.) the Senate Finance Committee moved toward agreement on a more modest plan to provide "catastrophic" coverage only.

Catastrophic insurance was the core of Carter's "first-phase" national health plan, and administration officials were working closely with Finance Committee Chairman

Russell B. Long (D La.) and other key members to develop the legislation.

Kennedy and his allies, principally organized labor, opposed catastrophic coverage for fear it would reduce pressure for a more comprehensive national health program. Catastrophic insurance would cover only "catastrophically" high medical bills, those remaining after a family had already paid several thousand dollars out of its own pocket in a year, or after private insurance coverage had been exhausted.

But many in Congress and the administration believed the country could not afford a comprehensive health plan and opted to go for "50 percent of something," rather than hold out for "100 percent of nothing," as Sen. Abraham Ribicoff (D Conn.) a longtime backer of catastrophic insurance, put it.

Long opened the 1979 action in February, when he announced that he planned to "push and agitate a bit" for catastrophic insurance — "about as much as we can afford to enact in this Congress." He introduced legislation and began hearings and markup in March.

The Finance Committee worked on the legislation off and on throughout the year, and seemed on the verge of reporting it in November. But several committee members and the administration insisted on substantial new health benefits for the poor; Long and some other members objected, and further action was postponed so that committee staff could try to work out an acceptable compromise.

Kennedy unveiled his comprehensive national health plan May 14. He made several concessions to Carter administration positions, and called on the president to join him and the coalition of labor, black, religious, elderly and farm groups that supported comprehensive national health care, in an effort to guarantee complete health coverage for all Americans.

President Carter announced his plan June 12, after administration officials had spent months honing it into shape. It was considerably scaled down from his 1976 campaign commitment to comprehensive national health insurance, but Carter said the United States could only afford a gradually phased in program. *(1978 action, p. 63-A)*

Without naming his opponents, he noted that 30 years' "rigid" pursuit of "the idea of all or nothing at all" had failed to get a comprehensive health plan out of Congress. It was time, he said, to "rise above the differences that have created that stalemate and act now" on his first-phase program.

Administration officials denied that pressure from Kennedy had pushed the president into backing a more liberal program than he originally had planned.

Carter's plan would increase federal health care spending, in the first year of benefits, by about $18 billion over existing levels, and private (employer) expenses for health care by $6 billion, the administration estimated. Kennedy said his plan would add about $29 billion to the federal budget and $11 billion to expenditures by businesses and workers the first year.

Reactions, Pro and Con

Testimony before the Finance Committee early in the year indicated broad political support for insurance against catastrophic medical costs.

Three Republican senators, Robert Dole (Kan.), John C. Danforth (Mo.) and Pete V. Domenici (N.M.), introduced their own catastrophic bill (S 748), with a deductible of $5,000 and 60 days' hospitalization, and improved Medicare benefits.

Another Republican senator, Bob Packwood (Ore.), suggested that passage of catastrophic insurance would help stave off demand for a "British-style, or Kennedy-style, national health service."

There was qualified support from much of organized medicine for catastrophic coverage, if government's role were kept to a minimum. Medical and insurance industry spokesmen also expressed support for an all-federal Medicaid program.

Then-HEW Secretary Joseph A. Califano Jr. made clear that the administration would support catastrophic insurance only if it was accompanied by cost control legislation and improved benefits for the poor and elderly.

A spokesman for the American Association of Retired Persons objected that catastrophic legislation would simply heat up health care inflation further if it did not include meaningful cost controls.

The AFL-CIO flatly rejected catastrophic coverage without other improvements, and the National Urban League said such coverage would do nothing to help the estimated 8 million poor people who had neither private nor public health coverage or the one in five Americans who had inadequate coverage.

Finance Committee Action

The Finance Committee began its markup with three bills before it (S 350, S 351, S 760), but essentially it made up its catastrophic health insurance plan as it went along. By the end of the year, the committee had made most of the critical decisions.

The panel decided to make it mandatory, not optional, for employers to provide catastrophic insurance for workers. It set the deductible at $3,500, but also provided a lower, income-related deductible for lower-paid workers, a proposal advanced by Ribicoff, Robert Dole (R Kan.) and Daniel Patrick Moynihan (D N.Y.).

These were the general specifications of the plan agreed to by the committee:

Benefits, Coverage. All employers would be required to offer full-time employees health insurance covering the same benefits now provided by Medicare: physicians' fees and hospitalization, limited drug, durable medical equipment and mental health benefits, home health visits and up to 100 days of nursing home care.

Outpatient drugs and extended nursing home care, the two major exclusions of Medicare, would also be excluded from the minimum benefit package. The committee also excluded prenatal, maternity and infant care in the first year of life, with no cost-sharing — a feature the administration especially wanted included.

The plans would pay for specified benefits after an individual or family had spent a substantial amount themselves, either out of pocket or under a supplementary insurance policy, on medical bills.

All full-time employees (those working 25 hours a week or more) would have to join their employers' plans unless they were already covered through a second job or a spouse's or parent's job. No one could be excluded because of pre-existing health conditions. The plans also would have to cover children, students and other dependents of insured individuals; dependent survivors, for at least one year after the insured person's death; a spouse and other dependents, for 30 days after divorce

Dioxins Study Bill

President Carter Jan. 2, 1980, vetoed a bill (S 2096) requiring the Department of Health, Education and Welfare (HEW) to study the health effects of dioxins, the chemicals used in Agent Orange and other herbicides. Congress had cleared the bill Dec. 19, 1979.

Carter said he supported efforts to investigate the effects of dioxins, but disapproved S 2096 because it required that HEW's design for the study be approved by Congress' Office of Technology Assessment (OTA). Such a "legislative veto device" was an "unconstitutional intrusion" into the executive branch's administrative authority, he said. The bill was unnecessary anyway, he added, because HEW already planned to conduct a study of dioxins.

Carter signed another bill (HR 3892 — PL 96-151) that contained an identical provision with regard to a Veterans Administration (VA) study of dioxins, because that bill also extended authorizations for veterans' health benefits and contained provisions on staffing of VA hospitals that had been worked out in lengthy negotiations with Congress. However, Carter said he would tell the VA administrator not to consider the provision requiring OTA approval of its study legally binding.

S 2096 was the result of a compromise between the House and Senate Veterans' Affairs committees on what agency should study the health effects of Agent Orange, a defoliant used in Vietnam, on U.S. soldiers who served there. The House panel insisted the VA should do it, and that was authorized in HR 3892. *(Details, Veterans Health chapter)*

In return, the House committee agreed to S 2096, which required HEW to study the health effects of dioxin exposure on agricultural, Forest Service and chemical workers and other civilians who had come in contact with dioxins, and to review existing scientific studies of the long-range health effects of dioxin exposure. The Senate passed the bill Dec. 6, the House Dec. 19.

or legal separation from the insured; unemployed former employees, for a certain period after they left a job, and employees of employers who had failed to pay their premiums, for at least 30 days. All these persons with temporary coverage would have the option to convert to individual coverage if they wished.

Self-employed individuals would not be required to buy coverage, but could do so if they wished from an industry "pool." State and local governments also could have their employees covered by the pool.

Cost-Sharing. Individuals or families earning $14,000 a year or more would have to pay up to $3,500 of medical bills annually before insurance coverage began; the deductible would be adjusted periodically for inflation. Workers earning less than $14,000 a year would pay 25 percent of their annual income as a deductible, or $3,500, whichever was less. Insurance carriers would fully pay claims for these persons, periodically billing the federal government for their costs.

Employees could also be required to pay up to one-fourth the cost of their insurance premiums, although employers could pay the full cost or reduce the employees' share if they wished.

Medicare beneficiaries would not have to pay more than $1,000 a year in co-payments and deductibles for hospitalization and doctor bills; above that figure, Medicare would pay all "reasonable" costs or charges for covered services, including, for the first time, drugs to treat life-threatening or chronic illnesses.

Employer Subsidy. Employers could get a tax credit for the cost of providing new, mandated benefits. The credit would be a declining percentage of an employer's new costs for the first few years of the program. Employers could also continue to claim the tax deduction currently allowed for existing health insurance plans. State and local governments choosing to upgrade existing plans to conform with the new catastrophic minimum package could get a rebate from the federal government for their new costs.

"Pool" Coverage. To qualify for the catastrophic program, insurance companies would have to participate in state or regional insurance pools, as would health maintenance organizations and self-insured persons. The pools would sell the basic catastrophic plan to any individual or firm, at no more than 150 per cent of the average cost for small employer groups. The pools were intended to be a source of insurance for part-time workers, the self-employed, high-risk individuals and others.

Medigap Certification. The committee agreed to create a voluntary federal certification program for so-called "Medigap" insurance — private plans to supplement Medicare. The committee provided penalties of $25,000 or five years' imprisonment for falsifying information to obtain certification, falsely posing as an agent of the federal government to sell the insurance, knowingly selling duplicative policies or advertising or selling by mail policies not approved by state insurance commissioners.

Health Planning

Congress Sept. 21, 1979, completed action on a three-year, $987 million extension of the controversial federal-state-regional health planning system, which allocated health resources such as hospital beds and expensive diagnostic machines.

The health planning system was intended to block excess hospital expansions and duplication in services and major medical equipment. It had been criticized both for being ineffective and for having a potential to "ration" health services. But advocates such as Sen. Edward M. Kennedy (D Mass.) argued that "rational planning" was needed to "assure the provision of quality health care at reasonable cost," as Kennedy told the Senate Sept. 21.

S 544 included provisions dealing with several major planning controversies. For the first time, it extended the requirement for state approval of major medical equipment (by "certificate-of-need" programs) to equipment located in doctors' offices, if the equipment was to be used on hospital inpatients.

It also postponed a cutoff of federal funds to states that had not yet enacted mandatory certificate-of-need programs and, reflecting pressure for less federal interference in local planning decisions, eliminated a requirement in the original law that state and local planning decisions must conform to national guidelines issued by

the Department of Health, Education and Welfare (HEW). This provision was a direct response to a 1977 furor over national planning guidelines that were widely interpreted as an HEW move to shut down hospitals and services not meeting the guidelines. *(Guidelines, p. 61-A)*

To promote competition among providers of health care, the bill largely exempted prepaid group health plans from the state approval requirement. To deal with the highly emotional question of underused hospital facilities, it provided incentives rather than penalties, creating a new $155 million program of grants to encourage hospitals to shut down unneeded acute-care beds or convert them to needed uses. In the past, decertification of underused facilities had been suggested.

Overall, the bill added no new regulatory authority for health planning agencies, but considering the controversy surrounding the planning system, advocates were pleased that the three-year extension made it through Congress at all. *(See Health Planning chapter)*

Emergency Medical Services

Congress Nov. 29, 1979, cleared legislation (S 497) continuing a popular federal program that subsidized regional emergency medical services (EMS). Although it had been rumored that President Carter might veto the measure because it more than doubled what the administration wanted to spend, he signed it Dec. 12 (PL 96-142).

The final version authorized a total of $196 million over three years, continuing at about existing appropriations levels federal support for organizing and upgrading regional emergency transportation and communications systems, and for training specialists in emergency care.

The final compromise also included, unchanged, a Senate provision that extended for two years federal research and public information programs on sudden infant death syndrome, also known as "crib death." *(See Emergency Services chapter)*

Nurse Training Aid

President Carter and the nurses' lobby each scored a partial victory in 1979 in the long-running legislative battle over federal aid to the nation's nursing schools.

Carter Sept. 29 signed into law a one-year, $103 million extension of federal aid for nursing education (S 230 — PL 96-76) — half as much money, and for half the period of time, as the program approved by Congress in 1978. Carter had pocket vetoed the 1978 bill, a two-year, $206 million reauthorization, saying the funding levels were excessive and that there was no longer a need for most federal support for nurse training. *(1978 action, p. 68-A; see also Rural Health chapter)*

The one-year extension was intended to continue the aid long enough to permit a general congressional review in 1980 of federal aid to all health professions training. Federal aid to medical and other health professions schools was to expire in 1980. *(See Manpower chapter)*

S 230 also authorized $45 million over three years for disease prevention and health promotion programs in the Department of Health, Education and Welfare (HEW) and an extra $12 million for the National Health Service Corps.

The Senate had passed its version of S 230 (S Rept 96-101) by voice vote May 7, and the House passed a similar nurse training bill July 27 (HR 3633 — H Rept 96-183). The Senate approved the conference report on the bill (H Rept 96-419) Sept. 7 and the House approved it Sept. 20.

Development of the Programs

Although some nurse traineeships were authorized by Congress in 1956, comprehensive federal aid to nursing education dated from 1964. It included construction grants for new schools, project grants to upgrade training, and financial aid for students, with loan forgiveness for nurses who worked in health care shortage areas.

The programs were reauthorized in 1968; 1971, when general-purpose "capitation" (per-student) grants were added, and 1975, when a series of presidential vetoes of nurse training bills began. President Ford vetoed two reauthorizations because he thought they were too expensive; Congress overrode a third veto.

Like Ford, President Carter also wanted to abolish most federal aid to nursing schools. He said more than a decade of federal aid had greatly increased the numbers of nurses graduating each year and that further help for nursing schools was no longer warranted. In his fiscal 1980 budget he called for minimal funding, to continue aid only for programs training specialized nurse practitioners.

As in the past, the nurses took their case to Congress, arguing that many areas, particularly rural regions and inner cities, still had acute shortages of nurses.

Only 15 of the nation's 1,339 nursing schools did not receive some form of federal aid, according to HEW.

Provisions

As signed into law, PL 96-76:

Nurse Training. Extended through fiscal 1980 authorization for capitation, construction and other types of grants to nurse training schools, and loans and other financial aid for students. Authorized $103 million, including $2 million for a new program of grants for training nurse anesthetists.

● Required the HEW secretary to study national nursing needs and related subjects, including the need for continued federal support to nurse education programs.

Other Health Professions. Permitted the secretary to raise to $15,000, from $10,000, the maximum amount individual students in schools of medicine, osteopathy and dentistry could borrow each year in federally insured loans. The total indebtedness allowed these students was raised to $60,000, from $50,000.

● Authorized the secretary to extend National Health Service Corps service deferrals for individuals needing more time to complete residencies or other advanced clinical training before beginning their service.

● Authorized an additional $12 million for fiscal 1980 for the National Health Service Corps, for a total one-year authorization of $82 million.

● Doubled the amount HEW could set aside for financial distress grants to health professions schools, and eliminated a requirement that second-year grants under the program be 25 per cent less than first-year grants. These changes were intended primarily to aid several predominantly black health professions schools with severe financial problems.

● Barred medical or other health professions schools receiving federal funds from discriminating against applicants on the basis of their views on abortion or sterilization.

● Permitted a waiver for dental schools of mandatory increases in class sizes as a condition of eligibility for capitation grants.

● Revised certain area health education center participation requirements.

● Authorized a series of administrative changes in the Public Health Service, including authority to promote enrollment of physicians' assistants and other mid-level practitioners.

● Extended for three years, through fiscal 1982, disease prevention and health promotion programs in HEW; authorized a three-year total of $45 million for these programs.

Doctors Unionization

By a 60-vote margin, the House Nov. 28, 1979, rejected a bill (HR 2222) to permit medical interns and residents in hospitals to unionize.

Unfortunate timing and opposition by two notably successful lobby groups, representing hospitals and medical schools, were cited as reasons for the rejection of the bill to bring hospital "housestaff" — young doctors in advanced training programs who cared for patients — under the National Labor Relations Act (NLRA). The vote was 167-227.

The bill would have reversed a 1976 National Labor Relations Board (NLRB) finding that the young doctors were "students" and thus not entitled to coverage under the labor act.

As reported by the Education and Labor Committee Oct. 10, HR 2222 (H Rept 96-504) simply declared that young doctors, with college and medical school degrees, licensed or otherwise legally authorized to treat patients in hospitals, were to be considered employees for purposes of NLRA coverage. The measure would have applied to an estimated 60,000 persons participating in advanced clinical training programs in non-profit, non-public hospitals.

Military Doctor Bonuses

In an effort to alleviate a shortage of doctors and dentists in the armed forces, Congress moved in 1979 to boost special pay bonuses and provide other financial incentives for them to join and remain in the military services. However, the bill fell victim to President Carter's budget-cutting campaign; he vetoed it March 11, 1980.

The bill would have created a permanent new system of four types of bonuses to retain doctors on active duty and reward them for becoming certified by medical specialty boards. It also ended the pay differentials between obligated doctors — those who were "paying back" federal loans for medical education with years of active-duty service — and unobligated physicians, who earned more. Under the bill, a military doctor could have earned as much as $63,000 a year, plus up to $8,000 more for practicing a specialty in short supply in the military medical corps. Under existing law, military physicians' salaries peaked at $59,000. Civilian doctors' earnings averaged $70,000, according to the Defense Department.

The House passed the bill (HR 5235 — H Rept 96-517) Nov. 13, 1979, and the Senate passed its version (S 523 — S Rept 96-507) Dec. 20. Both chambers approved the conference report (H Rept 96-754) in February 1980. Congress made no effort to override the veto.

Drug Law Revision

Revision of federal drug laws had been under consideration for many years, but it was not until 1979 that Congress — and only one chamber — acted to revise the statute, with the Senate clearing a bill, (S 1075), sponsored by Sen. Edward M. Kennedy (D Mass.) that made major changes in the way drugs were marketed and tested. The bill was a re-written version of a 1978 Carter administration proposal and aroused considerable controversy. The House did not act on the legislation in 1979, and, as of mid-1980, the fate of the bill remained unclear. *(Details, Drug Law Revision chapter)*

Saccharin Ban Moratorium

The House voted overwhelmingly in 1979 to permit diet foods and soft drinks sweetened with saccharin to stay on the market for two more years.

By a 394-22 vote July 24, it passed a bill (HR 4453 — H Rept 96-348) extending through June 30, 1981, the moratorium on Food and Drug Administration (FDA) efforts to ban saccharin-sweetened products. The Senate followed suit in June 1980. *(See Food Law Revision chapter)*

Drug Abuse Programs

Congress Dec. 19, 1979, agreed to continue federal drug abuse efforts for two more years, but refused President Carter's request to fold funds for state drug abuse programs into single, consolidated grants for mental health, drug and alcohol abuse services.

Although the consolidation plan might have streamlined administration of the three programs, "the unique aspects of drug abuse and addiction" might have been neglected by "the bureaucracy," said Sen. Donald W. Riegle Jr. (D Mich.), chairman of the Senate Labor and Human Resources Subcommittee on Alcoholism and Drug Abuse.

Congress cleared the $444 million reauthorization (S 525) Dec. 19 by voice votes in both houses, and the president signed the bill into law (PL 96-181) Jan. 2, 1980.

The Senate had passed a one-year extension of the drug abuse programs May 7, with an automatic continuation for a second year unless there was congressional action to prevent it (S 525 — S Rept 96-104). The House approved its one-year version Oct. 16 as part of a bill (HR 3916 — H Rept 96-193) that also continued federal alcoholism programs. Differences between the two bills were worked out in staff-level negotiations, without a formal conference. The alcoholism reauthorization (S 440) cleared Congress as a separate bill. *(Story, below)*

Provisions

As signed into law, S 525:

● Extended through fiscal 1981 authorizations for federal drug abuse programs; authorized $214 million in fiscal 1980 and $230 million in fiscal 1981.

● Required state drug abuse advisory councils to include women and elderly members, and to recognize special needs of these groups in state drug abuse plans. Required states to coordinate their treatment and prevention services for drug abuse with those for alcohol abuse, to coordinate state efforts with those of local governments, and to receive local government comments on state drug abuse plans. Also required states to promote drug abuse programs in the workplace, through local governments and private businesses.

● Required preferential treatment for prevention and treatment proposals targeted on drug problems of women, the elderly and children under age 18. Stipulated new special guidelines for federally funded projects, such as availability to the handicapped or persons speaking little English.

● Directed the National Institute on Drug Abuse to develop model prevention and treatment programs for use in the workplace, to be disseminated through state programs.

Alcohol Abuse Programs

President Carter Jan. 2, 1980, signed into law a reauthorization of federal alcoholism and alcohol abuse programs that some members of Congress said cleared the way for the government to begin requiring health warning labels on liquor bottles.

Sens. Strom Thurmond (R S.C.) and Donald W. Riegle Jr. (D Mich.) maintained that compromise language in the two-year, $416.5 million measure (S 440 — PL 96-180) was structured so as to "permit and encourage" federal agency action on liquor health warnings as early as June 1980.

But opponents of mandatory labeling, such as Sen. Wendell H. Ford, a Democrat from bourbon-producing Kentucky, insisted the compromise didn't mean that at all.

The Senate had attached an amendment requiring health warnings on liquor in its bill (S 440 — S Rept 96-103), passed May 7, 1979; the House bill (HR 3916 — H Rept 96-193) passed Oct. 16, had no such provision. The compromise version was negotiated informally, without a conference, and approved by voice votes in both houses Dec. 19. The House bill also had included a one-year extension of federal drug abuse programs, which cleared Congress as separate legislation (S 525) Dec. 19. *(Story, above)*

In passing the separate bills, Congress rejected the president's request to consolidate alcoholism, drug abuse and mental health grants to states into single, multi-purpose grants at reduced funding levels. Alcohol and drug abuse professionals had feared their programs would be downgraded if they lost their separate legislative identities.

Provisions

As signed into law, S 440 (PL 96-180):

Federal Programs. Extended federal alcoholism and alcohol abuse programs through fiscal 1981. Authorized $199.5 million in fiscal 1980 and $217 million in 1981.

● Required the director of the National Institute on Alcohol Abuse and Alcoholism to make programs for underserved populations such as women and adolescents a high priority.

● Created a National Commission on Alcoholism and Other Alcohol-Related Problems, with a two-year, $1 million authorization. Directed the commission to recommend national alcohol abuse policy to the president.

● Added members from the Departments of Labor, Treasury and Education to the interagency committee on federal alcoholism programs.

● Extended eligibility in alcohol abuse programs for federal civilian employees to families of those employees.

● Required the secretaries of the Treasury and HEW to report jointly to Congress and the president, by June 1, 1980, on the nature and extent of birth defects and other health hazards associated with alcohol consumption by pregnant women and other individuals. Required the secretaries to recommend actions they could take under the Federal Alcohol Administration Act and the Federal Food, Drug and Cosmetic Act to inform the public of such hazards.

State Programs. Required state alcoholism advisory councils to include as members women and elderly persons, and required state alcoholism plans to estimate the needs of these groups.

● Required states receiving formula grants to coordinate their alcoholism and drug abuse activities and to encourage development of alcoholism programs in state and local government, private business and industry.

● Extended authorizations for grants and contracts to states adopting a model statute designed to treat alcoholism as a disease rather than a crime, and to public or private entities conducting alcoholism prevention and treatment programs.

Medicare-Medicaid Benefits

The Senate Finance Committee July 12, 1979, voted to kill President Carter's hospital cost control proposal (S 570) and approved instead a bill that would limit only federal payments to hospitals for Medicare and Medicaid patients. The full Senate did not act in 1979.

The bill was thought by many observers to be the only type of hospital cost control that stood a chance of passage in the 96th Congress. However, as a form of cost control its enactment would be something of a hollow victory, since the Department of Health, Education and Welfare (HEW) had already moved administratively in 1979 to adopt the substance of the committee's changes in hospital payments. *(See Medicare/Medicaid chapter)*

HEW warned that limiting cost-cutting to the two federal programs not only would save less than the administration's cost control plan, but also would risk discrimination against Medicare and Medicaid patients as federal hospitalization payments for them dropped further below those of private insurance plans.

The House Ways and Means Committee also approved a package of Medicare-Medicaid changes in 1979, mainly making minor benefit improvements for Medicare, providing incentives to encourage prepaid medical plans such as health maintenance organizations to enroll more elderly members, and establishing a voluntary federal certification program for private "Medigap" insurance plans, sold as a supplement to Medicare coverage. The House had passed similar legislation in 1978, but the Senate took no action and it died at the end of the 95th Congress. *(1978 action, p. 72-A)*

Child Health Program

The House Dec. 11, 1979, voted to expand and upgrade a preventive health care program for poor children under the state-federal Medicaid program. Sponsors said the new Child Health Assurance Program (CHAP) could provide health care to as many as five million additional children, as well as 220,000 low-income women pregnant for the first time — at a possible cost of nearly $2 billion a year by 1984. The Senate Finance Committee reported a less expensive version in 1979, but the full chamber did not consider the legislation that year. In his fiscal 1981 budget revisions, Carter scaled down his original request considerably, and the program's future was still in doubt as of mid-1980. *(Details, Child Health chapter)* ∎

Health Policy: A Selected Bibliography

Books

Abel-Smith, Brian. *Value for Money in Health Services: A Comparative Study.* New York: St. Martin's Press, 1976.

American Enterprise Institute for Public Policy Research. *Comprehensive National Medical Care: Should the Federal Government Provide a Program for all U.S. Citizens?* Washington, D.C.: 1972.

Braverman, Jordan. *Crisis in Health Care.* Washington, D.C.: Acropolis Books, 1978.

Brown, J. H. U. *The Health Care Dilemma.* New York: Human Science Press, 1978.

Brown, J. H. U. *The Politics of Health Care.* Cambridge, Mass.: Ballinger, 1978.

Campbell, Alastair V. *Medicine, Health and Justice: The Problem of Priorities.* New York: Longman, 1978.

Carlson, Rick J. and Cunningham, Robert, eds. *Future Directions in Health Care: A New Public Policy.* Cambridge, Mass.: Ballinger, 1978.

Davis, Karen. *Health and the War on Poverty.* Washington, D.C.: Brookings Institution, 1978.

Davis, Karen. *National Health Insurance: Benefits, Costs, and Consequences.* Washington, D.C.: Brookings Institution, 1975.

Eckholm, Erik P. *The Picture of Health: Environmental Sources of Disease.* New York: Norton, 1977.

Fedder, Judith et al. *National Health Insurance: Conflicting Goals and Policy Choices.* Washington, D.C.: The Urban Institute, 1980.

Fein, Rashi, *The Doctor Shortage.* Washington, D.C.: Brookings Institution, 1967.

Feingold, Benjamin F. *Why Your Child is Hyperactive.* New York: Random House, 1975.

FitzPatrick, Malcolm S. *Environmental Health Planning: Community Development Based on Environmental and Health Precepts.* Cambridge, Mass.: Ballinger, 1978.

Friedman, Kenneth M. and Rakoff, Stuart H., eds. *Toward a National Health Policy: Public Policy and the Control of Health-Care Costs.* Lexington, Mass.: D. C. Heath, 1977.

Fuchs, Victor. *Who Shall Live?* New York: Basic Books, 1975.

Grossman, Howard. *For Health's Sake: A Critical Analysis of Medical Care in the United States.* Palo Alto, Calif.: Pacific Books, 1977.

Jonas, Steven et al. *Health Care Delivery in the United States.* New York: Springer, 1977.

Kallet, Arthur and Schlink, F. J. *100,000,000 Guinea Pigs: Dangers in Everyday Foods, Drugs, and Cosmetics.* New York: Vanguard Press, 1932.

Kane, Robert et al. *An Overview of Rural Health Care Research.* Santa Montico, Calif.: Rand Corporation, 1978.

Kennedy, Edward M. *In Critical Condition: The Crisis in America's Health Care.* New York: Simon & Schuster, 1972.

Knowles, John H., ed. *Doing Better and Feeling Worse.* New York: W. W. Norton, 1977.

Lewis, Charles E., et al. *A Right to Health: The Problem of Access to Primary Medical Care.* New York: Wiley, 1976.

Marmor, Theodore R. *The Politics of Medicare.* Chicago, Ill.: Aldine, 1973.

Mechanic, David. *Future Issues in Health Care: Social Policy and the Rationing of Medical Services.* New York: Free Press, 1979.

Meyer, Jack A. *Health Care Cost Increases.* Washington, D.C.: American Enterprise Institute for Public Policy Research, 1979.

National Academy of Science. *How Safe Is Safe? The Design of Policy on Drugs and Food Additives.* Washington, D.C.: 1974.

Paine, Leslie H. W., ed. *Health Care in Big Cities.* New York: St. Martin's Press, 1978.

Paringer, Lynn, et al. *Health Status and Use of Medical Services: Evidence on the Poor, Black, and the Rural Elderly.* Washington, D.C.: Urban Institute, 1979.

Roemer, Milton. *Rural Health Care.* St. Louis, Mo.: Mosby, 1976.

Sigerist, Henry E. *Civilization and Disease.* Ithaca, N.Y.: Cornell University Press, 1943.

Sorkin, Alan L. *Health Manpower: An Economic Perspective.* Lexington, Mass.: D. C. Heath, 1977.

Turner, James S. *The Chemical Feast.* New York: Grossman, 1970.

Verrett, Jacqueline and Carper, Jean. *Eating May Be Hazardous to Your Health.* New York: Simon & Schuster, 1974.

Government Documents

Ahearn, Mary C. *Health Care in Rural America.* Washington, D.C.: U.S. Department of Agriculture, 1979.

Roberts, Steven A., ed. *Proceedings of the National Conference on the Environment and Health Care Costs, August 15, 1978.* Springfield, Va.: National Technical Information Service, 1978.

U.S. Congress. Congressional Budget Office. *Controlling Rising Hospital Costs.* Washington, D.C.: Government Printing Office, 1979.

U.S. Congress. House. Committee on Interstate and Foreign Commerce. Subcommittee on Health and Environment. *Child Health Care: Oversight: Hearings, May 16, 1979.* 96th Cong., 1st sess. Washington, D.C.: Government Printing Office, 1979.

U.S. Congress. House. Committee on Interstate and Foreign Commerce. Subcommittee on Health and Environment. *Community Support for Mental Patients; Hearings, October 11, 1979.* 96th Cong., 1st sess. Washington, D.C.: Government Printing Office, 1979.

U.S. Congress. House. Committee on Interstate and Foreign Commerce. Subcommittee on Health and the Environment. *Development of Primary Health Care Services: Hearings, August 10, 1978.* 95th Cong., 2nd sess. Washington, D.C.: Government Printing Office, 1978.

U.S. Congress. House. Committee on Interstate and Foreign Commerce. Subcommittee on Health and the Environment. *Health Research: Future Directions: Hearings, November 14, 1979.* 96th Cong., 1st sess. Washington, D.C.: Government Printing Office, 1979.

U.S. Congress. House. Committee on Interstate and Foreign Commerce. Subcommittee on Health and the Environment. *Infant Mortality: Oversight: Hearings, Oc-*

tober 5, 1979. 96th Cong., 1st sess. Washington, D.C.: Government Printing Office, 1980.

U.S. Congress. House. Committee on Interstate and Foreign Commerce. Subcommittee on Health and the Environment. *President's Hospital Cost Containment Proposal: Hearings, March 12, 1979, part I; Hearings, April 2, 9, 30, May 21, 23, 1979, part II.* 96th Cong., 1st sess. Washington, D.C.: Government Printing Office, 1979.

U.S. Congress. House. Committee on Interstate and Foreign Commerce. Subcommittee on Health and Environment. *Programs of the Public Health Service Act. Oversight: Hearings March 15, 1979.* 96th Cong., 1st sess. Washington, D.C.: Government Printing Office, 1979.

U.S. Congress. House. Committee on Interstate and Foreign Commerce. Subcommittee on Health and the Environment. *Saccharin Ban: Oversight: Hearings, April 11, 1979.* 96th Cong., 1st sess. Washington, D.C.: Government Printing Office, 1979.

U.S. Congress. House. Committee on Interstate and Foreign Commerce. Subcommittee on Oversight and Investigations. *Infant Formula: Our Children Need Better Protection. Committee Print #96-IFC 42.* 96th Cong., 2nd sess. Washington, D.C.: Government Printing Office, 1980.

U.S. Congress. House. Committee on Interstate and Foreign Commerce. Subcommittee on Oversight and Investigations. *Man-In-The-Plant: FDA's Failure to Regulate Deceptive Drug Labeling. Committee Print #95-73.* 95th Cong., 2nd sess. Washington, D.C.: Government Printing Office, 1978.

U.S. Congress. House. Committee on Interstate and Foreign Commerce. Subcommittee on Oversight and Investigations. *Regulation of Over-the-Counter Drugs: Hearings, June 22, 1979.* 96th Cong., 1st sess. Washington, D.C.: Government Printing Office, 1979.

U.S. Congress. Senate. Committee on Finance. *Catastrophic Health Insurance and Medical Assistance Reform: Hearings,* March 27-29, 1979. 96th Cong., 1st sess. Washington, D.C.: Government Printing Office, 1979.

U.S. Congress. Senate. Committee on Finance. *Health Care Cost Containment and Other Proposals. Report #96-9.* 96th Cong., 1st sess. Washington, D.C.: Government Printing Office, 1979.

U.S. Congress. Senate. Committee on Finance. *Presentation of Major Health Insurance Proposals: Hearings, June 19, 21, 1979.* 96th Cong., 1st sess. Washington, D.C.: Government Printing Office, 1979.

U.S. Congress. Senate. Committee on Finance. *Proposals for Medicare-Medicaid Reform and Overall Hospital Revenues Limitation. Report #96-10.* 96th Cong., 1st sess. Washington, D.C.: Government Printing Office, 1979.

U.S. Congress. Senate. Committee on Finance. Subcommittee on Health. *Findings of Permanent Subcommittee on Investigations on Health Maintenance Organizations; Hearings May 18, 1978.* 95th Cong., 2nd sess. Washington, D.C.: Government Printing Office, 1979.

U.S. Congress. Senate. Committee on Finance. Subcommittee on Health. *Health Assistance for Low-Income Children: Hearings, June 25, 1979.* 96th Cong., 1st sess. Washington, D.C.: Government Printing Office, 1979.

U.S. Congress. Senate. Committee on Finance. Subcommittee on Health. *S 505 and Other Health Care Cost Containment Proposals. Report #96-6.* 96th Cong., 1st sess. Washington, D.C.: Government Printing Office, 1979.

U.S. Congress. Senate. Committee on Labor and Human Resources. *Final Report of the Joint Commission on Prescription Drug Use, Inc.* 96th Cong., 2nd sess. Washington, D.C.: Government Printing Office, 1980.

U.S. Congress. Senate. Committee on Labor and Human Resources. *Special Needs and Problems of Older Americans in Rural and Small Communities: Hearings, July 28, 1978.* 95th Cong., 2nd sess. Washington, D.C.: Government Printing Office, 1978.

U.S. Congress. Senate. Committee on Labor and Human Resources. Subcommittee on Health and Scientific Research. *Drug Regulation Reform Act of 1979: Hearings, May 17, 18, 1979.* 96th Cong., 1st sess. Washington, D.C.: Government Printing Office, 1979.

U.S. Congress. House. Committee on Ways and Means. *National Health Insurance. Joint Staff Analysis Prepared with CRS Assistance by the Subcommittee on Health, House Interstate and Foreign Commerce Committee, Subcommittee on Health and the Environment. Committee Print #96-40.* 96th Cong., 1st sess. Washington, D.C.: Government Printing Office, 1979.

U.S. Congress. Senate. Committee on Labor and Human Resources. Subcommittee on Health and Scientific Research. *Preclinical and Clinical Testing by the Pharmaceutical Industry: Hearings, October 11, 1979.* 96th Cong., 1st sess. Washington, D.C.: Government Printing Office, 1979.

U.S. Congress. Senate. Committee on Veterans' Affairs. *National Academy of Sciences Study of Health Care for American Veterans and the VA Response: Hearings, September 30, October 17, November 16, 1977, part I; Hearings, January 11, February 6, March 6, 1978, part II.* 95th Cong., 1st sess.; 95th Cong., 2nd sess. Washington, D.C.: Government Printing Office, 1979.

Articles

Behn, Robert D. and Sperduto, Kim. "Medical Schools and the 'Entitlement Ethic.'" *Public Interest,* Fall 1979, pp. 48-68.

Birnbaum, Howard, et al. "Focusing on the Catastrophic Illness Debate." *Quarterly Review of Economics and Business,* Autumn 1979, pp. 17-33.

Bisogni, Carole. "The Widening Debate Over Food Additives. *Human Ecology Forum,* Fall 1979, pp. 15-18.

Blumberg, Mark S. and Gentry, Douglas W. "Routine Hospital Charges and Intensity of Care: A Cross-Section Analysis of Fifty States." *Inquiry,* March 1978, pp. 58-73.

Burney, Ira L. et al. "Medicare and Medicaid Physician Payment Incentives." *Health Care Financing Review,* Summer 1979, pp. 62-78.

Cantwell, James R. "Implications of Reimbursement Policies for the Location of Physicians." *Agricultural Economics Research,* April 1979, pp. 25-35.

"Child and Family Health." *Public Health Reports,* September/October 1979, pp. 399-437.

Christianson, Jon B. and McClure, Walter. "Competition in the Delivery of Medical Care." *New England Journal of Medicine,* vol. 301, 1979, pp. 295-316.

"Cost of Disease and Illness in the United States in the Year 2000." *Public Health Reports*, September/October 1978, pp. 493-588.

Davidson, Stephen M. "The Status of Aid to the Medically Needy." *Social Service Review*, March 1979, pp. 92-105.

Daly, Patricia A. "The Response of Consumers to Nutrition Labeling." *Journal of Consumer Affairs*, Winter 1976, pp. 170-178.

Demkovich, Linda E. "Cutting Health Care Costs: Why Not Let the Market Decide?" *National Journal*, October 27, 1979, pp. 1796-1800.

Demkovich, Linda E. "FDA in Hot Water Again Over Cost of Proposed Drug Labeling Rule." *National Journal*, September 22, 1979, pp. 1568-1570.

Demkovich, Linda E. "Last Year It Was Saccharin, This Year It's Sodium Nitrite." *National Journal*, September 1978, pp. 1468-1470.

Demkovich, Linda E. "Who Can Do A Better Job of Controlling Hospital Costs?" *National Journal*, February 10, 1979, pp. 219-223.

Enthoven, Alain C. "Health Care Costs: Why Regulation Fails, Why Competition Works, How to Get There From Here." *National Journal*, May 26, 1979, pp. 885-889.

Feldstein, Martin S. "The High Cost of Hospitals and What to Do About It." *Public Interest*, Summer 1977, pp. 40-54.

"Focus on Medical Costs and How to Control Them." *Management Focus*, November/December 1979, pp. 10-25.

Fuchs, Victor R. "The Economics of Health in a Post-Industrial Society." *Public Interest*, Summer 1979, pp. 3-20.

Gaus, Clifton R. et al. "Contrasts in HMO and Fee-For-Service Performance." *Social Security Bulletin*, May 1976, pp. 3-14.

Gifford, James F., Jr. and Anlyan, William G. "The Role of the Private Sector in an Economy of Limited Health Care Resources." *New England Journal of Medicine*, vol. 300, 1979, pp. 790-793.

Ginzberg, Eli. "Health Reform: The Outlook for the 1980s." *Inquiry*, December 1978, pp. 311-326.

Greene, James. "Drug Testing in Children." *FDA Consumer*, June 1978, pp. 11-13.

Greenspan, Ronald. "Hospital Cost Control: Single-Edged Initiatives for a Two-Sided Problem." *Harvard Journal on Legislation*, April 1978, pp. 603-668.

Hall, Charles P. Jr. et al. "Medicaid and Cash Welfare Recipients: An Empirical Study." *Inquiry*, March 1977, pp. 43-50.

"Health Care Symposium." *Harvard Journal on Legislation*, April 1978, pp. 431-684.

"Health Facility Regulation." *North Carolina Law Review*, August 1979, pp. 1163-1479.

Herder-Dorneich, Phillipp. "Social Control in Health Economics." *Review of Social Economy*, April 1978, pp. 1-17.

Herzlinger, Reginia. "Can We Control Health Care Costs?" *Harvard Business Review*, March/April 1978, pp. 102-110.

Holahan, J. et al. "Paying for Physicians' Services Under Medicare and Medicaid." *Milbank Memorial Fund Quarterly/Health and Society*, Spring 1979, pp. 183-211.

"How the FDA Rates Prescription Drugs." *Consumer Reports*, October 1978, pp. 578-581.

Judd, Leda R. "Federal Involvement in Health Care After 1945." *Current History*, May/June 1977, pp. 201-206.

Kennedy, Donald. "The Food and Drug Administration and the Backward Motion Toward the Source." *Public Health Reports*, November/December 1978, pp. 607-615.

Lairson, David R. et al. "Catastrophic Illness in an HMO." *Inquiry*, Summer 1979, pp. 119-130.

Leepson, Marc. "Food Additives." *Editorial Research Reports*, May 12, 1978, pp. 343-360.

Leepson, Marc. "Medical Education." *Editorial Research Reports*, November 25, 1977, pp. 891-908.

Leepson, Marc. "Rural Health Care." *Editorial Research Reports*, November 23, 1979, pp. 841-860.

de Lesseps, Suzanne. "Controlling Health Costs." *Editorial Research Reports*, January 28, 1977, pp. 63-80.

Leveson, Irving. "Some Policy Implications of the Relationship between Health Services and Health." *Inquiry*, Spring 1979, pp. 9-21.

Levin, Arthur, ed. "Regulating Health Care: The Struggle for Control." *Proceedings of the Academy of Political and Social Science*. #4, 1980, pp. 1-244.

Luft, Harold S. "How Do Health Maintenance Organizations Achieve Their Savings? Rhetoric and Evidence." *New England Journal of Medicine*, vol. 298, 1978, pp. 1336-1343.

Margolis, Richard J. "Doctors for Sale." *New Leader*, March 13, 1978, pp. 14-15.

Marmor, Theodore et al. "The Politics of Medical Inflation." *Journal of Health Politics, Policy and Law*, Spring 1976, pp. 69-84.

Maynard, Alan. "The Medical Profession and the Efficiency and Equity of Health Service." *Social and Economic Administration*, Spring 1978, pp. 3-19.

Mead, Lawrence M. "Health Policy: the Need for Governance." *Annals of the American Academy of Political and Social Science*, November 1977, pp. 39-57.

Milch, Robert A. "An Overview of the Economics of Health Care." *World*, Autumn 1976, pp. 3035.

"The Money in Curing Hospitals." *Business Week*, August 6, 1979, pp. 54-56.

Mushkin, Selma J. et al. "Cost of Disease and Illness in the United States in the Year 2000." *Public Health Reports*, September/October 1978, pp. 493-588.

Nesbitt, Tom E. "How to Curb Medical Costs Without Surrendering Free Choice." *Enterprise*, July 1978, pp. 1012.

"Physicians and New Health Practitioners: Issues for the 1980s." *Inquiry*, Fall 1979, pp. 195-229.

Pines, Wayne L. "New Prescription for Drug Regulation." *FDA Consumer*, June 1978, pp. 6-10.

Reed, Ben. "The Struggle for the People's Health Needs." *Political Affairs*, March 1978, pp. 28-34.

Robeson, Franklin E. "Health Costs: Savings in the Private Sector." *California Management Review*, Summer 1979, pp. 49-56.

Sacks, P. "Are You Paying Too Much for Your Prescriptions?" *Family Health*, April 1978, pp. 8-10.

Seidman, Laurence S. "Hospital Inflation: A Diagnosis and Prescription." *Challenge*, July/August 1979, pp. 17-23.

Shapiro, Sidney A. "Limiting Physician Freedom to Prescribe a Drug for Any Purpose: The Need for FDA

Regulation." *Northwestern University Law Review,* December 1978, pp. 801-872.

Smith, R. J. "Ever So Cautiously, the FDA Moves Toward a Ban on Nitrites." *Science,* September 8, 1978, pp. 887-891.

Stambler, Howard V. "Health Manpower for the Nation: A Look Ahead at the Supply and the Requirements." *Public Health Reports,* January/February 1979, pp. 3-10.

"Unhealthy Costs of Health Care." *Business Week,* September 4, 1978, pp. 58-61.

Wilson, Ronald W. et al. "Continuing Trends in Health and Health Care." *Annals of the American Academy of Political and Social Science,* January 1978, pp. 140-156.

Zaratzian, Virginia L. "Cancer Hazards in Food." *Ecologist,* January/February 1977, pp. 12-21.

Weinstein, Milton C. "Decision Making for Toxic Substance Control: Cost-Effective Information Development for the Environmental Carcinogens." *Public Policy,* Summer 1979, pp. 334-383. ∎

Index

XYZ